Pre-publication REVIEWS, COMMENTARIES, EVALUATIONS...

"This is a wonderful and important book that very effectively provides us with practical applications of medical family therapy. Linville and Hertlein provide an excellent pragmatic guide with creative interventions for mental health professionals working with families facing illness, disability, loss, or bereavement. It is a terrific resource for practitioners, educators, and students."

John S. Rolland, MD
Professor of Psychiatry and Co-Director,
Center for Family Health,
University of Chicago;
Author, *Families, Illness, & Disability:
An Integrative Treatment Model*

"As a professional, I have several roles that are directly impacted by many of the health care issues covered in this book. I have provided treatment to many of the populations covered in this book, served an administrative role at Gilda's Club Chicago, and now oversee the training of future clinicians. I find the theory and practical information contained in the book useful in all three settings. As a clinician, the information and practical tools are useful in treating and addressing the myriad issues presenting with issues related to cancer, including the grief that is experienced and the stress such a diagnosis has on the entire family system. As a trainer of future clinicians the text offers a pragmatic approach to preparing trainees to work with these populations. The tools are useful in helping them to understand the issues that may arise during their careers. It takes the information from the purely theoretical and provides hands-on ways of working with individuals, couples, and families that are touched by illness."

Torrey Wilson, PhD
Doctoral Program Director,
Adler School of Professional Psychology,
Chicago, Illinois

NOTES FOR PROFESSIONAL LIBRARIANS AND LIBRARY USERS

This is an original book title published by The Haworth Press, Inc. Unless otherwise noted in specific chapters with attribution, materials in this book have not been previously published elsewhere in any format or language.

CONSERVATION AND PRESERVATION NOTES

All books published by The Haworth Press, Inc., and its imprints are printed on certified pH neutral, acid-free book grade paper. This paper meets the minimum requirements of American National Standard for Information Sciences-Permanence of Paper for Printed Material, ANSI Z39.48-1984.

DIGITAL OBJECT IDENTIFIER (DOI) LINKING

The Haworth Press is participating in reference linking for elements of our original books. (For more information on reference linking initiatives, please consult the CrossRef Web site at www.crossref.org.) When citing an element of this book such as a chapter, include the element's Digital Object Identifier (DOI) as the last item of the reference. A Digital Object Identifier is a persistent, authoritative, and unique identifier that a publisher assigns to each element of a book. Because of its persistence, DOIs will enable The Haworth Press and other publishers to link to the element referenced, and the link will not break over time. This will be a great resource in scholarly research.

The Therapist's Notebook for Family Health Care
*Homework, Handouts, and Activities
for Individuals, Couples, and Families
Coping with Illness, Loss, and Disability*

HAWORTH Practical Practice in Mental Health
Lorna L. Hecker, PhD
Senior Editor

101 Interventions in Family Therapy edited by Thorana S. Nelson and Terry S. Trepper

101 More Interventions in Family Therapy edited by Thorana S. Nelson and Terry S. Trepper

The Practical Practice of Marriage and Family Therapy: Things My Training Supervisor Never Told Me by Mark Odell and Charles E. Campbell

The Therapist's Notebook for Families: Solution-Oriented Exercises for Working with Parents, Children, and Adolescents by Bob Bertolino and Gary Schultheis

Collaborative Practice in Psychology and Therapy edited by David A. Paré and Glenn Larner

The Therapist's Notebook for Children and Adolescents: Homework, Handouts, and Activities for Use in Psychotherapy edited by Catherine Ford Sori and Lorna L. Hecker

The Therapist's Notebook for Lesbian, Gay, and Bisexual Clients: Homework, Handouts, and Activities for Use in Psychotherapy by Joy S. Whitman and Cynthia J. Boyd

A Guide to Self-Help Workbooks for Mental Health Clinicians and Researchers by Luciano L'Abate

Workbooks in Prevention, Psychotherapy, and Rehabilitation: A Resource for Clinicians and Researchers edited by Luciano L'Abate

The Psychotherapist as Parent Coordinator in High-Conflict Divorce: Strategies and Techniques by Susan M. Boyan and Ann Marie Termini

The Couple and Family Therapist's Notebook: Homework, Handouts, and Activities for Use in Marital and Family Therapy by Katherine A. Milewski Hertlein, Dawn Viers, and Associates

The Therapist's Notebook for Integrating Spirituality in Counseling: Homework, Handouts, and Activities for Use in Psychotherapy edited by Karen B. Helmeke and Catherine Ford Sori

The Therapist's Notebook for Integrating Spirituality in Counseling II: More Homework, Handouts, and Activities for Use in Psychotherapy edited by Karen B. Helmeke and Catherine Ford Sori

Interactive Art Therapy: "No Talent Required" Projects by Linda L. Simmons

Therapy's Best: Practical Advice and Gems of Wisdom from Twenty Accomplished Counselors and Therapists by Howard Rosenthal

The Christian Therapist's Notebook: Homework, Handouts, and Activities for Use in Christian Counseling by Philip J. Henry, Lori Marie Figueroa, and David R. Miller

The Therapist's Notebook, Volume 2: More Homework, Handouts, and Activities for Use in Psychotherapy by Lorna L. Hecker, Catherine Ford Sori, and Associates

The Group Therapist's Notebook: Homework, Handouts, and Activities for Use in Psychotherapy edited by Dawn Viers

The Therapist's Notebook for Family Health Care: Homework, Handouts, and Activities for Individuals, Couples, and Families Coping with Illness, Loss, and Disability by Deanna Linville, Katherine M. Hertlein, and Associates

Introduction to Complementary and Alternative Therapies edited by Anne L. Strozier and Joyce Carpenter

The Therapist's Notebook for Family Health Care
Homework, Handouts, and Activities for Individuals, Couples, and Families Coping with Illness, Loss, and Disability

Deanna Linville, PhD, LMFT
Katherine M. Hertlein, PhD
and Associates

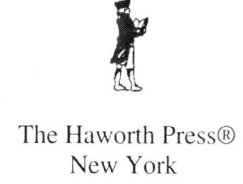

The Haworth Press®
New York

For more information on this book or to order, visit
http://www.haworthpress.com/store/product.asp?sku=5420

or call 1-800-HAWORTH (800-429-6784) in the United States and Canada
or (607) 722-5857 outside the United States and Canada

or contact orders@HaworthPress.com

Published by

The Haworth Press, Inc. 10 Alice Street, Binghamton, NY 13904-1580.

© 2007 by The Haworth Press, Inc. All rights reserved. No part of this work may be reproduced or utilized in any form or by any means, electronic or mechanical, including photocopying, microfilm, and recording, or by any information storage and retrieval system, without permission in writing from the publisher. Printed in the United States of America.

PUBLISHER'S NOTE
The development, preparation, and publication of this work has been undertaken with great care. However, the Publisher, employees, editors, and agents of The Haworth Press are not responsible for any errors contained herein or for consequences that may ensue from use of materials or information contained in this work. The Haworth Press is committed to the dissemination of ideas and information according to the highest standards of intellectual freedom and the free exchange of ideas. Statements made and opinions expressed in this publication do not necessarily reflect the views of the Publisher, Directors, management, or staff of The Haworth Press, Inc., or an endorsement by them.

Cover design by Kerry E. Mack.

Library of Congress Cataloging-in-Publication Data

The therapist's notebook for family health care : homework, handouts, and activities for individuals, couples, and families coping with illness, loss, and disability / [edited by] Deanna Linville, Katherine Milewski-Hertlein, and associates.
    p. cm.
  Includes bibliographical references and index.
  ISBN: 978-0-7890-2696-5 (soft : alk. paper)
  1. Family psychotherapy. 2. Adjustment (Psychology) 3. Loss (Psychology) I. Linville, Deanna. II. Hertlein, Katherine M.
[DNLM: 1. Family Therapy-methods. WM 430.5.F2 T3979 2007]

RC488.5.T4548 2007
616.89'156-dc22

2006102538

To my family who has taught me about the true meaning of loving each other "in sickness and in health." **DL**

To Eric with love, to whom I owe my achievements to his enduring emotional (and technical!) support. **KH**

CONTENTS

About the Editors	xi
Contributors	xiii
Foreword *Wayne Denton, MD, PhD, LMFT*	xix
Preface	xxi
Acknowledgments	xxiii

SECTION I: INTERVENTIONS FOR WORKING WITH FAMILIES AND CHRONIC ILLNESS

1. The Biopsychosocial-Spiritual Interview Method   3
   Jennifer Hodgson
   Angela L. Lamson
   Lauren Reese

2. A "FAST" Approach to Health Care   13
   Thomas M. Gehring
   Katherine M. Hertlein

3. Increasing Social Support to Manage Chronic Illness   19
   Claudia Grauf-Grounds

4. Doctor's Bag of Coping Skills   25
   Miriam Claire Godwin

5. Coping and Adapting to Developmental Changes, Challenges, and Opportunities Using a Patient Education Tool in Family Therapy   31
   Layne A. Prest
   Heath Grames

6. An Adaptive World Model for Meeting the Demands of Chronic Illness   41
   W. David Robinson
   Layne A. Prest
   Jason S. Carroll

7. Positive and Negative Feelings Boxes   49
   Miriam Claire Godwin

8. Extraordinary Parts: The Wife, Mother, and Survivor 53
    Katherine M. Hertlein
    Deanna Linville

9. The Healthy Families Project 59
    Lisa Lavelle

SECTION II: INTERVENTIONS FOR WORKING WITH CHILDREN AND ILLNESS

10. Fun with Bubbles: Relieving Childhood Pain and Physical Symptoms 67
    Olivia Chiang
    Jeri Hepworth
    Susan McDaniel

11. The Superhero in All of Us 73
    Deanna Linville
    Michelle R. Ward

12. The Angry Feelings Toolbox 77
    Michelle R. Ward
    Deanna Linville

13. Why Is My Kid Doing This and What Can I Do? Facilitating Family Problem Solving Using Scatterplots 83
    Theodore A. Hoch

14. The ANGELS (*A Neighbor Giving Encouragement, Love, and Support*): A Collaborative Project for Teens with Diabetes 91
    Tai J. Mendenhall
    William J. Doherty

15. Facilitated Mirroring: Building Perspective in Clients with Asperger's Syndrome 103
    Nan Gray Lester

SECTION III: ILLNESS-SPECIFIC INTERVENTIONS FOR FAMILIES

16. Adaptation of the Family Systems Illness Model for HIV/AIDS Patients and Their Partners 113
    G. Bowden Templeton
    Shayne R. Anderson
    Stephanie R. Burwell

17. Quilting As a Meaning-Making Intervention for HIV/AIDS 119
    Shoshana D. Kerewsky

18. Family-Oriented Diabetes Management: Good Nutrition and Portion Control 125
    Carol Pflaffly

19. Steps to an Ecology of Treatment: A Handout for Clients with Diabetes 131
    Shoshana D. Kerewsky

20. Every Woman's Problem: Self-Assessment for Disordered Eating and Body Image Despair 141
    Margo D. Maine

21. Put a Wrench in It 149
    Nicole M. Childs
    Stephanie R. Burwell

22. Women Caring for Partners with Dementia: A Contextual Model 157
    Christine A. Fruhauf
    Jennifer T. Aberle

23. Inviting Resiliency to Join the Family's Journey with Cancer 167
    Anne Prouty Lyness

24. Exploring Mood Differences: Sports Car and K-Car Metaphor 175
    Nancy Taylor Kemp

SECTION IV: INTERVENTIONS FOR WORKING WITH GRIEF AND LOSS

25. Story Squares: Creating a Dialogue with Grieving Children 187
    Tiffany B. Brown

26. Open Up a Window 195
    Miriam Claire Godwin

27. Threading the Strengths of Families Through Loss and Grief 201
    Miriam Claire Godwin
    Angela L. Lamson

28. A Creative Encounter with Anticipatory Loss 207
    Claudia Grauf-Grounds

29. Aging Parents and End-of-Life Decisions: Helping Families Negotiate Difficult Conversations 211
    Nathalie L. Kees
    Jennifer T. Aberle
    Christine A. Fruhauf

BONUS SECTION: PROFESSIONAL DEVELOPMENT WITH ILLNESS AND LOSS

30. Achoo!: Treating Clients When the Therapist Faces a Chronic Illness   219
    Katherine M. Hertlein

31. Building Your Home Project   225
    Angela L. Lamson
    Patrick L. Meadors

Index   233

ABOUT THE EDITORS

Deanna Linville, PhD, LMFT, is an assistant professor in the Marriage and Family Therapy Program in the School of Education at the University of Oregon. She also serves as the clinical director for the Center for Family Therapy and the lead therapist for RainRock, an eating disorder residential treatment program. She serves on the editorial board for the *Journal of Family Relations* and is a reviewer for the *Journal of Marriage and the Family* and has published in journals such as *Journal of Marriage and Family Therapy, Journal of Feminist Family Therapy, Journal of Youth and Adolescence,* and *Families, Systems, & Health.* Her research interests include domestic violence, eating disorders, collaborative family health care, and international adoption. She can be reached via e-mail at Linville@uoregon.edu.

Katherine M. Hertlein, PhD, is an assistant professor in the Department of Marriage, Family, and Community Counseling at the University of Nevada, Las Vegas. She received her PhD in marriage and family therapy from Virginia Tech. She has published in several journals including *Journal of Couple and Relationship Therapy, American Journal of Family Therapy, Contemporary Family Therapy, Journal of Feminist Family Therapy,* and *Journal of Clinical Activities, Assignments, and Handouts in Psychotherapy Practice.* She serves as reviewer for several journals, as a co-editor for a book on therapy interventions for couples and families, and as a co-editor on a book for the clinical treatment of infidelity. Her areas of interest include infidelity treatment, research methodology and measurement, and training in marriage and family therapy. She can be reached via e-mail at katherine.hertlein@unlv.edu.

Contributors

Jennifer T. Aberle, MS, is a doctoral student in the School of Education and adjunct instructor in the Human Development and Family Studies Department at Colorado State University. She teaches in the area of death, dying, and grief as well as family studies and human development courses. She is also a clinician in the University Drug and Alcohol treatment program and has a small marriage and family therapy private practice in the community. She has served as the managing editor for the *Journal of Feminist Family Therapy* and has written and presented in the areas of grief and loss, feminist and social justice teaching, and curricular development. She may be reached at 102 Gifford Building, Colorado State University, Fort Collins, CO 80523; 970-491-3520; jtaberle@cahs.colostate.edu.

Shayne Anderson, MS, is a doctoral student in child and family development with a specialization in marriage and family therapy at the University of Georgia. He works primarily with couples and Latino families using an attachment-based model of therapy. His research focuses on the process of change in couples therapy.

Tiffany B. Brown, MEd, is a doctoral student in the Marriage and Family Therapy Program at Texas Tech University. She recently received her master of education degree in marriage and family therapy from the University of Oregon. She currently provides medical family therapy at a children's hospital within the children's oncology and pediatric intensive care units. She has been working with children and grief for seven years as a leader of support groups for children and families and as a core staff member at an annual four day residential children's grief camp.

Stephanie R. Burwell, PhD, is an assistant professor at the University of Georgia in the Department of Child and Family Development. Her clinical and research interests are in medical family therapy, with an emphasis in behavioral oncology. Her recent publications have focused on the quality of life among younger women diagnosed with breast cancer, including depressive symptoms, sexual function following surgical treatment, and relationships with partner and children. She is an AAMFT clinical member and approved supervisor and was recently awarded an Early Career Membership to the American Family Therapy Academy.

Jason S. Carroll, PhD, is an assistant professor in the Marriage, Family and Human Development Program in the School of Family Life at Brigham Young University. Dr. Carroll specializes in couple assessment and family adaptation to adversity. He can be reached at School of Family Life, 2092-C JFSB, Brigham Young University, Provo, UT 84602; (801) 422-7529; jcarroll@byu.edu.

Olivia Chiang, PsyD, is a pediatric/family psychology fellow at the University of Rochester Medical Center. Her clinical interests include helping families cope with medical illnesses, grief and bereavement, and chronic pain.

Nicole M. Childs, MS, is a doctoral student at the University of Georgia in the Department of Child and Family Development. She is currently completing her clinical internship at Mercer

University, serving as instructor and clinician. Her clinical and research interests are in medical family therapy, sexuality, and female-related concerns. Her recent publications have focused on posttraumatic stress associated with the trauma of hurricanes, and the impact mothers' breast cancer has on adolescents. She has been an AAMFT student member since 2000. Her anticipated goal of graduation is August 2007.

William J. Doherty, PhD, LMFT, is a professor in the Department of Family Social Science and director of the Marriage and Family Therapy Program at the University of Minnesota. His scholarly and clinical interests include fatherhood; families and health; professional, family, and community partnerships; professional practice patterns of marriage and family therapists; and moral and community issues in therapy.

Christine A. Fruhauf, PhD, is an assistant professor in the Department of Human Development and Family Studies and the associate director of the Center on Aging at Colorado State University. Her research interests include family caregiving, grandparent-grandchild relationships, and quality of life for individuals who have Alzheimer's disease or a related disorder. She has published in the *Journal of Family Issues, Journal of GLBT Family Studies, Gerontology & Geriatrics Education, Geriatrics & Aging,* and the *Qualitative Report.* She may be reached at 112 Gifford Building, Colorado State University, Fort Collins, CO 80523; 970-491-1118; cfruhauf@cahs.colostate.edu.

Thomas M. Gehring, PhD, clinical psychologist, supervisor, and psychotherapist, is the author of the FAST. He is professor of psychology at the University of Basle, Switzerland and chief psychologist at the Swiss Federal Ministry of Defense, Department of Human Resources.

Miriam Claire Godwin, MS, LMFT, is an outpatient child and family therapist with PORT Human Services in Greenville, North Carolina, and part-time instructor for the Department of Child Development & Family Relations at East Carolina University. She earned a BA in psychology and a MS in marriage and family therapy at East Carolina University. Her research and clinical interests include working with at-risk adolescents and their families (in-home and collaboratively with their school), and families who have a member with a physical and/or mental disability. Her clinical specialty is incorporating the use of art into family therapy interventions. She has presented posters at the North Carolina Association of Marriage and Family Therapists and at the North American Society of Adlerian Psychology Conferences.

Heath Grames, PhD, LMFT, is director of behavioral health and a family therapist at the OneWorld Community Health Center and an assistant professor in family medicine, training family medicine residents and teaching in the medical family therapy program. Dr. Grames has a special interest in medical family therapy, depression, and cultural diversity. He can be reached at OneWorld Community Health Center 4920 South 30th St., Ste. 103, Omaha, NE 68107; hgrames@unmc.edu.

Claudia Grauf-Grounds, PhD, LMFT, is chair and associate professor for marriage and family therapy at Seattle Pacific University. She also holds clinical faculty status at the University of Washington's School of Medicine in the Department of Family Medicine. Dr. Grauf-Grounds obtained a BA from Stanford University in psychology, an MA from Fuller Theological Seminary in theology and counseling, and an MA and PhD from the University of Southern California in sociology with a certificate in family therapy. Prior to her joining the faculty of SPU, she taught and supervised at the University of San Diego and SHARP Family Practice Residency. A licensed marriage and family therapist in California and Washington and approved supervisor through the American Association for Marriage and Family Therapy, she has authored several articles on collaborative family health care and family therapy training.

Jeri Hepworth, PhD, a family therapist, is professor and vice-chair of family medicine. Her masters and doctoral degrees are from the University of Connecticut, and her professional work has focused on families and health, psychosocial issues in medicine, and managing personal and professional stress. Among her publications, she is co-author of three books: *Medical Family Therapy, The Shared Experience of Illness,* and the about-to-be-released *Family Oriented Primary Care.* She has consulted internationally and held leadership positions in multiple professional associations. Her professional commitment is to promote more effective collaboration between families, physicians, and other clinicians as they care for patients with health crises and chronic disease.

Theodore A. Hoch, EdD, is a psychologist, counselor, and board certified behavior analyst who serves as director of psychological services at Northern Virginia Training Center. He also serves as an adjunct assistant professor of special education and affiliate associate professor of psychology at George Mason University, both in Fairfax, Virginia. His clinical interests include functional assessment and treatment of problem behaviors in adults and children with developmental disabilities, and counseling and therapy for children and adults with developmental disabilities and their families.

Jennifer Hodgson, PhD, LMFT, is an assistant professor and AAMFT approved supervisor in the Department of Child Development & Family Relations and program director for the Marriage and Family Therapy Program at East Carolina University. Her research and clinical interests include working with families who have experienced a medical diagnosis, particularly Parkinson's Disease or other progressive illnesses; cross training and collaborative models; and changes due to medical technology. She has published in the Journals of *Families, Systems, and Health, Marital and Family Therapy, Journal of Trauma Practice, Journal of Feminist Family Therapy,* and *Journal of Family Psychotherapy* to name a few. Her published works have included the following topics: medical family therapy, Parkinson's Disease and the family, spirituality and Alzheimer's Disease, later life couples and breast cancer, and family therapy research.

Nathalie L. Kees, EdD, LPC, is an associate professor in the Counseling and Career Development Program in the School of Education at Colorado State University. She has served as guest editor for the *Journal for Specialists in Group Work Special Issue on Women's Groups* and for the *Journal of Counseling and Development Special Issue on Women and Counseling.* She has recently co-authored a book on group facilitation skills for managers for Praeger Publishing. She founded the American Counseling Association's Women's Interest Network and is published in the areas of women issues in counseling, women's groups, and women's spirituality. She may be reached at 224 Education, Colorado State University, Fort Collins, CO 80523; 970-491-6720; Nathalie.Kees@colostate.edu.

Nancy Taylor Kemp, PhD, is a licensed psychologist in private practice in Eugene, Oregon, and is an instructor of psychopharmacology in the Counseling Psychology doctoral program at the University of Oregon. Dr. Kemp has been in private practice for sixteen years, with specialties in the treatment of bipolar disorder, post-traumatic stress disorder, attention deficit hyperactivity disorder, and psychosocial issues related to physical disability. She has provided groups for individuals with bipolar disorder in the community and at University of Oregon while clinical director at the Counseling and Testing Center. Dr. Kemp has provided numerous presentations on bipolar disorder and on issues related to disability. She is president-elect of Lane County Psychologists' Association and a member of the International Society for Bipolar Disorders.

Shoshana D. Kerewsky, PsyD, is an adjunct assistant professor of counseling psychology and human services at University of Oregon. She is also a licensed psychologist in private practice.

Her clinical specialties include grief and loss, adjustment to chronic illness, cultural issues, and lesbian/gay/bi/trans development and concerns. She may be reached at the Counseling Psychology and Human Services Department, 5251 University of Oregon, Eugene, OR 97403-5251; kerewsky@uoregon.edu.

Angela L. Lamson, PhD, LMFT, CFLE, is an associate professor and AAMFT approved supervisor in the Department of Child Development & Family Relations Medical Family Therapy Program at East Carolina University. Her research and clinical interests include working with families who have experienced a miscarriage, stillbirth, or the death of a child in the neonatal intensive care unit; Alzheimer's; or changes due to medical technology. She has published in the *Journal of Marital and Family Therapy, Families, Systems, & Health,* and *Journal of Systemic Therapies* and presented at the American Association for Marriage and Family Therapy, Collaborative Family Healthcare Association, the International Society for Traumatic Stress Studies, and National Council on Family Relations.

Lisa Lavelle, LCSW, is a research assistant for the Center for Families and Health at the Ackerman Institute for the Family as well as a faculty member at the Ackerman Institute for the Family. She has a special interest in working with families, couples, and individuals around social justice issues and the impact of illness on families/relationships and how those relationships impact an illness. She may be reached at the Center for Families and Health at the Ackerman Institute for the Family, 149 E. 78th Street, New York, NY 10021; 212-879-4900 x145; lisalavelle@yahoo.com.

Nan Gray Lester, MS, of Eugene, Oregon, founded the Asperger Advocacy Coalition following her son's diagnosis in 1999. Her advocacy lead to major changes in regional school districts, including the development of a publicly funded, freestanding middle and high school program for students with Asperger's Syndrome that is now considered a national model. Nan holds an interdisciplinary masters degree in psychology, public policy, and education. She is currently in private practice providing support groups, counseling, and mediation services to individuals and families affected by Asperger's Syndrome, Autism Spectrum Disorder, and related disabilities.

Margo D. Maine, PhD, cofounder of the Maine & Weinstein Specialty Group, is a clinical psychologist who has specialized in the treatment of eating disorders for over twenty-five years. Author of *The Body Myth: Adult Women and the Pressure to Be Perfect* (with Joe Kelly, John Wiley, 2005), *Father Hunger: Fathers, Daughters and the Pursuit of Thinness* (Gurze, 2004), and *Body Wars: Making Peace With Women's Bodies* (Gurze, 2000), she is a senior editor of *Eating Disorders: The Journal of Treatment and Prevention* and board member of the Eating Disorders Coalition for Research, Policy, and Action, and of Dads and Daughters. A founding member and fellow of the Academy for Eating Disorders and a member of the Founder's Council and past president of the National Eating Disorders Association, she is a member of the psychiatry departments at the Institute of Living/Hartford Hospital's Mental Health Network and at Connecticut Children's Medical Center, having previously directed their eating disorder programs. She may be reached at Maine & Weinstein Specialty Group, 970 Farmington Ave., West Hartford, CT 06107; 860-313-4431; mdm@mwsg.org.

Susan McDaniel, PhD, is a professor of psychiatry and family medicine, associate chair for the Department of Family Medicine, and director of Wynne Center for Family Research in the Department of Psychiatry, at the University of Rochester School of Medicine & Dentistry. She is nationally and internationally known for her publications in the areas of medical family psychology and family systems medicine. Her special areas of interest are mental health in primary care, family dynamics and genetic illness, and gender and health. She is a frequent speaker at meetings of both health and mental health professionals. Dr. McDaniel has been recognized by the American Psychological Association as the 1995 Family Psychologist of the Year; she received the award for Innovative Contributions to Family Therapy from the American Family Therapy Academy in 2000; and the Award for Distinguished Contribution to Education from the Association of Medical School Psychologists in 2004. Dr. McDaniel was chair of the Commission on Accreditation for Marriage and Family Therapy Education in 1998, president of the Division of Family Psychology of the American Psychological Association in 2000, and chair of the APA Publications and Communications Board in 2003. Dr. McDaniel was the first psychologist, representing APA, to complete the Bureau of Health Professions Primary Care Policy Fellowship in 1998. Dr. McDaniel is co-editor with Thomas Campbell, MD, of the multidisciplinary journal, *Families, Systems & Health*. She co-authored or co-edited the following books: *Systems Consultation* (1986), *Family-Oriented Primary Care* (1990 and 2005), *Medical Family Therapy* (1992), *Integrating Family Therapy* (1995), *Counseling Families with Chronic Illness* (1995), *The Shared Experience of Illness* (1997), the *Casebook for Integrating Family Therapy* (2001), *Primary Care Psychology* (2004), and *The Biopsychosocial Approach: Past, Present, and Future* (2004). She is completing a book now titled *Individual, Families, and the New Genetics: A Biopsychosocial Perspective*.

Patrick L. Meadors, MS, is a doctoral student in the medical family therapy PhD program at East Carolina University. He is currently an associate member of AAMFT and student member of Collaborative Family Health Care Association. He was a full-time visiting instructor for two years in the Child Development and Family Relations department at East Carolina University before pursuing his doctoral education in the Medical Family Therapy program. He is currently involved in the interdisciplinary teaching of clinical interviewing skills to first year medical students at the Brody School of Medicine at East Carolina University. His research interests include working with individuals, couples, and families who have experienced loss, specifically the loss of a child due to miscarriage, and traumatic illness/injury. He is interested in self-of-the-provider issues on intensive care units who frequently experience losses.

Tai J. Mendenhall, PhD, LMFT, is an assistant professor in the Department of Family Medicine and Community Health at the University of Minnesota Medical School, and the director of behavioral medicine at the UMN's St. John's Hospital/Family Medicine residency program. His principal investigative and clinical interests include community-based participatory research (CBPR); citizen health care; and individual and family-oriented interventions for diabetes.

Carol Pfaffly, PhD, LMFT, is the associate director of Behavioral Health at the Fort Collins Family Medicine Residency Program in Fort Collins, Colorado. She manages the behavioral medicine curriculum for family medicine residents and directs the behavioral services provided to patients in the residency's medical clinic. She co-coordinates the services for an integrated mental health project implemented in collaboration with the local health district. She has published in journals such as *Family Medicine, Journal of Collaborative Family Healthcare,* and *American Family Physician.* Her research interests include child sexual abuse, collaborative family health care, and interagency health care partnerships. She may be reached at Fort Collins Family Medicine Center, 1025 Pennock Place, Fort Collins, CO, 80524; 970-495-8839; cjp1@pvhs.org.

Layne A. Prest, PhD, LMFT, is an associate professor and director of behavioral medicine in the Medical Family Therapy Program. In his practice, Dr. Prest specializes in collaborative care and medical family therapy. He has contributed to a previous Therapist's Notebook, writing on the role of spirituality in dealing with chronic illness. He may be reached at Department of Family Medicine, University of Nebraska Medical Center, 983075 Nebraska Medical Center, Omaha, NE 68198-3075; (402) 559-5393; laprest@unmc.edu.

Anne Prouty Lyness, PhD, LMFT, is associate professor and director of clinical training in the Marriage and Family Therapy program within the Department of Applied Psychology at Antioch New England Graduate School in Keene, New Hampshire. Anne attended two-and-one-half years at the University of South Carolina School of Medicine prior to switching to family therapy. She earned her masters degree in marriage and family therapy from East Carolina University in 1993 and her doctorate from the Purdue University in 1996. She has a lifelong interest in feminism and her writing reflects her clinical and research interests in women's health and the importance of focusing on human diversity and marginalized voices in therapy, training, and research. She has served in divisional and national offices within the American Association for Marriage and Family Therapy of which she is a clinical member and approved supervisor. She is also the current editor of the *Journal of Feminist Family Therapy,* and a partner in an interdisciplinary group private practice in Keene, New Hampshire.

Lauren Reese, MS, did her undergraduate work at the University of Georgia with a degree in child and family development. She then worked as the coordinator of the Family Solutions Program in Athens, Georgia, for two years. Lauren completed her master's in Marriage and Family Therapy at East Carolina University in May 2005. She lives in Atlanta, Georgia, with her family.

W. David Robinson, PhD, LMFT, is an assistant professor and associate director of behavioral medicine and the Medical Family Therapy Program. Dr. Robinson has contributed to a previous Therapist's Notebook, writing on the role of spirituality in dealing with chronic illness. He may be reached at Department of Family Medicine, University of Nebraska Medical Center, 983075 Nebraska Medical Center, Omaha, NE 68198-3075; (402) 559-5868; wdrobins@unmc.edu.

G. Bowden Templeton, MS, LMFT, is a doctoral student in Department of Child and Family Development at the University of Georgia specializing in marriage and family therapy. He received a master's degree in marriage and family therapy from Mercer University School of Medicine where he developed clinical and research interests in medical family therapy.

Michelle R. Ward, MS, LPC, LMFT, is in private practice with Creative Therapy Associates in Fairfax, Virginia. She earned her masters degree in marriage and family therapy from Virginia Tech University in 2000. She specializes in play and expressive art therapy with children and adolescents, and family therapy with children and their families. She is a clinical member of the American Association for Marriage and Family Therapy, the American Counseling Association, and the Association for Play Therapy.

Foreword

While the earliest origins of family therapy were in medical settings (e.g., Bateson, Jackson, Haley, & Weakland, 1956), the fields of family therapy and medicine long had an uneasy relationship (e.g., Denton, 1990; Haley, 1976, 1980; Minuchin, 1974). Eventually, addressing the inherent connection between families and illness became unavoidable and the "medical family therapy" movement began to take shape (e.g., McDaniel, Hepworth, & Doherty, 1992). Medical family therapy was initially only a niche area of interest within family therapy. Accompanied by a growing interest of family therapists to move into the mainstream of health care (Shields, McDaniel, Wynne, & Gawinski, 1994), the ideas of medical family therapy slowly began to take hold within the larger practice of family therapy. Today, aspects of medical family therapy have been incorporated into the curriculum of most, if not all, marriage and family therapy programs (e.g., Denton, Patterson, & Van Meir, 1997), and specialization is even beginning to be offered in some settings. The growth of medical family therapy has been both in conjunction with and parallel to the related movement of collaborative health care (e.g., Doherty, 1995; McDaniel, Campbell, & Seaburn, 1995).

As a domain of clinical practice matures, the development of professional resources for providers must develop alongside. Medical family therapy has benefited from seminal texts (e.g., McDaniel, Hepworth, & Doherty, 1992; Rolland, 1994), innovative academic instruction (e.g., Patterson & Magulac, 1994; Patterson & Van Meir, 1996), and the development of internships (e.g., Brucker et al., 2005; Edwards, Patterson, Grauf-Grounds, & Groban, 2001). The field is also now ready for additional resources for medical family therapy practitioners. Therapists working in medical settings or with families facing medical conditions can benefit from readily implementable ideas that will be beneficial to these families. Drs. Linville and Hertlein have succeeded in compiling such a resource—one of the first of its kind for medical family therapy.

The present text provides a wide range of practical interventions that will be immediately useful in working with families coping with a multitude of medical conditions. The first section presents interventions that will be applicable to nearly any family coping with a chronic condition. Specific interventions for working with children (an often overlooked group in family therapy) are age-appropriate and constitute another section. Illness-specific interventions are provided in another section for many of the most common illnesses encountered in clinical practice. An entire section is provided for interventions related to grief and loss; grief and loss are everyday aspects of the practice of medical family therapy and will be of great benefit to therapists and families alike. Finally, medical family therapy can be emotionally draining to the therapist and a bonus section addressing the "self-of-the-medical family therapist" offers thoughtful suggestions for self-care.

This work has numerous strengths. Many of the established and emerging leaders of the medical family therapy movement are contributors and practitioners can benefit from their accumulated years of experience and apply clinically tested interventions in their own practices. Although there are multiple authors, each chapter follows the same outline which helps give the book one "voice." The interventions are applicable to therapists from a wide variety of theoretical backgrounds and, in many cases, actual handouts are provided or descriptions of materials needed are carefully listed.

This book is important in representing the growth and development of medical family therapy but, most significant, it provides useful ideas and tools for clinical medical family therapists. It is a book that the practicing medical family therapist will want to own, read, and refer back to.

Wayne Denton, MD, PhD, LMFT

References

Bateson, G., Jackson, D. D., Haley, J., & Weakland, J. (1956). Toward a theory of schizophrenia. *Behavioral Science, 1,* 251-264.

Brucker, P. S., Faulkner, R. A., Baptist, J., Grames, H., Beckham, L. G., Walsh, S., et al. (2005). The internship training experiences in medical family therapy of doctoral-level marriage and family therapy students. *American Journal of Family Therapy, 33,* 131-146.

Denton, W. H. (1990). A family systems analysis of DSM-III-R. *Journal of Marital and Family Therapy, 16,* 113-125.

Denton, W. H., Patterson, J. E., & Van Meir, E. S. (1997). Use of the DSM in marriage and family therapy programs: Current practices and attitudes. *Journal of Marital and Family Therapy, 23*(1), 81-86.

Doherty, W. J. (1995). The why's and levels of collaborative family health care. *Family Systems Medicine, 13,* 275-281.

Edwards, T. M., Patterson, J. E., Grauf-Grounds, C., & Groban, S. (2001). Psychiatry, MFT, & family medicine collaboration: The Sharp Behavioral Health Clinic. *Families, Systems, & Health, 19,* 25-35.

Haley, J. (1976). *Problem solving therapy.* San Francisco: Jossey-Bass Inc.

Haley, J. (1980). *Leaving home.* New York: McGraw-Hill.

McDaniel, S. H., Campbell, T. L., & Seaburn, D. B. (1995). Principles for collaboration between health and mental health providers in primary care. *Family Systems Medicine, 13,* 283-298.

McDaniel, S. H., Hepworth, J., & Doherty, W. J. (1992). *Medical family therapy: A biopsychosocial approach to families with health problems.* New York: Basic Books.

Minuchin, S. (1974). *Families and family therapy.* Cambridge, MA: Harvard University Press.

Patterson, J. E., & Magulac, M. (1994). The family therapist's guide to psychopharmacology: A graduate level course. *Journal of Marital and Family Therapy, 20,* 151-173.

Patterson, J. E., & Van Meir, E. (1996). Using patient narratives to teach psychopathology. *Journal of Marital and Family Therapy, 22,* 59-68.

Rolland, J. S. (1994). *Families, illness, and disability: An integrative treatment model.* New York: Basic Books.

Shields, C. G., McDaniel, S. H., Wynne, L. C., & Gawinski, B. A. (1994). The marginalization of family therapy: A historical and continuing problem. *Journal of Marital and Family Therapy, 20*(2), 117-138.

Preface

The effects of illness, disability, and loss in our everyday lives can be profound. Such physical and emotional experiences can alter our daily routines, influence our decision-making processes, deplete our resources (financial and emotional), and generate a wide variety of perceptions and emotions. In addition to individual repercussions, these challenges also mark the lives of the family members and social networks of those individuals experiencing them. Some common problems faced by couples and families with health care issues include changes to familiar roles, adjustment to a new stage within the couple or family lifecycle, increased conflict and communication problems, potential financial difficulties, and managing caretaking responsibilities.

While many books and journals present a wide variety of interventions for relationships, couples and families managing chronic illness, disability, and/or loss often present with unique clinical issues which may not be best served by typical interventions. Special considerations for this population are warranted, given the specific way a health care issue might manifest itself within a particular family system. In order to be most effective, therapists treating clients with health care or loss issues (even when such issues are not identified as the presenting problem) should be well-versed in the effects of health care and bereavement issues on systems, as well as have some knowledge of specific illnesses such as cancer, diabetes, and HIV/AIDS to be able to fully understand their clients.

The purpose of this book is to offer family therapists many creative resources (homework, handouts, or activities) designed for working with clients dealing with illness, loss, and disability. This is accomplished by introducing readers to field-tested theoretical interventions. It allows counselors the benefits of reading about effective activities that have helped clients struggling with health care or grief issues. This book is a primary resource for providing a comprehensive guide of interventions for working with specific issues affecting individuals, couples, and families dealing with illness, loss, and disability. In addition to information about specific family dynamics and topics, it also provides practical therapeutic activities for the use in the practice of mental health clinicians providing health care to families.

Organization

This book is organized into five sections: interventions for working with families and chronic illness, interventions for working with children and chronic illness, illness-specific interventions for families, interventions for working with grief and loss, and a bonus section devoted to professional development. The first chapter of the first section, devoted to interventions for families, highlights the biopsychosocial-spiritual information within a client system by describing an interview structure for gaining such information. The next two chapters in this section provide interventions devoted to assessing the impact of the social network of clients. These are followed by four chapters that present various ways to cope with illness, loss, or disability and also focus on how to adapt to the circumstances that these health care challenges may bring. The last two chapters in this section present an application of IFS to working with illness, and an application of a wellness-oriented family group to a low-income population.

The chapters in the next section are allocated to those interventions specifically geared toward children and adolescents. In some cases, the focus of these interventions is on the child or adolescent experiencing the illness; in other cases, the child or adolescent is adjusting to or coping with the diagnosis or the loss of an important figure in their lives. The interventions for children include activities that focus on relieving symptomology, helping children to process their emotions related to illness or loss, and cultivating problem-solving strategies. The next chapter highlights a unique intervention for teens with diabetes, and the last chapter is devoted to children and teens with a diagnosis of Asperger Syndrome.

The third section contains interventions for specific illnesses. The first two chapters focus on HIV/AIDS patients and their families. These are followed by two more chapters presenting creative ideas for the treatment of clients with a diabetes diagnosis. The treatment of eating disorders is the topic of the next two chapters. These are followed by a contextual model for working with female partners of those who suffer from dementia. The subsequent chapter relates to interventions for cancer patients and their families. This section is completed by a chapter discussing a specific intervention for families who struggle with a bipolar member.

Grief and loss comprise the interventions for the fourth section. Here, the chapters are organized in a manner consistent with life-cycle development. For example, the first chapter provides an intervention for children who are struggling with managing grief and loss, followed by one couple and two family activities. The last chapter in this section details an intervention for working with aging parents and making end-of-life decisions. Finally, in the last section, we provide readers with two chapters that can help them navigate illness, disability, and loss in their clinical practice, whether it be their own issue or that of their clients.

Creativity with Unique Challenges

Individuals and families dealing with medical illness, disability, and loss may have unique needs warranting interventions that are responsive to the particular challenges that they face. Many of the interventions in this book capitalize on the roles creativity and generativity play in addressing the unique struggles of clients dealing with illness, disability, and loss. Medical family therapists can have an important role in delivering effective systems-oriented health care that values interactions between the mind and body as well as among the family, the health care team, and the greater community.

Acknowledgments

We have been most fortunate to have been influenced by many wonderful people. With a special thanks to our families, specifically Eric Knobelspiesse and Eric Hertlein, for putting up with our schedules and believing in us. Thanks to the staff at The Haworth Press for their enthusiasm and willingness to support this project, especially Dr. Lorna Hecker, series editor, for offering us the opportunity to be involved in a project that benefits the practitioners that believe in the spirit and benefits of collaborative health care. Wayne Denton has provided us with a wonderful forward, and we would like to thank him for taking the time out of his busy schedule to support this project. We also would like to thank our numerous authors who have contributed to this book and who have made this project a success. It has been an excellent opportunity to work with such a talented pool of clinicians and authors; we have learned so much from their stories and their creative ingenuity, and believe that clients are lucky to have these thoughtful and effective clinicians in the field.

SECTION I:
INTERVENTIONS FOR WORKING WITH FAMILIES AND CHRONIC ILLNESS

Chapter 1

The Biopsychosocial-Spiritual Interview Method

Jennifer Hodgson
Angela L. Lamson
Lauren Reese

Type of Contribution: Activity/Intervention

Objective

Conducting an initial interview can be a challenging task even for the seasoned mental health professional. Initial interviews are typically time limited. The objective is to get to know as much as possible about the client/patient in a short period of time, while effectively joining and communicating empathy. To support the acquisition of a comprehensive patient/family profile, the authors have taken the biopsychosocial ideas of Engel (1977, 1980) and combined them with attentiveness to spirituality (Wright, Watson, & Bell, 1996) to form the Biopsychosocial-Spiritual (BPSS) Interview method. The BPSS interview consists of questions regarding the client/patient's physical symptoms, diagnosis, and medical treatment (Biomedical aspect); the thoughts, feelings, and state of mental health associated with the illness/treatment (Psychological aspect); the sources of support and relationship to and with others (Social/Environmental aspect); and the client/patient's system of beliefs (Spiritual aspect). This method can help professionals gain insight as to how the client/patient physically and emotionally copes with the illness, as well as the support systems that are available to him or her. Using this method with the family members of the identified patient also helps in the assessment of resources and support, and the impact that the illness has on the family system. Please note that from this point on, the term *patient* is synonymous with *client* and refers to the person(s) receiving services.

Rationale for Use

As McDaniel, Hepworth, and Doherty wrote in their groundbreaking 1992 text titled, *Medical Family Therapy: A Biopsychosocial Approach to Families with Health Problems:*

> The days of innocence are over. We now know that human life is a seamless cloth spun from biological, psychological, social, and cultural threads; that patients and families come with bodies as well as minds, feelings, interaction patterns, and belief system; that there are no biological problems without psychosocial implications, and no psychosocial problems without biological implications. Like it or not, therapists are dealing with biological problems, and physicians are dealing with psychosocial problems. The only choice is whether to do integrated treatment well or do it poorly. (pp. 1-2)

Therefore, as family therapists gain access to primary, secondary, and tertiary care settings, being armed with a structured comprehensive interview method is imperative to their work.

Engel noted (1977, 1980) that from the subatomic to the biosphere levels we are all connected. The smallest abnormal cell mutation may have global impact as patients go for second and third opinions, families wrestle with the potential loss of a family member to an unknown illness, providers struggle with how or whether or not to quarantine the afflicted, communities search for the source and tout theories about the meaning for its presence, and scientists feverishly work to identify its lethality and race for a cure. Viruses such as HIV fit this description. To focus only on the psychological impact would ignore the social and spiritual ramifications that may be feeding the presence of depressive or anxious symptoms. It is therefore impossible to separate any part of the illness experience without losing sight of the whole. Whether it is a first, fourth, or last session, medical family therapists are aware of the power of each dimension and never lose sight of any of them throughout the course of therapy.

Biologically we are enigmas; much of what happens underneath the surface of the skin is a mystery. Patients come to providers describing symptoms that may or may not fit a known cause. Medical family therapists may gain intimate access to biological symptoms as patients fear or do not see the importance of mentioning them to their medical providers. Loss of muscle strength, aches and pains, changes in libido, loss of or increase in appetite and sleep, and gastrointestinal discomfort are examples of such symptoms. To many mental health providers these symptoms may be relegated to the territory of medical providers and deemed outside one's scope of practice, but as the conductor of a symphony, all parts are meaningful even if we do not understand how to fix a broken instrument. The key is to be inquisitive and unassuming. The objective is to collect information and assemble the puzzle with the patient, family, and health care team.

Psychologically, patients are most open to mental health providers regarding emotions or the way they feel, think, and behave. Alert to the subtle changes in how they approach life's challenges or react to stressors, newly diagnosed patients or those overcome by chronic illness find the uneasiness of psychological distress somewhat unbearable. While many desire a rapid fix toward relief, many accept the idea that it took two weeks, two years, two decades, two generations to develop the problem, and that it will not go away overnight. However, most will not share the deeper layers of the onion with the therapist during the initial sessions. This is reserved for a time when trust has been established. In the beginning, most are inclined to talk outside of the obvious reasons they are entering into a therapeutic relationship.

Socially, many think that their problem is their responsibility and therefore their duty to amend *it*. It is unrealistic to assume that extracting the person from his or her natural environment and interacting with him or her as an isolated part without connection to a larger system will give therapists a complete understanding of how the problem is perpetuated or perhaps how the problem is a solution in and of itself that may lead to deeper and more protected issues. Whether it is a broken leg, traumatic brain injury, or diagnosis of a terminal disease, the individual who is the recipient of the diagnosis will need people in their natural environment to help him or her though out the healing process. Many therapists and medical professionals have failed to ask about the impact of the social system only to find out later that it is a large contributor to the patient's noncompliance with medications or the designated treatment plan. It is easier to claim patient resistance than to admit to trying to force a round puzzle piece into a square space.

Spiritually, the beliefs and meaning that patients and family members ascribe to an illness may have grand implications for treatment plan adherence or strategy. Beyond the dramatic stories of refusal of medical procedures or pharmaceuticals, some believe that illness is the result of bad karma, failed attempts to know Jesus, a disrespect for the environment, trapped demons, or past sins that have finally caught up to the perpetrator. Regardless of affiliation with an organized religion, everyone has beliefs and meaning that they ascribe to why they are hurt, ill, disabled, or facing death. These beliefs may in turn have a direct impact on the person's or family's willingness to make necessary changes toward wellness.

In isolation, each of these variables is enough for any one person to manage. However, we cannot continue to ignore the interrelatedness of these variables or our responsibility for organizing treatment that is comprehensive. Therefore, the proposed Biopsychosocial-Spiritual Interview Method can assist clinicians in obtaining a comprehensive understanding of their patient's constellation of symptoms, beliefs, meaning, and strengths. This helps patients recognize that details fused together as a whole make greater sense than telling a story without intimate knowledge of all the significant characters.

Instructions

The BPSS Interview is designed to facilitate the gathering of information about a patient for the purpose of building rapport, understanding his or her illness experience, and establishing a sense of his or her social network. The following format may be adopted for the purpose of gathering information and detail for the benefit of the patient, caregivers, and larger system. Interviewers may gather data using a pencil and paper but not allow that or the recommended questions to sterilize the process and interfere with joining with the interviewee. Interviewers should jot down notes and also construct a narrative summary of the interview experience later and place a copy in the patient's file. Summaries should be clear and succinct for members of the treatment team to read.

The interview was developed for use in an inpatient rehabilitation unit of a major medical hospital and has also been used in hospice, nursing homes, assisted living environments, and community homes of individuals over the age of sixty-five. It may be amended for use in primary, secondary, and/or tertiary care settings. The interview is for an initial visit that may or may not lead to a formal therapy agreement. Medical family therapists often assess the patient prior to the medical provider visiting them. This interview format could be used for that situation as well as a triage or initial interview assessment.

Opening/Building Rapport

Purpose: The opening of an interview is critical. It is not recommended that the interviewer approach the interview with the intent to gather as much data as possible. Although this is a wonderful secondary gain, the most important task is to build trust and let the interviewee know that you are interested in him or her and want to be helpful. It is also important that the interviewer explain the purpose (e.g., part of initial intake, triage for services, etc.) and intent of the BPSS interview experience and how it may be helpful to the patient and/or family once it is complete. In our training program we use it as a training guide for newer therapists to assist them in learning how to ask questions about each area of the human experience. However, we firmly believe that this should be standard care for all therapists who practice medical family therapy. Depending on the context and situation, some of the following statements may need modification. We propose the following as a possible opener to the interview experience:

Statement: Hello Mr./Mrs./Ms./Dr. {name}. My name is {your name} and I am here to talk with you a little bit about your overall health. I am a {insert profession} who is invested in making sure that you get the best care possible and believe that by collecting the following information I can begin to understand the strengths and struggles that you have experienced prior to our meeting today. If it is okay, I would like to talk with you about your biomedical and psychological health, as well as information about your social network and the beliefs and meaning you attribute to your current health status. If at any time the questions I am asking make you uncomfortable, or you tire from talking, just let me know. I am here to learn from you and to assist you by obtaining information that may be helpful to you as you make decisions about your health care.

General Questions

Purpose: As with any initial interview it is important to obtain basic demographic information. Depending on your place of employment you may be required to obtain certain facts (e.g., insurance information, diagnosis history, place of birth, current medications, etc.). Feel free to tailor the next part of the BPSS interview to your unique setting. If more than one person is in the room, you may want to obtain this information from them as well, particularly if they are family (as defined by the object of the interview) or part of the caregiving system. NOTE: some restrictions may exist in your work environment regarding the request of information from non-patients; following accreditation standards and federal guidelines supersedes the involvement of non-patients in the interview process. We recommend that you initiate this part of the interview with the following statement, "I am going to ask you a few general questions to get an idea of who you are and a little bit about your social and occupational history." The following represent a few questions that may be useful in your data collection process. The initial question is intentionally open-ended and is designed to allow the interviewee(s) to guide the process. The sequence of questions after that point is irrelevant.

Questions:

1. Could you tell me a little bit about yourself (such as age, marital status, children, occupation)?
2. Who do you currently live with in your household (names, ages)?
3. What is your present employment status? If on leave of absence or disability from your job, do you plan to return to it?
4. If you could choose anywhere in the world to live where would it be and why?
5. What do you do for pleasure and relaxation?

Biomedical

Purpose: Depending on the context and nature of the person's medical/mental health visit, this section may be more or less intense for the individual and his or her loved ones. If in a secondary or tertiary care setting, the severity of the individual's health may be more obvious; if so, then this section may need to be approached more gingerly or directly. It is recommended that if the client/patient is not new to the system, but is new to you, that you first ask the nurses, physicians, etc. about the best way to initiate this section. The last question is designed to serve as a transitional aid into the next section of the interview and may also result in powerful theories that the patient/family holds about the interrelatedness of their biomedical and psychological well-being.

Possible Questions:

1. Could you tell me a little bit about the status of your health, illness/injury experience? What symptoms are you concerned about? Which ones did you notice first? What procedures or treatments have you had to help manage it/remedy it?
2. Can you tell me a little bit about your relationship with your medical providers? For example, what have they done that has been helpful to you and what are the more difficult parts of working with the medical system?

3. What has surprised you most about how your body has responded to what it has been through?
4. Have you, or any of your family members, ever needed medical attention for an illness or injury in the past? If yes, how will it or how has it influenced your current experience?
5. How do you notice that your physical symptoms impact your emotions, thinking, and behavior?

Psychological

Purpose: The psychological experience of a patient may be closely guarded unless it is the focus for his or her visit. The interviewer is encouraged to ask questions that appear to fit the patient's/family's experience and level of comfort. This interview tool is useful for an initial assessment and as a potential alert to items in need of follow-up. If during the course of the interview it is determined that the interviewee/family member is at risk for harm to self or others, the obvious course of action is to move into crisis management mode and discontinue the interview method as prescribed. Interviewees must understand that as mental health providers they are bound to the same legal mandates regardless of being an assigned mental health provider or of simply conducting an initial assessment. The following questions are designed to help understand the mental, emotional, and behavioral changes that may have accompanied the reason for the visit. Again, the last question is designed to serve as a transitional aid to the next section.

Possible Questions:

1. How do you think that your illness experience has impacted you (e.g., emotionally, mentally)?
2. What has been the emotion that has surprised you the most throughout this experience? Why?
3. Has anything changed regarding the way you think about yourself, your family, and your other activities (e.g., work, hobbies, etc.) since your diagnosis? If so, what?
4. What thoughts can you bring up that make you feel good about yourself? What thoughts tend to deplete you of the vital energy needed to take care of yourself?
5. What comments have your family and/or friends made to you about how you are handing life, your relationships, the reason for your visit?

Social/Environmental

Purpose: Oftentimes the patient is alone and the interview is conducted from only his or her perspective. Tailor this section as appropriate to those in attendance. The interview may be interventive as issues or details are brought to the surface. Help the people in the room understand that this interview is designed to gather information and not necessarily be a direct path to change. If during the course of the interview people get upset and the interview context becomes unsafe or too intense, discontinue the interview with the family system and ask to continue it only with the identified patient. Offer up the explanation that it is important to have as much information as possible to assist the person coming in for care, but over time we hope to help resolve or initiate change with the issue(s) that seem to be important to all of the family system. The purpose of this section is to understand the impact that the health visit and/or illness/injury experience has had on one's social network (e.g., spouse, children, siblings, parents, close friends, coworkers, etc.) and the environmental conditions that may impact their health and well-being.

Possible Questions:

1. Beside yourself, who would you say worries most about your health? What worries him or her?
2. Who are the members in your support system who have done the most to assist you (emotionally, mentally, physically, etc.) throughout this experience? What have they done? Who do you wish would do more and why?
3. What challenges, related or unrelated to the reason for your visit today, are present with your social support system? How have you been dealing with them?
4. How does your family show one another that they care or are concerned (particularly in an illness/injury situation)?
5. What other stressors (e.g., financial, transportation, occupational, legal, educational, etc.) are weighing on you and complicate how you are able to manage your health?

Spiritual

Purpose: This is often the topic that clinicians seem to have the most difficulty asking about during the interview process. It is important for the interviewee to understand that this section is not designed to judge one's beliefs or convince others to become religious or spiritual. Rather, it is designed to understand the beliefs and meaning that may be attributed to the reason for the health concerns/visit. By working within the belief structure of the interviewee, one may understand the challenges present when making a change, accepting medical intervention, or following up with a recommended treatment plan. It may also be a source of hope and strength for the patient and family members during a time when answers may not be readily available and time is moving along at a relentless pace.

Possible Questions:

1. Why do you believe that you have had this illness experience, health crisis, or pattern of remarkable health?
2. What meaning has (reason for visit) given to your life?
3. Is there a person, place, or thing beyond you that helps you to cope with the reason for your visit? If so, how is this helpful for you?
4. Has your health experience influenced your thoughts about spirituality? If yes, how?
5. What parts of your health do you believe are beyond your control?

Closing

Purpose: It is important that the person participating in this interview knows what will happen with the information that has been shared. If it will become part of his or her chart, this needs to be stated in the beginning as well as restated at the conclusion of the interview. If the person conducting this interview remains part of the treatment team, it is important that the patient and family members present have an opportunity to summarize this experience (e.g., what it was like, anything they may want to add, what will they remember most about it), as well as note what goals they have as a result of the information shared.

We recommend that to close the interview you thank your interviewee(s) by name for the time spent and information shared. Let them know that you will be sharing what you learned with (whomever will have access to their chart and/or who is the object of a signed release) and that if used as a class assignment, research instrument, or vehicle for a conference presentation any identifying information will be removed to maintain privacy and confidentiality. If appropriate shake interviewee(s) hand and return furniture (e.g., chair) where it was before you entered the room.

Brief Vignette

The following is a condensed version of a BPSS Interview conducted between a master's level marriage and family therapy student and a patient receiving care at an outpatient surgical clinic. Some information has been changed to protect the interviewee's identity.

General Patient Information. Patient is a single Caucasian female in her late forties. Patient worked as a teacher for many years then later as a nurse. Patient is currently working as an energy or healing touch therapist. She currently lives alone and has two grown children. Her son is thirty-one years old and is described as being very intuitive and a smart man. Patient stated that her daughter has Down syndrome and is deaf. Patient stated that her daughter lives on her own with the help of an aide and volunteers at a local soup kitchen. Patient describes her daughter as a challenge but she also stated that she feels as though she has learned so much about herself from her daughter.

Biomedical. Patient stated she has had some serious bouts with illness over the past twenty years. Patient stated she was diagnosed with Guillain-Barré syndrome[1] in 1980 and then went into remission a few years later. In 1991, she was hospitalized for pneumonia. Then in 2000, patient stated she could hear her spleen talking to her and she knew something was wrong but she kept ignoring it. Then one night she went to the movies and bowling with her friends. During the course of the night her friends kept telling her that she looked "yellow." Patient went to the hospital that night and was admitted because when the doctors checked her hemoglobin it was only 3.2. On average, a normal hemoglobin range should be between 12 and 18 g/dL (grams per deciliter of blood). The doctors told her that he was surprised she was still standing. Patient was then diagnosed with cirrhosis (liver disease). That night the doctors told her that she needed to stop drinking and the patient replied, "I don't drink." Patient stated that she had always eaten healthy foods and taken care of her body. When asked about her relationships with her medical providers, patient stated that she has always had good relationships with her doctors and nurses and felt support from them.

Psychological. When asked how the patient felt she has been dealing emotionally with her illness, patient stated she feels that even though she has faced many challenges, she believes she is here on earth for a reason. In addition, she said she felt that it is not her time to go yet. Patient feels joy and strong sense of self. Patient stated that she keeps herself positive and strong with the use of daily affirmations, meditation, and deep breathing exercises. Patient also stated that her morning routine helps her to stay strong throughout the day.

Social. When asked about the members of her support system, the patient stated she has a very strong social support network. She said she feels blessed because she has so many wonderful friends and great relationships with both her parents and her children. When asked who she was most proud of in her family, patient stated the she was very proud of her son for being strong willed, intuitive, and intelligent.

Spiritual. Patient was asked what role she believed her spirituality has played in her health and well-being and she replied that her spirituality has had a major impact on her life. She stated that her faith has been instrumental in managing her illnesses. Patient also stated that her faith has been the most important part of her life and it greatly influences her outlook on life.

---

1. Guillain-Barré syndrome (GBS) is a rare medical condition involving a person's immune system and nerves. It causes the muscles to not function as they are supposed to, and in severe cases, the patient may be paralyzed. Most victims are hospitalized for it but usually make a full and complete recovery.

The following is a personal reflection from the student who conducted the interview:

This experience has been a very positive learning process for me. After she [the patient] agreed to complete the interview she immediately began to tell me about her children and work history. I was just so amazed at how willing she was to open up to me. I thought we would just talk about this on a surface level but she really seemed to feel comfortable and we just began talking.

I thought it was interesting because before the interview, I had gone through the interview form and marked the questions I wanted to ask. I had brought the form with me and was planning to take some notes so that I would not forget any important information. However about three to four minutes into the conversation I set the paper aside and relaxed into my seat and I was able to give the patient my full attention. I suppose I realized that I did not need to write anything down. I recognized that I would remember the important parts. What was more important at that moment was that I gave my full attention to the patient.

I was incredibly amazed by this woman's strength. She is an unbelievable person who has weathered so much in her life. I just sat there and listened to her in awe of her vitality and accomplishments. It was remarkable to me that I could feel so much positive energy in the room even though she was talking about such difficult times in her life.

Completing this interview was a very positive growth experience for me. I think I will feel much more comfortable talking with clients about illnesses or injuries now. At the end of the interview, I began to scan my interview outline to see if I had forgotten to ask any important questions and I realized that we had covered every item I had checked off. I never even had to look at the paper. A really important lesson I learned from this experience is to let the client/patient take me where he or she needs to go. I discovered that if I can do this, then we are probably going to get much further than we would if I tried to lead the client/patient on my agenda.

Suggestions for Follow-Up

Reflection is essential for developing a treatment plan that accommodates the patient's unique personality and needs. Reflect on what therapy skills, interventions, or psychoeducation may be important for this patient/family given the information obtained in the interview. You may be able to take into account what theoretical approach, evidence-based research, or clinical information is most appropriate to share at follow-up sessions or prior to discharge. Make sure to collaborate first with the other medical provider(s) involved in his or her care so that you are all consistent with the overall treatment plan.

Give a typed summary back to patient/family to review and edit (much like member checking in qualitative methodology). This way the interviewer is able to capture whether personal biases influenced the way that questions were asked or the way that answers were written. A dictation device may assist with maintaining the integrity of the interview and transcript.

Contact other personal/professional collaborators relevant to the patient's care to assist you in fulfilling the goals discussed in the BPSS Interview summary. If possible, assemble a biopsychosocial-spiritual team to maximize care and treatment outcomes.

Use a summary of the BPSS Interview as a treatment team opener/impetus for initiating collaboration. This will give all of the team members an idea for who the patient is and the systemic issues surrounding the health issues at hand. Do not forget to include the patient and members of his or her support system on this team too!

Revisit the BPSS interview every fourth visit (if on a weekly basis), or once a month for more infrequent visits, to see if any changes have emerged. This will insure that the appropriate treatment plan and team are in place and involved and that goals are being adequately addressed. A summary of any changes should be documented in the patient's chart.

Use scaling questions to note improvements and changes in areas of growth. It may be important to use a scaling question (rating change on a scale of 1 to 10) for each of the BPSS subsections and then a scaling question for overall well-being.

Contraindications for Use

Some medical contexts make obtaining BPSS interview information a challenge (e.g., acute care situations, semiprivate rooms). Although a more thorough one can be obtained at a later date, some acute care situations require medial or mental health stabilization before this information can be collected. Some rooms contain other patients and families separated simply by a thin curtain and confidentially cannot be insured.

If information about suicide, homicide, child maltreatment, or domestic violence emerges then the collection of information in subsequent sections is inappropriate until the crisis is resolved or a plan of safety is put into place. Also, if the interviewee refuses participation, then the use of this intervention is contraindicated. It is imperative that the patient be present and that consent is provided. Other family members or support system members may also be present but the patient must be there and give consent for anyone else to participate. Likewise, if the interviewee is under the age of eighteen, then consent obtained from the parental unit or legal guardian consent is required. Finally, certain health conditions may make complying or recognition of full compliance challenging to ascertain (e.g., traumatic brain injury, dementia, substance abuse). In these situations it is best to wait until the patient has medical clearance or is determined to be cognitively intact.

References and Resources for the Professional

Blount, A. (Ed). (1998). *Integrated primary care: The future of medical and mental health collaboration.* New York: W. W. Norton.

Cummings, N. A., Cummings, J. L., & Johnson, J. N. (Eds). (1997). *Behavioral health in primary care: A guide for clinical integration.* Madison, WI: Psychological Press.

Engel, G. L. (1977). The need for a new medical model: A challenge for biomedicine. *Science, 196,* 129-136.

Engel, G. L. (1980). The clinical application of the biopsychosocial model. *American Journal of Psychiatry, 137,* 535-544.

McDaniel, S. H., Hepworth, J., & Doherty, W. J. (1992). *Medical family therapy: A biopsychosocial approach to families with health problems.* New York: Basic Books.

Patterson, J. Peek., C. J., Heinrich, R. L., Bischoff, R. J., & Scherger, J. (2002). *Mental health professionals in medical settings.* New York: W. W. Norton.

Rolland, J. S. (1994). *Families, illness, & disability: An integrative treatment model.* New York: BasicBooks.

Seaburn, D. B., Lorenz, A. D., Gunn, W. B., Gawinski, B. A., & Mausch, L. B. (1996). *Models of collaboration: A guide for mental health professionals working with health care practitioners.* New York: BasicBooks.

Wright, L., Watson, W. L., & Bell, J. M. (1996). *Beliefs: The heart of healing in families and illness.* New York: BasicBooks.

Bibliotherapy Sources for the Client

Clark, C. C. (2002). *American holistic nurses' association guide to common chronic conditions: Self-care options to complement your doctor's advice.* Hoboken, NJ: Wiley.

Keene, N. (1998). *Working with your doctor: Getting the healthcare you deserve.* Sebastopol, CA: O'Reilly & Associates, Inc.

Korsch, B. M., & Harding, C. (1997). *The intelligent patient's guide to the doctor-patient relationship: Learning how to talk so your doctor will listen.* New York: Oxford University Press.

Pettus, M. C. (2004). *The savvy patient: The ultimate advocate for quality health care.* Herndon, VA: Capital Books.

Thomas, L., Oster, N., & Darol, J. (2000). *Making informed medical decisions: Where to look and how to use what you find.* Sebastopol, CA: O'Reilly & Associates, Inc.

Tolson, C. L., & Koenig, H. G. (2003). *The healing power of prayer: The surprising connection between prayer and your health.* New York: Baker Books.

Chapter 2

A "FAST" Approach to Health Care

Thomas M. Gehring
Katherine M. Hertlein

Type of Intervention: Activity

Objective

The purpose of this intervention is to use the Family System Test (FAST) (Gehring, Debry, & Smith, 2001) to explore clients' experiences with their health care system and providers. It can be used for both assessment and intervention with individuals, couples, and families whose lives are significantly intertwined with the health care system.

Rationale for Use

Families are affected by many systems, on both the micro and macro levels. In addition to the systems and subsystems that affect one another in the home, couples and families interact with external systems on a daily basis. For example, adults employed outside the home are affected by their work environment, including co-workers, management, workload demands, and the structure of the workday. Children and adults who attend schools are also influenced by their academic environment, including interactions with peers, teachers, and larger social issues. Systems thinkers ascribe to the concepts of circularity and recursiveness, meaning that just as one's attitudes, cognitions, and behavior are influenced by external systems (or macro levels), one's characteristics also have a marked impression on these macro levels.

Although therapists typically assess for the impact macro levels have with their clients, the importance of this assessment is especially pronounced when working with clients who present with a health care issue. The relationship between the client, family, and health care system is a critical component to one's healing process. Using the FAST (see Figure 2.1) is one important way to identify the extent to which couples and families are affected by their health care concerns.

The FAST (Family System Test) is an assessment and treatment tool developed to assess clients' views of their family, specifically their views on family cohesion and hierarchy within the family (Gehring, Debry, & Smith, 2001). The goals of the FAST include identifying the extent of any health-related or psychosocial issues within the family; assessing the family's conceptualization of their relationships; and to measure change within the family structure and cohesion. In the FAST, clients are encouraged to (take blocks and place them) place symbolic figures on a board in relation to one another, representing how cohesive they feel toward the other family members. In addition, they are also encouraged to place family members who have greater positions of hierarchy within the system atop other blocks, towering over other members. In this

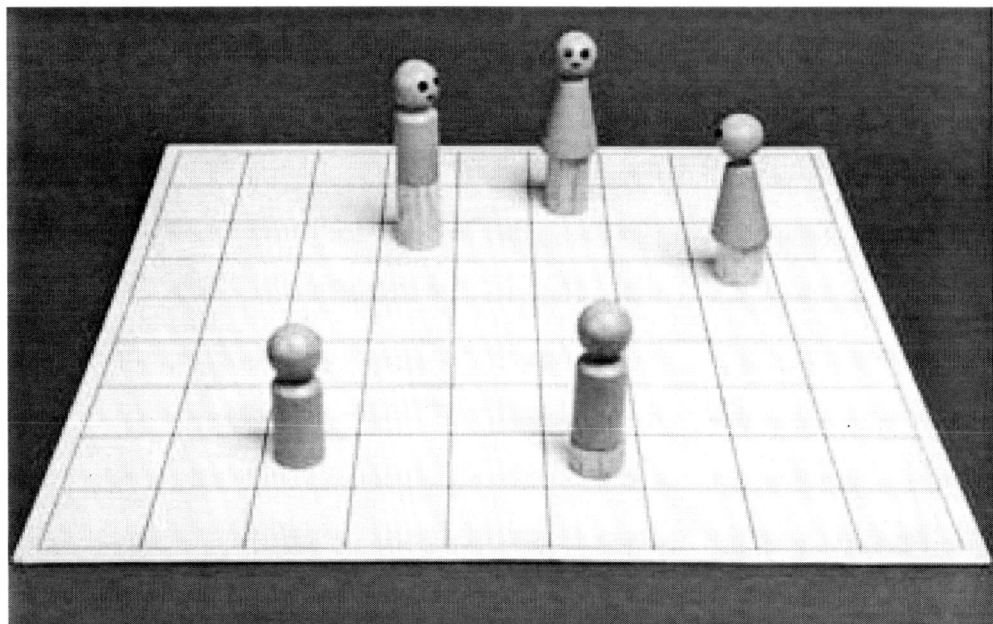

FIGURE 2.1. *Source:* From Gehring, T.M., Debry, M., & Smith, P.K. (Eds.) (2001). *The Family System Test: Theory and Application.* Sussex, England: Brunner-Routledge.

way, including cohesion and hierarchy, one's position and structure in the family is represented in relation to other family members. The FAST is based on three theoretical frameworks. First, it is underscored by structural family therapy (Minuchin, 1974) (families are encouraged to place characters higher and lower than other characters as a way to represent hierarchy) which stresses the negative impact of unclear generational boundaries such as cross-generational coalitions and reverse hierarchies. Second, it is influenced by developmental family psychology in that family relationships may change whether the family is experiencing a transition or managing a difficult developmental stage. Finally, the family psychopathology framework influences the FAST, as it can provide a window to assess healthy and disturbed members of the family in their perception of the family (Gehring, Debry, & Smith, 2001).

In addition to the three frameworks on which the FAST is based, this specific intervention related to health care is also based on two other frameworks: Bronfenbrenner's ecological model and symbolic-experiential therapy. Bronfenbrenner believed that people are affected and influenced by three levels of ecosystems: microsystem, exosystem, and macrosystem. Microsystems operate in the closest proximity to us and are composed of our immediate family, group of friends or peers, neighborhoods in which we live and possibly including places of worship. The next level is the exosystem, which comprises schools, mass media, employment, community, and medical agencies. The macrosystem is politics, societal values, and economics. Specifically related to this intervention, therapists can use the FAST to assess and enhance the relationship between the microsystem (individual and family) and the exosystem (health care) in a symbolic manner.

Symbolic-experiential therapy is a framework that allows clients to explore their world in greater detail through the use of symbols (Connell, Mitten, & Whitaker, 1993). People use symbols to represent their experiences. More specifically, this activity has its roots in the Kvebaek Family Sculpture Technique. The Kvebaek Technique is a family sculpture technique that asks family members to symbolically represent how close they feel to one another (Berry, Hurley, & Worthington, 1990; Hernandez, 1999). The therapist invites family members to identify themselves as a block, and then to place these blocks on a standard grid as a way to demonstrate closeness to one another. Once the family members place themselves either near or far from one another, they may use this arrangement as a metaphor throughout the course of therapy (Connell, Mitten, & Whitaker, 1993).

In our adaptation of the FAST, the therapist encourages the family to select figures (pieces) to represent the members of their family, but also pertinent people in the health care profession related to their current condition. Such people might include but are not limited to: primary care physicians, specialists, nurses, pharmacists, and/or insurance company representatives. Further, the symbolic representation of the family may be altered during different developmental stages of illness identified by Rolland (1994).

Instructions

The FAST evaluation consists of three different types of materials for the client: a monochromatic board, six male and six female characters, and eighteen cylindrical blocks of different heights (Gehring & Marti, 2001). The evaluator also needs a four-part test form, a tool explaining the scoring of the instrument, and a protocol for the follow-up interviews that should be conducted. These materials can be ordered from Hogrefe and Huber Publishers. The Web site is: http://www.hhpub.com (see Figure 2.1.).

Although there are several specific steps to the FAST, it is easy to conduct, takes a short time to complete (approximately ten minutes for individuals and thirty minutes for families or other groups), and demonstrates good reliability and validity. When using the FAST, the therapist first shows the client(s) how to place figures on the board, how to show hierarchy, and explains the meaning of the various representations. The therapist then turns the task over to the clients who place the figures in relation to one another per their perspective, as well as in hierarchical positions. The therapist records the height of each figure as well as distance from one another and conducts a follow-up interview per FAST protocol. After clearing the board, the therapist asks the family to depict the family as they would like to see it, clears the board, and again conducts a follow-up interview. Finally, the therapist asks the family to place the figures in a way representative of the family structure in a conflict. Related to health care, the therapist would also ask the family to include figures representing the pertinent people related to their health care issue.

Brief Vignette

Nicole and Jordan came to therapy citing communication problems. The couple had been married for fourteen years. They came to therapy after Nicole's diagnosis with multiple sclerosis. The couple had two small children, ages five and seven. Jordan was also becoming increasingly concerned with Nicole's reduced mobility. In the past two years, her mobility was so impaired that she was spending most of her days on the couch. Nicole was upset because she would ask Jordan to do more around the house and he was constantly forgetting. She indicated that it was difficult for her to get around the house and accomplish the small tasks, and that she felt ignored when Jordan "did not care enough" about her or their family to maintain the housework while she was ill. At this point in their communication, the couple indicated that these conversations about household responsibilities would escalate into fights.

The therapist initially had the couple depict where they currently saw each other and where they would like to be. Jordan depicted Nicole in a higher position in the family, and put himself in her shadow, facing her back. Nicole depicted Jordan as being turned away from her. When the therapist had the couple place the pieces where they would like to be, Nicole and Jordan positioned themselves in higher places over their children, but turned toward and close to each other. When the therapist instructed the couple to depict how they would represent their struggle with the MS, an interesting pattern emerged. Nicole picked a piece which she labeled "symptoms."

She put this piece atop several blocks and demonstrated how this piece towered over her. She also put the piece close to Jordan, and the two pieces faced her. Nicole placed the piece representing herself in a far corner of the board. When it was Jordan's turn to complete the activity, he placed Nicole on several blocks, and in between he and Nicole, placed the children, her physician, and her mother. He placed everyone else on blocks with the exception of himself.

The therapist encouraged Jordan to discuss what stood out the most in Nicole's representation. He stated that the symptoms stood out the most, and it almost felt like Nicole was a "slave" to her symptoms. Nicole told Jordan that was accurate and that she really wanted to do what she used to do around the house, but that she was at the mercy of the severity of her symptoms. Nicole did not realize that Jordan felt last in her life and she asked him to do things not because she viewed him as last, but because she felt she could depend on him as she had so many other times in her life.

This conversation was the first the couple had about household management that did not escalate into an argument. The therapist encouraged both Nicole and Jordan to select one thing they could do each day over the next week to bring themselves symbolically closer to where they wanted to be. Jordan admitted that he was worried the symptoms would eventually take over Nicole and that he would effectively lose his wife. Nicole reassured him that she was still the same person despite the illness, and suggested that they start spending time focusing on aspects of their relationship that had not changed.

After this session, the therapist continued to use the FAST regularly as a way to track the changes in the couple's life. Nicole reported that she liked seeing how she and Jordan were getting closer together because it reinforced their process even more. Jordan stated that if he could not communicate what he wanted to say to Nicole, he could use the representation as an example.

Suggestions for Follow-Up

As mentioned, this game-like activity is an intervention as well as an assessment. The therapist should make note of the positions of the pieces. As therapy progresses, the therapist can use this tool as a way to evaluate how close the family is getting to their ideal picture. Under what circumstances or after which interventions/discussions in therapy did members significantly change their positions? Did some members grow closer while others grew farther apart? Another suggestion for the families is to have the family perform some homework task related to the representations they made in session, such as journaling. Some prompts for journaling might include:

- What was difficult about this activity? What was rewarding for you?
- Were you surprised by any of the representations that your family members made? Why or why not?
- What things do you want to be different in your family? What things do you want to see the same?
- Who determined who went first? Why?
- Did you learn anything you did not know before about your mother? Father? Daughter? Son? If so, what?

Contraindications for Use

As family members depict their perceptions about the family, it is imperative that each family member maintains an environment of safety and security. The therapist must be able to ensure that family members are respectful to one another as opposed to attacking one another for how they each depict the family. It is imperative that the therapist use this intervention only if he or she is certain the family members will act in a respectful way toward one another.

References

Berry, J. T., Hurley, J. H., & Worthington, E. L. (1990). Empirical validity of the Kvebaek Family Sculpture Technique. *American Journal of Family Therapy, 18*(1), 19-31.

Connell, G. M., Mitten, T. J., & Whitaker, C. A. (1993). Reshaping family symbols: A symbolic experiential perspective. *Journal of Marital & Family Therapy, 19*(3), 243-251.

Gehring, T. M., Debry, M., & Smith, P. K. (Eds.). (2001). *The Family System Test: Theory and application.* Sussex, England: Brunner-Routledge.

Gehring, T.M. & Marti, D. (2001). Concept and psychometric properties of the FAST. In: T.M. Gehring, M. Debry, & P.K. Smith (eds.), The Family System Test (FAST): Theory and Application. London and Philadelphia: Routledge, pp. 3-27.

Hernandez, S. (1999). The emotional thermometer: Using family sculpting for emotional assessment. *Family Therapy, 25*(2), 121-128.

Minuchin, S. (1974). *Families and family therapy.* Cambridge, MA: Harvard Press.

Rolland, J. (1994). *Families, illness, and disability: An integrative model.* New York: Basic Books.

Readings and Resources for the Professional

Gehring, T. M., Debry, M., & Smith, P. K. (Eds.) (2001). *The Family System Test: Theory and application.* Sussex, England: Brunner-Routledge.

Kaduson, H. G., & Schaefer, C. E. (2001). *101 more favorite play therapy techniques.* Northvale, NJ: Jason Aronson, Inc.

Marston, D. C., & Szeles-Szecsei, H. (2001). Using "play therapy" techniques with older adults. *Clinical Gerontologist, 22*(3-4), 122-124.

Mitten, T., & Piercy, F. P. (1993). Learning symbolic-experiential therapy: One approach. *Contemporary Family Therapy, 15*(2), 149-168.

Chapter 3

Increasing Social Support to Manage Chronic Illness

Claudia Grauf-Grounds

Type of Contribution: Homework, Intervention

Objective

Families dealing with chronic illness often experience a depletion of emotional and practical resources overtime. As resources dwindle, secondary illness related to the chronic illness (e.g., depression) can be found in other family member as well as the primary patient. The objective of this intervention is to remind the family that they have social resources that can be accessed, and to facilitate the connection to these resources.

Rationale

A key dimension in positively coping with illness is access to social support. Family stress theory (McCubbin & Patterson, 1983) and resiliency theory and research (Walsh, 1998) speak to the need to increase social support in order to adapt well to stressful life events. Several reviews of the literature emphasize how higher levels of social support relate to better health outcomes for those suffering with a wide range of chronic illnesses (Rowe, 1996; Kaplan & Toshima, 1990; House, Kahn, McLeod, & Williams, 1985).

Chronic illnesses bring a host of new time-consuming lifestyle requirements. Commonly, the patient and his or her family must shift old patterns of functioning and relate to one another in different ways. As demands on time are increased in one area, resources become drained and even simple tasks can become overwhelming (e.g., buying groceries). Increasing practical support in maintaining daily activities can significantly decrease stress in the family. The emotional needs of family members can also heighten and a wide range of grief responses are common. When families have emotional support with the variability of responses over time, they are able to function more effectively (Walsh, 1998).

Families who face chronic health issues need to reorganize themselves for both short-term and long-term concerns of individual members and the family as a whole. More closed family systems might have ability to respond well to a health crisis in the short term, but can show burnout in the long run. Rolland (1994) addresses how families vary in the tasks that are needed at different stages of an illness. Families that are able to access resources flexibly often do better than families that treat problems as fixable in a time-limited way.

Central to the exercise explored in this chapter is the capacity for family members to bring in resources when there is need and to recognize that the needed resources are both practical and emotional. The impact of chronic illness is often unpredictable, so a good day can easily be followed by a bad day. Therefore, resources must be practical. Family members sometimes report preferring to talk to someone on the outside of daily activity (Farmer, Marien, & Clark, 2004). A person listening and caring for one's emotional responses associated with chronic illness can be as much of a gift as someone picking up one's children from school. The coping theme of "letting others help" is difficult for many independent or isolated persons; patients and their families clearly benefit when they allow others to assist them.

Instructions for Homework

If this exercise is done as *homework*, the patient (and his or her family) is asked to write down the names of extended family or friends who might be willing to assist the patient/family in a specific practical or emotional way. Offering examples to the patient/family is useful. You might ask them to consider: *"Who in your family or friendship network might be willing to take care of the kids for awhile?"* or *"Who might you take a walk with?"* or *"Who might make a healthy meal for you?"* or *"Who in your family might lend a shoulder to lean on if you are having a bad day?"* or *"Who might be able to drive you to a medical appointment?"* What is important here is to simply list the names of persons who might be interested in becoming a support. Do not be concerned about how they would help.

The next part of the homework is to gather addresses for the persons listed. These can either be residential or e-mail addresses. (If the patient is not functioning very well, have family members or friends assist in this aspect of the exercise so it does not become too burdensome.) If the addresses are residential, purchase 4 × 6 index cards, envelopes to fit one index card, and stamps for the number of names listed.

Place the following note inside the envelope along with the index card, replacing the patient name and contact information with your own or type this note in the text portion of the e-mail. This is known as the "model letter."

> As a friend or family member of Joan Wood, you are being asked to write down one to two ways that you might be able to help her in the next year. Joan needs support to work on some of her health issues right now and we believe you would like to encourage this. Try to be very, very specific, such as: "I would be willing to cook a dinner for Joan and her family," or "I would be willing to talk to Joan on the phone for a half hour when she is feeling stressed," or "I would be willing to run an errand for Joan that will take an hour" or "I would be willing to take care of your kids for one weekend a year."
>
> On one side of the enclosed index card, please list that best way to contact you and on the other side list the specific activity you would be willing to contribute. Mail this card back to Joan at the following address: 245 Elm Street Quincy, WA 97440. It you cannot help at this time, please feel free to send the card back noting this. Thank you for the gift of considering this kind of support.

The final part of the exercise is for the patient to collect the cards he or she receives back from the "support persons" and place them in a visually prominent and central location of the home. For example, several patients who did this exercise chose to place their cards in a photo album and placed this on top of their bedroom dresser. The patient is directed to read the index cards on a regular basis and to use the offered resource when needed or at least once during the year.

Instructions for Intervention

When this exercise is done as an *intervention*, the therapist and/or physician requests that the patient actually invite extended family members and friends into the clinical setting. Sometimes a conference room needs to be found to accommodate the number of persons who attend. If a physician is present, he or she can briefly explain the impact of chronic illness on the patient and some behaviors that could be helpful in addressing the specific chronic illness (e.g., reduce stress, low-fat diet, exercise, feeling emotional support from family/friends). The therapist/physician can facilitate the previous exercise, passing out an index card to each person and asking him or her to write on one side, a specific way he or she might be able to assist the patient, and on the other side, his or her contact information. The patient collects the index cards and places them in a central location in the home.

Brief Vignette

Gina, age thirty-three, received a diagnoses of diabetes and chronic hypertension from her primary care physician about a year ago. Divorced for five years, Gina has primary custody for her two children ages nine and six, although the children visit their father during holidays and during the summer. The oldest has been diagnosed with attention deficit disorder, but seems to be doing well with medication and meeting with a school counselor. In general, Gina functions adequately, and works full-time as a nurse. The children's father pays child support fairly regularly; however, he struggles with his alcohol use and sometimes calls Gina in the middle of the night after he has had too much to drink and asks her to take him back. Most of her extended family and her ex-husband live in the neighboring state. There are many days in Gina's life that are stressful, exacerbating her chronic illness conditions.

Gina is overweight, monitors her blood sugars regularly, but has not been able to address her hypertension. Her physician has strongly recommended a regimen of medication and exercise to address her high blood pressure. Some weeks Gina binges on sugar and overeats; during these times, she does not check her glucose levels. Her father also has diabetes and has had serious circulatory problems in his feet, with the threat of amputation.

The therapist working with Gina noted that she was continuing to do less and less self-care regarding her health issues, and mild depressive symptoms were developing. The therapist had worked with Gina since Gina had moved to the area two years after her divorce, and determined that this would be a good time to attempt to increase Gina's social resources. For a homework assignment, Gina is asked to develop a list of persons including neighbors, church connections, friends at work, children's school connections, and extended family who might be willing to provide some intermittent help with the children, the house, or her health issues. Names of persons who might be easy to talk with about her family situation are also requested. Gina returns the assignment to the therapist two weeks later. Eight names are listed and briefly reviewed. Gina is given a "model letter" to use as a template and she is asked to modify and copy the letter as she wishes, purchase index cards, envelopes, and stamps for the eight persons. She then is asked to mail the letters.

Two weeks later Gina has five index cards in her hand, and with tears in her eyes, states that she is feeling hopeful again. Her work friend offered to walk with her on a regular basis during lunch. Two extended family members wrote that they would love to take the kids for a weekend while she visited her father; they also stated that they would be willing to "talk anytime" about the family situation. A church friend said that she would place Gina on her "prayer concern list" and pray for her everyday; she also suggested that they take a cooking class together for people with diabetes. Finally, a neighbor and school-related friend of Gina's children invited Gina to use their home as a "drop off" anytime so that Gina could do some exercise or just get some "time alone at home."

Gina decided to purchase a small photo album with a daisy on the cover to put the index cards into, and then placed the album by her bed stand. In this way she said she was reminded each day of the support she had around her.

Suggestions for Follow-Up

Follow-up depends on the context of care. If a medical office has a behavioral specialist, the therapist and/or primary care physician can ask how well the patient is accessing his or her social support during regular primary care visits used to monitor the diabetes and hypertension. In a psychotherapy clinic setting, social support can be reviewed at regular intervals. Questions can also be asked if new needs have developed and if new persons might be needed to help the patient and his or her family better manage the chronic illness. In this way, a continuing pattern of bringing in resources from the outside is punctuated and encouraged.

Contraindications for Use

In general, this exercise works well with those with few social contacts, since it tends to shape acquaintances into friends. However, those who have limited abilities to choose healthy relationships must be cautioned in this exercise. For example, if clients choose partners with domestic violence histories for social support, the cost of these relationships might outweigh their benefits. Assist clients in selecting those who can offer assistance without jeopardizing their safety.

References and Readings for the Professional

Farmer, J. E., Marien, W. E., & Clark, M. J. (2004). Primary care supports for children with chronic health conditions: Identifying and predicting unmet family needs. *Journal of Pediatric Psychology, 29*(5), 355-367.

Gagnon, L. M., & Patten, S. B. (2002). Major depression and its association with long-term medical conditions. *Canadian Journal of Psychiatry, 47*(2), 149-153.

Glasgow, R. E., Strycker, L. A., Toobert, D. J., & Eakin, E. (2000). A social-ecologic approach to assessing support for disease self-management: The chronic illness resources survey. *Journal of Behavioral Medicine, 23*(6), 559-583.

House, J. S., Kahn, R. L., McLeod, J. D., & Williams, D. (1985). Measures and concepts of social support. In S. Cohen and S. L. Symes (Eds.), *Social support and health* (pp. 83-108). San Diego: Academic Press.

Kaplan, R. M., & Toshima, M. T. (1990). The functional effects of social relationships on chronic illnesses and disability. In B. S. Sarason, I. G. Sarason, & G. R. Pierce (Eds.), *Social support: An interactional view* (pp. 427-453). New York: Wiley.

McCubbin, H., & Patterson, J. (1983). The family stress process: The double ABCX model of adjustment and adaptation. In H. McCubbin, M. Sussman, & J. Patterson (Eds.), *Social stress and the family: Advances and developments in family stress theory and research* (pp. 7-37). Binghamton, New York: The Haworth Press.

Moldin, S. O., Scheftner, W. A., Rice, J. P., Nelson, E., Knesevich, M. A., & Akiskal, H. (1993). Association between major depressive disorder and physical illness. *Psychological Medicine,* (23), 755-761.

Riess-Sherwood, P., Given, B. A., & Given, C. W. (2002). Who cares for the caregiver: Strategies to provide support. *Home Health Care Management & Practice, 14*(2), 110-121.

Rolland, J. (1994). *Families, illness, and disability: An integrative treatment model.* New York: Basic Books.

Rowe, M. A. (1996).The impact of internal and external resources on functional outcomes in chronic illness. *Research in Nursing & Health, 19*(6), 485-497.

Schein, L. A., Bernard, H. A., Spitz, H. I., & Muskin, P. R. (Eds). (2003). *Psychosocial treatment of medical conditions: Principles and techniques.* New York: Brunner Routledge.

Tichon, J. G., & Shapiro, M. (2003). With a little help from my friends: Children, the Internet and social support. *Journal of Technology in Human Services, 21*(4), 73-92.

Uchino, B. N., Cacioppo, J. T., & Kiecolt-Glaser, J. K. (1996). Relationship between social support and physiological processes: A review with emphasis on underlying mechanisms and implications for health. *Psychological Bulletin, 119,* 488-531.

Walsh, F. (1998). *Strengthening family resilience.* New York: Guilford Press.

Bibliotherapy Sources for the Client

Fennell, P. A. (2001). *The chronic illness workbook: Strategies and solutions for taking back our Life.* Oakland: New Harbinger Publications.

Register, C. H. (1999). *The chronic illness experience: Embracing the imperfect life.* Center City, MN: Hazelden.

Rossman, M. D. (2002). *The art of getting well: Maximizing health and well-being when you have a chronic illness.* Alameda, CA: Hunter House Publishers.

Wells, S. M. (2000). *A Delicate Balance: Living Successfully with Chronic Illness.* New York: HarperCollins Publishers.

Chapter 4

Doctor's Bag of Coping Skills

Miriam Claire Godwin

Type of Contribution: Activity

Objective

The purpose of this activity is to assist clients in developing numerous coping skills that can be used when they are faced with challenges associated with their illness or disability or that of a family member. The activity can also be used with families to demonstrate their capability to cope appropriately with challenges posed by illness or disability. This activity can be used in conjunction with treatments prescribed by medical professionals.

Rationale for Use

Illness, loss, or disability can be stressful for patients and their family members because of the sometimes complex and/or unpredictable changes and challenges they can pose. Realigning family roles and understanding the loss of functioning due to the illness, loss, or disability can be stressful because of the adaptation it requires (Rolland, 1994). Any event (such as a medical diagnosis) can be perceived as stressful by a family because of the variable amount of change it can require in the family's system. Any change to a family's sense of equilibrium can result in an increased level of stress (McKenry & Price, 2000). The sense of a loss of control over one's health or the health of a loved one can be very stressful and result in unhealthy coping mechanisms. Parents can feel stressed when their child is diagnosed with an illness or disability because they want to "fix it" or protect their child and they may be unable to do so due to the nature of the diagnosis. Siblings can feel stressed because they feel ignored by their parents or other family members when the attention is on the ill or disabled family member.

Clients faced with their own illness or disability or that of a family member may need to develop appropriate coping skills to support healthy functioning as individuals and as part of a family system. The development of healthy coping skills can reduce stress by utilizing appropriate outlets for feelings that may otherwise manifest in ways that are hurtful (i.e., angry outbursts or violent acts). Unmanaged stress can negatively influence health and further exacerbate the physical symptoms of the client experiencing the illness or disability, or it can negatively influence the health of family members who are not diagnosed with the illness or disability (Campbell, 2000). When caring for a loved one who has an illness or disability, the physical health of the caregiver is important because he or she needs to be able to provide care and cannot do so if he or she falls ill. Managing stress can support the client and their family members in speeding the recovery process by promoting good emotional and physical health. Likewise, reducing stress can help lower the intensity, duration, and presence of many physical symptoms because stress tends to exacerbate physical symptoms of all kinds (Campbell, 2000). Effectively managing stress can support a family in returning to a new, healthy equilibrium so that they can function as a system once again (McKenry & Price, 2000).

Clients develop coping skills in many ways. They may have been using the same coping skill for years because it worked in reducing stress when it was utilized (e.g., a client may draw every time she feels stressed because it has worked for her since she was a young child). Some clients develop coping skills by talking to others and discovering what they use as tools for reducing stress (e.g., a client may find that her friend walks around the block when she feels stressed and may try the same activity when experiencing stress herself). Resources available to family members in the community can support the development of appropriate coping skills. Support groups can be a very useful resource for clients in managing stress and developing coping skills. The group meetings may share coping skills or have open discussions about coping skill development to aid in the reduction of stress. Sometimes, just sharing thoughts and feelings in a support-group setting can be a tremendous stress reducer because it provides clients the opportunity to express themselves. Taking part in a support group allows clients to build connections to others that are experiencing similar situations and creates a sense of normalcy. Building connection between family members can also serve as a coping skill. According to Olson, Russell, & Sprenkle (1980), families that are high in cohesion are more successful in adjusting to stressful events.

This activity was designed to encourage clients to develop coping skills that they can draw from in times of stress. This activity is different from what is predominantly seen in literature relating to stress because it links coping skills directly to medical illness or disability. It can be tailored to meet the needs related to coping with a specific illness or disability. This activity focuses on identifying and building off of the preexisting appropriate coping skills of the client and identifying and eliminating inappropriate coping skills.

Clients dealing with an illness or disability often become very familiar with medical professionals during their treatment. The "Doctor's Bag" concept builds off of the client's familiarity with medical professionals and the tools professionals use in treating illness or disability. The activity was derived from the theoretical base of Experiential Family Therapy. Experiential theorists believed that, "a healthy family deals with stress by pooling its resources and sharing problems, not dumping them all on one family member" (Nichols & Schwartz, 2001, p. 178). Using resources to manage stress is the focus of this activity. Healthy expression of feelings (often through appropriate coping skills) can facilitate mental health, according to experiential thought (Nichols & Schwartz, 2001).

Instructions

The clinician should share with the client that doctors frequently have a bag of tools or instruments they use when treating patients. They should ask the client if he or she has ever seen a doctor or other medical professional use a bag to carry their tools or instruments. The clinician should discuss with the client when he or she has seen a doctor use the tools in his or her bag to treat a patient, themselves, or an ill family member. All family members present should be encouraged to share feedback on what items might be in a doctor's bag.

The clinician should take time to process with the client what the term "coping skills" means to him or her and in what situations coping skills could be employed. The clinician should establish a clear understanding with the client under what circumstances he or she should use coping skills. Questions that could be asked are, "What feelings have you experienced in relation to the illness/loss/disability that have been negative? What are some challenges you have faced in relation to the illness/loss/disability?" The clinician should process with the client how he or she would know when it is time to use a coping skill. The clinician could ask, "When would it be most helpful to use a coping skill? What feelings or situations would warrant the use of a skill to help you cope in a healthy way?" The clinician should process with the client specific feelings (e.g., sadness, anger, anxiety, or stress) and specific situations (e.g., increased arguing in the house, increased intensity or duration or presence of a physical symptom) that could warrant the use of a coping skill.

The clinician should ask the client when or if he or she has experienced these feelings or situations and ask, "How have you handled those feelings or situations? What is something you could do to assist you in handling that emotion or situation in a healthy way?"

The clinician should focus the client on the coping skills he or she is currently using when faced with challenges associated with personal illness/loss/disability or that of a family member. The client should be engaged in listing the coping skills currently used on separate, small sheets of paper (i.e., "writing in my journal" or "listening to music"). The clinician should assess with the client what coping skills listed are adaptive and effective. The client should not be listing ineffective or maladaptive skills (smoking cigarettes, hitting the family pet, etc.).

The clinician should encourage the client to think of new coping skills and list them as well (i.e., "talking to my mom" or "taking a walk"). The clinician could ask questions such as, "In that situation, what needs to be done to help you function in a healthy and positive way?", "The last time you felt that way, what could you have done differently to handle it in an appropriate way that was not harmful to yourself or others?", "What are some things you could do to release negative feelings in a way that will not harm yourself or others?" With each coping skill named, the clinician should instruct the client to write the coping skill on a separate piece of paper, fold it, and set them all aside to be placed in the "Doctor's Bag."

The clinician should engage the client in decorating his or her "Doctor's Bag" in any manner he or she chooses. If there is more than one client present, they should each be provided a bag, as each individual's coping skills may differ. They should be instructed to complete the decoration process all at one time. The bag should be completed during the session, but left to dry (if paint or glue was used) someplace secure until the next session. If the bag is taken home, the risk of damaging the decorations is very high and should be avoided.

The client or clients should be encouraged to use positive colors, words, or pictures to decorate the bag and help them visually recognize it as a positive tool for them. Positive words could include: hope, faith, patience, love, peace, etc. Positive pictures could include: a religious symbol, smiley faces, hearts, animals, etc. Anything representing positive feelings for the individual client will be ideal for decorating the bag.

The clinician should encourage the client to think of actual materials to include in the "Doctor's Bag" for use as a coping skill (i.e., a stress ball to squeeze or an actual journal he or she writes in) and ask him or her to place these materials in the bag.

The clinician should challenge the client to make his or her "Doctor's Bag" readily available and to pull coping skills from it when feeling stressed, anxious, angry, etc. The clinician could provide storage examples such as: beside the bed, in the car, in a child's backpack, in the family room, etc. The bag should be kept wherever the client can easily access it when needed.

Supplies

The bag used for this activity should be a blank, canvas bag available at a local craft store. The bags are usually cream in color, which allows the client to cover the material with any desired decoration. The bag could also be one that the client already has that has special meaning to him or her (an old purse or a small duffle bag). If the client provides his or her own bag and it is already decorated, he or she can add iron-on decals, ribbons, or buttons to add to its decoration. These materials can also be purchased at a local craft store.

If using the blank, canvas bag for the activity, decoration supplies such as fabric paints, fabric markers, and/or glitter glue should also be provided. These can be purchased at a local craft store or craft department. When using paints, markers, or glitter, a smock should be provided to protect the client's clothing from damage.

The clinician should also provide paper (ordinary notebook paper will suffice) to write the coping skills on, and/or the actual materials used for the coping skill. Some of the materials could include: play dough (used to manipulate with the hands when feeling frustrated), a stress ball made from sand and balloons or purchased at a local store, crayons and paper used for drawing if that has been identified as a coping skill, or a list of directions for relaxation breathing techniques.

Brief Vignette

Laurel, age ten, came to therapy with the presenting concern that she was having angry outbursts when her brother, Ben, age four, exhibited symptoms of the cerebral palsy he had been diagnosed with two years earlier. Her therapist explored the specific situations that influenced her angry outbursts. The therapist encouraged Laurel to share the emotions she was having difficulty handling. He gave her an opportunity to express the concerns about her brother's behavior and how it influenced her behavior.

The therapist processed with Laurel what "coping skills" were and under what circumstances they should be used. They worked together in exploring what coping skills Laurel already possessed, assessed them for effectiveness and appropriateness, and made a list of alternative and new coping skills.

Laurel was provided a blank, canvas bag, fabric paints, markers, and glitter glue to create her "Doctor's Bag of Coping Skills." The therapist discussed with Laurel what a "Doctor's Bag" was and instances in which she had witnessed a medical professional use tools or instruments to work with her brother and his illness. The therapist helped Laurel understand how she could create her own "Doctor's Bag" and fill it with activities that would support her in effectively coping with her brother's illness.

Laurel used the fabric paints to write "love, happiness, patience, and family" on her bag. She said those words helped her remember the good things about her brother. She also created drawings of their family pet and a cross that symbolized her religious beliefs. Laurel set aside the bag to dry and worked with her therapist in creating coping skills to fill the bag. They added play dough to use when Laurel felt frustrated with her brother, and she agreed to manipulate it with her hands to work out her feelings, rather than hit her brother as she had done in the past. They included a journal for Laurel to write in when she felt like communicating her feelings, instead of yell at her parents as she had done in the past. They also added crayons and paper for her to use to draw, which she said she often did when she felt alone and scared.

Laurel discussed the bag and its contents with the therapist. They agreed she would keep the bag in the family room because that is where she often encountered her brother's stress provoking behavior and where she often had her angry outbursts. Laurel discussed with her therapist how and when she would use the bag and discussed what she could do if the bag was not readily available (such as taking a walk).

After a few additional sessions, the therapist discussed with Laurel how she had been using the "Doctor's Bag" and what had been most helpful about the activity and the coping skills discussed. The therapist worked with Laurel in determining that one of her coping skills was no longer effective and they developed a more appropriate one to place in the bag.

Suggestions for Follow-Up

The clinician should process with the client what it was like to develop his or her "Doctor's Bag" and see how many coping skills the client already possessed. The clinician could ask, "What did you like about the activity? What did you not like about the activity? What feelings did you experience when you were creating the bag? Were you surprised how many coping skills you already had?"

Another follow-up suggestion is for the clinician to process with the client when he or she used the "Doctor's Bag" and how it was or was not helpful. "When was the first time you used the Doctor's Bag?" "When was a time you think you should have used the bag and didn't?" "What stopped you from using the bag at that time?" "What can you do in similar situations in the future?" "What has been the most helpful thing about the bag?" "What has been the least helpful?"

In addition, the clinician might challenge the client to continue adding to the bag as he or she thinks of new coping skills. Time should also be taken in future sessions to do a "check up" to see what coping skills are no longer effective. When the client describes times in which he or she was unable to cope with situations or feelings effectively, the clinician should do a "check up" to see what needs to be added or subtracted from the current list of coping skills in the "Doctor's Bag."

The clinician should also process with the client the difference between bags medical professionals use and the one the client developed. Encouraging the client to explore things other than medicine that can assist people in coping with illness/loss/disability is often helpful. By exploring this aspect of coping with an illness/loss/disability, the clinician is supporting the client in developing a sense of agency, or an active involvement in medical care. The client could develop a better sense of control over his or her environment and behavior, which will benefit not only the client, but the rest of the family as well.

This activity can be used with clients of all ages and developmental ranges, but may pose special challenges for people personally experiencing the illness or disability. If the client is missing limbs or is paralyzed, the clinician should physically assist the client in the creation of the bag. The client should give verbal instructions about how the bag should be created and what the contents will be. If the client is unable to communicate verbally, then written or computer generated instructions should be made available.

The clinician should take special precautions to make sure the bag is readily available to the client (e.g., fits securely on the back of the wheelchair for a client that has a broken ankle and leg) and that the coping skills in the bag will be effective for the client. Coping skills that are not appropriate for the client should not be included in the bag (e.g., if the client is missing a leg, the coping skill of "running around the block" would be inappropriate. If the client was in a wheelchair, the coping skill of "wheel around the block" would be more realistic).

The activity should only be used with clients who express a desire to utilize and increase coping skills when faced with challenges associated with an illness/loss/disability. Specifically, the clinician might not use this activity if the client has not requested that developing coping skills be one of the treatment goals. It is also important that clinicians are aware of maladaptive coping skills, suicidal ideations, or abuse that may be present in the client's life or home. Assessing for safety of the client is important at every stage in treatment.

References and Resources for the Professional

Campbell, T. (2000). Physical illness: Challenges to families. In P. McKenry & S. Price (Eds.), *Families and change* (pp. 154-182). Thousand Oaks, CA: Sage Publications, Inc.

Davey, M., Gulish, L., Askew, J., Godette, K., & Childs, N. (2005). Adolescents coping with mom's breast cancer: Developing family intervention programs. *Journal of Marital and Family Therapy, 31,* 247-258.

Forman, S. G. (1993). *Coping skills interventions for children and adolescents.* San Francisco: Jossey-Bass.

Jones, A. (1998). *104 Activities that build: Self-esteem, teamwork, communication, anger management, self-discovery, and coping skills.* Richland, WA: Rec Room Publishing.

McKenry, P., & Price, S. (2000). Families coping with problems and change: A conceptual overview. In P. McKenry & S. Price (Eds.), *Families and change* (pp. 1-21). Thousand Oaks, CA: Sage Publications, Inc.

Nichols, M., & Schwartz, R. (2001). *Family therapy: Concepts and methods.* Boston: Allyn and Bacon.

Olson, D. H., Russell, C. S., & Sprenkle, D. H. (1980). Marital and family therapy: A decade review. *Journal of Marriage and the Family, 42,* 239-260.

Rolland, J. S. (1994). *Families, illness, and disability: An integrative treatment model.* New York: Basic Books.

Bibliotherapy Source for the Client

Kleinke, C. L. (2002). *Coping with life challenges.* Prospect Heights, IL: Waveland Press.

Chapter 5

Coping and Adapting to Developmental Changes, Challenges, and Opportunities Using a Patient Education Tool in Family Therapy

Layne A. Prest
Heath Grames

Type of Contribution: Handout

Objective

This handout is used in the first stage of therapy as a tool for assessment, treatment planning, and intervention. The information on the handout reminds therapists of important issues to look for in assessing the reciprocal impact of illness and/or disability and the life cycle. As a psycho-educational handout, it is provided to assist patients and their families in understanding the interplay among individual and family developmental stage and illness and disability. It is also helpful in stimulating discussion among family members and with the therapist about their experiences. These discussions can allow for important perceptions and emotional experiences for both family members and therapists. Therapists are better able to assess where the patient and family members are in their adaptation to the illness and to then facilitate growth through altered perceptions, expectations, experiences, and/or behaviors.

Rationale for Use

The experience of illness and disability is complex. The impact of a disease, or what has become known as the "illness experience" (e.g., McDaniel, Hepworth, & Doherty, 1997), is influenced by the interaction among the characteristics of the disease, the patient, his or her family, and the social system. Helping professionals from a number of disciplines have come to know this perspective as the Biopsychosocial (BPS) Model (Engle, 1977). Family therapists, for example, generally attempt to understand clinical presenting problems from this holistic point of view by assessing, planning treatment, and intervening in a way that takes into consideration what is happening at a variety of system levels. The patient or client characteristics which are considered within the BPS model include gender, personality, coping and resources, comorbid conditions, culture, age, and developmental stage (Carter & McGoldrick, 1999; Marshak, Seligman, & Prezant, 1999; Prest, Robinson, & Chang, 2002). Also included is an awareness of the important characteristics of the disease or disability itself. These characteristics include onset (acute or gradual), course (progressive, relapsing, or stable), level of incapacitation ("real" versus "perceived"), and outcome (nonfatal, potentially fatal or life-shortening, or fatal) (Rolland, 1994).

With respect to the life cycle issues, it is helpful to recognize the importance of both the individual and family life cycle stages. The impact of a chronic illness or disability will vary according to the developmental stage of an individual and his or her family and their intellectual and emotional capacity (which is in turn connected to developmental stage) (Rolland, 1987). Compare, for example, an unmarried nineteen-year-old versus a fifty-seven-year-old with adult children in coping with a progressive neuromuscular disease. From a perspective that only considers developmental tasks and capacity, these two people will likely respond in very different ways because of life cycle expectations, experiences, and tasks (which may or may not have been accomplished).

The illness can be experienced and described as having its own life cycle, for example, those which have a progressive course (Rolland, 1987). Consequently, the confluence of the individual and family life cycle with the life cycle of the illness can be an important aspect of the family members' experience (Marshak et al., 1999). The two people mentioned may also respond differently throughout the course of their disease. This is especially true if one (e.g., the younger) contracts a more rapidly advancing form of the disease than the other.

A clear understanding of the reciprocal interaction among the various components in the BPS model help therapists gain an appreciation for the complexity of life with an illness or disability. The interplay among these issues affects people's efforts to manage the illness and their attempts at adopting a new world view (Robinson, Carroll, & Watson, 2005). As a result, patients and their family members can benefit from a discussion of these very same issues—providing their own perspectives on their experiences, but also hearing an "outsider's" (an experienced therapist) perspective. We find that treatment team members (including patient and family members) "educating" one another about the illness or disability is an important part of the therapy process. The handout described in this chapter is a tool that can facilitate this discussion and be the basis for normalizing, providing anticipatory guidance, and gaining new understandings or strategies for coping and change.

This tool can also function as a useful treatment planning guide and reminder to the therapist to regularly consider the family life cycle stages and transitional steps when assessing and developing a treatment plan. The handout highlights the intergenerational impact of illness and disability, as well as the potential for variations depending on the life cycle stage. Notes can be made by the therapist on the handout during the assessment process, to be included in the treatment plan.

Instructions

The handout Developmental Changes, Challenges, and Opportunities: A Tool for Family Education, Coping, and Adaptation can be used in two ways: (1) as an educational handout for patients and family members; and (2) as a guide in developing the treatment plan.

Educational Handout: This handout is used once the therapist has joined with the patient and any family members or friends who are able to meet together, in the process of assessment and the beginnings of intervention. The handout is distributed to those present and described in some detail (focusing on the stage of the family life cycle in which the family finds themselves). The therapist uses anecdotes from work with other families to illustrate the concepts in the handout (i.e., the reciprocal impact of illness/disability and life cycle development). The patient and significant others are then invited to educate helping professionals about their perspectives and experiences. Our "professional" perspectives include information about the illness, contributing or exacerbating factors, coping strategies, and so on. We use the handout as a psychoeducational tool to provide anticipatory guidance regarding the relationship among the life stage that the person and family members are in and various aspects of the illness, including: typical developmental transitions, diagnosis, type of onset, course, level of incapacitation, and expectations about outcome. Clients are asked to think about how their process of lived experience is being influenced by things that aren't "personal," i.e., developmental issues, and then asked to comment on these reflections in subsequent sessions. This process can serve to externalize blame, resentment, and frustration as the clients realize that normal developmental challenges can be exacerbated by disabilities or illness. Conversely, the opportunities for growth are also highlighted, with the therapist leading a discussion regarding the crucible that illness or disability can be for a person and his or her family members.

Brief Vignettes

To illustrate the use of the Developmental Changes, Challenges, and Opportunities handout, two clinical vignettes are briefly outlined and discussed. The first vignette explores issues related to chronic illness in adolescence and the systemic impact on the family. The vignette will emphasize the use of the handout as a tool for both educational purposes for the family and as a tool for developing a treatment plan. The second case outlines the impact of chronic illness in a young family with children; it illustrates the use of the handout as primarily an educational tool.

Vignette One: The Young Diabetic

The Jones family presented to therapy to get help for their "non-compliant" son/stepson. Seventeen-year-old Michael was diagnosed with Type I (insulin dependant) diabetes three years ago. Although early on in the process he was vigilant in taking care of himself, Michael was now rarely consistent in checking his blood-sugar levels and taking his insulin. This non-compliance had resulted in several hospitalizations. When his blood sugar levels were out of control and he refused help from his parents, his stepmother became upset, yelled at him, and compared him unfavorably to her own son who was the same age as Michael. Subsequently, she and Michael's father would frequently argue.

Family dynamics. Michael's parents divorced approximately five years prior to therapy. He had a good relationship with his mother, but she lived on the East Coast (Michael resided in the Midwest with his father and stepmother) and had limited contact with him. Michael had two younger stepsiblings. His father remarried approximately one year after the divorce and his stepmother had two children: a son, Jason, seventeen, and a daughter, eleven. Jason was sexually active, used marijuana often, and regularly returned home after curfew. Jason and Michael agreed that Jason rarely got in trouble for his behavior. Jason was also quite popular at school, whereas Michael had few friends and was withdrawn. Michael's father, an engineer, was often out of town. When at home, he and Michael rarely spoke, and when they did, it often ended in arguments. Michael described his relationship with his father as distant, although he reported feeling close to his father when he and his mother were still married. In addition, Michael felt resentful toward his father for remarrying so soon after divorcing his mother, especially to a woman whose attitude Michael perceived as punitive and unaccepting of him. He never felt like he measured up to his stepmother's children, even though they often broke family rules. He also felt that his stepmother did not care if he lived there or not, and in fact he believed that she only cared that he checked his blood sugar levels and cared for himself so that she wouldn't have to bother with him.

Developmental changes, challenges, and opportunities. It was clear from the clinical presentation that this family with adolescents (see handout) was struggling with some of the expected developmental issues at this stage in the family life cycle. Perhaps most evident were the struggles surrounding the family power and intimacy dynamics. Michael's father was physically and emotionally distant from Michael and the rest of the family, leaving his wife to manage much of the day-to-day functioning of the family. The strained family relationships and poor communication were not conducive to accommodating Michael's development and independence as a teenager. In fact, Michael spoke of his stepmother controlling his every move, but not those of her own children. Michael's stepmother agreed that she was very strict with him, but related that it was because he was disobedient and she was worried for his health. Due to the diabetes, Michael was faced with the threat of premature suffering and death almost daily, and his mortality had become the focus of many of his arguments with his stepmother.

Using the handout. The developmental changes, challenges, and opportunities handout was first used during the joining and assessment phase of therapy. The therapist used it to validate the family members' different developmental needs, normalize the family members' struggles, and identify the previously mentioned problem areas, without formally introducing the handout to the family. Specifically, the focus of sessions one and two included joining with the family, assessment, and developing treatment goals, which included increasing Michael's compliance in caring for himself and improving family relationships. During the third session, the handout was introduced to the family members. The therapist and the family reviewed the handout and identified some of the issues with which they were struggling. The stepmother identified as her greatest concern that she and her husband had failed to focus on the couple relationship. Her husband agreed, but also added that they (seeming to really mean his wife) had been too hard on, and controlling of, Michael. The therapist facilitated a discussion among family members about the different parenting approaches used with the three children, highlighting the impact of the illness on this process. Michael was reframed as being in the same life cycle stage as his younger stepsister. He angrily agreed, stating he did not like being treated "as a kid." But the therapist then validated the stepmother's concerns about his health, while challenging her to recognize how her approach was making things worse. The therapist also challenged Michael to consider that his defiance was only inviting increased "mothering" by his stepmother. To Michael's father, the therapist suggested that his defense of Michael might be actually putting him at risk. The parents were both assisted to move to a united stance regarding Michael's self-care, as well as their expectations about other behavioral concerns. With a more consistent, but developmentally appropriate action plan, Michael was able to earn more freedom and independence by being more responsible. He improved checking his blood sugar levels and taking insulin as needed. Meanwhile, his father and stepmother focused on improving their co-parenting and marital relationship, which in turn helped them to be more effective with Michael.

Throughout therapy, the handout was referred to in order to measure how the family was progressing in obtaining their therapy goals and also to normalize the difficulties they faced as they were dealing with a chronic illness. With this family, the handout was used by the therapist to join with the family and present to them a conceptual model from which they would work. The conceptual model served for the family as a way to normalize their experience with chronic illness and to give them tangible goals for changes they wanted to make.

Vignette Two: The Fear of AIDS

Mr. and Mrs. Gonzalez had been married for twelve years. They were from a small town in Guatemala and had lived in the United States for seven years. They had come to the United States to escape poverty and seek a better life. As the first family members to come to the United States, their families expected them to assist family in Guatemala by sending money when they could and to provide a place to live for other family members as they made their way to the United States. As such, Mrs. Gonzalez' younger brother was living with them. Due to financial obligations in the United States and Guatemala, the Gonzalez' were living well below the poverty level and had few resources. Mr. and Mrs. Gonzalez had one child, named Jose.

Therapy began in the hospital. Mr. and Mrs. Gonzalez were both in the hospital room when the attending physician, six residents, a pharmacist, and the bilingual therapist (who also took on the role as interpreter) entered the room to discuss Mr. Gonzalez's health. Five days previously, Mr. Gonzalez had entered the hospital very ill, unable to keep food down. On this particular day, the team found him lying in the hospital bed, looking frail and pallid, with IV's and tubes hooked up to him. He had been diagnosed with AIDS, and his prognosis was poor. Amidst the chaos, Mrs. Gonzalez leaned toward the therapist and, in Spanish, asked him if her test results had come back. Before rounds began, as the cases were discussed, a resident had reported that the first test had come back positive, indicating that Mrs. Gonzalez, too, was HIV positive. The residents, pharmacist, and therapist were told not to disclose this information until another, more expensive but more accurate, test was completed. As he notified Mrs. Gonzalez that another test would need to be run before they could be sure, the therapist noticed a small boy sitting slouched over in a large chair in the corner. The boy was Jose, Mr. and Mrs. Gonzalez' seven-year-old son. He said nothing with the doctors present. After the medical team left the room, the therapist stayed with the family briefly to discuss their well-being and to schedule an appointment to return and meet with them. As the therapist spoke with Mrs. Gonzalez, Jose stood up and tried to get on the bed with his father. As he leaned to give his father a hug, his father pushed him away and rolled over.

Family dynamics. Throughout their marriage, Mr. Gonzalez had had sexual contact with a number of different men, but he had not disclosed this information to his wife. Mrs. Gonzalez reported being faithful in her marriage, except one affair she had approximately one year prior to her husband's hospitalization. She reported being worried that she was infected with AIDS from her affair and that she had passed it on to her husband. Mrs. Gonzalez had not told her husband about the affair. Mrs. Gonzalez' twenty-five-year-old brother (who was living with them), was curious about what was going on, but had not asked many questions and did not know of the diagnoses. Besides Mrs. Gonzalez' brother, the family was isolated, reporting having no family friends. The rest of the Gonzalez' family was living in Guatemala and were practicing Catholics. Mr. Gonzalez reported that no one would accept him if disclosed how he got AIDS.

Developmental changes, challenges, and opportunities. This vignette represents a family in the stage with young children. One of the most difficult developmental issues in this family had been the process of adjusting the couple system to make space for children. Even without the presence of the developmental challenge and the presence of the chronic illness, Mr. and Mrs. Gonzalez' marital relationship was suffering (they described it as distant) due to the secrecy and deception that existed. The direct impact of the chronic illness and making space for children was evidenced as Mr. Gonzalez rejected every advance by his son to get close to him. In secret, Mr. Gonzalez disclosed that he did not touch his son because he was afraid he would transfer the AIDS virus to his son through his perspiration. With a tear running down his cheek, he acknowledged seeing the pain on his son's face when he was rejected. Another task at this family developmental stage is for the family to be able to change roles as needed to accommodate new members and family growth. This particular illness was sufficiently debilitating and life threatening that the family felt constrained in their abilities. The focus was on survival rather than on family growth. The family secrecy served to perpetuate the problem.

Using the handout. For this family, the handout was very useful in identifying the many developmental issues that were delayed due to the chronic illness. Although the handout was never formally presented to Mr. and Mrs. Gonzalez, these issues, as well as the secrets in the family, were addressed in several meetings with them during the time Mr. Gonzalez was hospitalized. The therapist made the choice to not present the handout to the family because the family was in shock, in crisis, and was not ready to actively work to meet therapy goals. The focus of the first meeting with the Gonzalez family was on crisis intervention, validating their fears, and to lay the foundation to help Mr. and Mrs. Gonzalez begin to talk about what was happening. Each family member had decided to suffer alone and in silence with his or her pain. They were not focused on improving or adapting their current roles to accommodate the chronic illness and current crisis. Therefore, the handout was used with this family as an educational tool to identify areas of problems concerning their family's developmental cycle.

Much of the time the therapist spent with the Gonzalez family was spent encouraging communication between the couple and educating the family about AIDS. Due to the AIDS diagnosis, misconceptions about the illness, and Mr. Gonzalez' fears, the developmental needs of Jose were being compromised. As stated in the handout, a challenge at illness onset for families with young children is that it can disrupt parenting functions and interfere with the psychosocial development of the child. When the therapist discussed this with the family, Mr. and Mrs. Gonzalez agreed and reported feeling very guilty for what Jose was experiencing. Mr. Gonzalez was encouraged to embrace his son. After the myths of HIV/AIDS were discussed, he embraced his son for a long time as they both wept. Mr. Gonzalez' health subsequently improved enough for him to be released from the hospital, but he was not given a good prognosis concerning long-term survival. He continued to be weak enough that he needed a lot of help to take care of himself. Mr. and Mrs. Gonzalez returned to Guatemala several weeks after the therapist first met with them. It is unknown whether they began talking about the secrets each kept guarded.

If therapy had continued, the handout would have become a more formal part of setting goals and would have been used throughout therapy. The issues pertaining to family life cycle development would have been discussed more directly and therapy goals would have been encouraged and set in respect to the family and illness life cycle. In addition, communication between the couple would have continued to be emphasized and the couple would have been encouraged to seek support.

Suggestions for Follow-Up

The clinical vignettes illustrate the value of the Developmental Changes, Challenges, and Opportunities handout as a reminder to assess family dynamics and plan interventions while keeping in mind the developmental context. The vignettes also emphasize the value of the handout as a tool to identify therapy goals, offer psychoeducation, and collaborate with the client family concerning treatment. As seen, the handout is versatile and can be tailored in its use, depending on patient needs. It is important to record in case notes the level of use so that when the client and family return to therapy, the therapist can track questions, needs, and improvement. When working with chronically ill patients, therapy goals should be prioritized. As illustrated in Vignette Two, depending on the severity of the illness, some clients may be lost to follow-up because of their need to change location as they seek help from family members, friends, or medical institutions.

Contraindications for Use

Any time patient education material is utilized, it is important to make sure it is available in a form and at a level that it is usable; assess your client/family's reading level. When therapists work with people who speak languages other than English, it is important to make sure these materials are well translated in a culturally competent manner. In addition, stage model frameworks conceptualizing complex concepts such as life cycle development are limited. New models have been developed over time to address variations in the life cycle due to such phenomena as divorce and remarriage, couples who cannot or choose not to have children, single-parent families, and so on. The handout can be revised according to the demographics and experiences of the population with whom the therapist is working.

Readings and Resources for the Professional

Carter, B., & McGoldrick, M. (1999). *The expanded family life* (3rd ed.). Boston: Allyn & Bacon.

Engel, G. L. (1977). The need for a new medical model: A challenge for biomedicine. *Science, 196,* 129-136.

Marshak, L. E., Seligman M., & Prezant, F. (1999). Disability and the family life cycle: Recognizing and treating developmental challenges. New York: Basic Books.

McDaniel, S. H., Hepworth, J., & Doherty, W. J. (Eds.). (1997). *The shared experience of illness: Stories of patients, families, and their therapists.* New York: Basic Books.

Newby, N. M. (1996). Chronic illness and the family life cycle. *Journal of Advanced Nursing, 23*(4):786-791.

Prest, L. A., Robinson, W. D., & Chang, C. L. (2002). "Tears in the Tapestry: Anxiety and Depression in Families." Presented at American Association for Marriage & Family Therapy Annual Conference. Cincinnati, Ohio.

Robinson, W. D., Carroll, J. S., & Watson, W. L. (2005). Shared experience building around the family crucible of cancer. *Families, Systems, & Health, 23*(2), 131-147.

Rolland, J. (1987). Chronic illness and the family life cycle: A conceptual framework. *Family Process, 26*(2), 203-221.

Rolland, J. (1994). *Families, illness, and disability: An integrative treatment model.* New York: Basic Books.

Shuman, R. (1996). *The psychology of chronic illness: The healing work of patients, therapists, and families.* New York: Basic Books.

Bibliotherapy Sources for the Client

Fennel, P. A. (2001). *The chronic illness workbook: Strategies and solutions for taking back your life.* Oakland, CA: New Harbinger.

Frank, A. W. (1991). *At the will of the body: Reflections on illness.* New York: Mariner Books.

HANDOUT 5.1.
Developmental Changes, Challenges, and Opportunities: A Tool for Family Education, Coping, and Adaptation

Developmental Stage	Developmental Transition	Specific Developmental Issues	Challenges Due to Onset, Relapse, or Progression	Opportunities
Single, young adult	Accepting physical separation, financial independence, and increasingly adult-adult relationship	Identity development; Peer relationships; Starting to work	Reinforcing attachment with parents; Produces confusion about individuation process; Impedes adapting identity as worker	Challenges young adult and parents to more clearly define self within the family; Fosters sense of interdependence; Skills for balancing roles
Joining of families through stable partnerships	Commitment to new relationships	Forming couple system; Realigning other family and social relationships	Complicates couple interactional patterns; Impairs of negotiation of power and roles; Confusion of boundary between couple and extended family	Creates a crucible within which to renegotiate roles, rules, boundaries, rituals
Family with young children	Incorporating new members into family	Adjusting couple system to make space for child(ren); Taking on parenting roles; Changing roles of other family members	Disrupts partnering and/or parenting role functioning; Interferes with psychosocial development of child	Facilitates greater awareness of and sensitivity to others; Development of meaningful role identity, instrumental skills, and partnering relationships
Family with adolescents	Accommodating teen's development, growing independence, relationships	Shifting roles, power dynamics, hierarchy, boundaries; Refocus on couple and career issues; Growing concern for older generation	Foreclosing on identity issues, purpose in life; Impedes development of peer relationships; Premature entrance into later stage expectations about mortality	Generates new meanings incorporated into developing identity; Development of interdependence rather than autonomy

Prest, L., & Grames, H. (2007). Coping and adapting to developmental changes, challenges, and opportunities using a patient education tool in family therapy. In D. Linville, K. Hertlein, and Associates, *The therapist's notebook for family health care: Homework, handouts, and activities for individuals, couples, and families coping with illness, loss, and disability* (pp. 31-39). Binghamton, NY: The Haworth Press.

HANDOUT 5.1 (continued)

Developmental Stage	Developmental Transition	Specific Developmental Issues	Challenges Due to Onset, Relapse, or Progression	Opportunities
Launching	Exits and re-entries of young adults	Continued renegotiation of couple relationship; Development of parent-child, adult-adult relationships; Realignment to include in-laws and grandchildren	Complicates emancipation process; Taxes partners ability to juggle multiple roles	Deepens relationships among family members in spite of separation; Increases flexibility and adaptability
Family in Later Life	Accepting shifting generational roles and power dynamics	Shifting balance of care giving and receiving; Renegotiation of power; Dealing with disability and loss; Preparation for own death; Life review and integration	Accentuates anticipatory grief and possibly generates hopelessness	Heightens appreciation for the time that is left to the members of family in its current form; Helps members to see into the future, visualizing relationships continuing despite loss
Family at End of Life	Accepting loss of family members through death	Grief and reorganization of family system	Aborted, complicated, or unending grief	Healthy grieving process and deepened sense of meaning and connection with others

Prest, L., & Grames, H. (2007). Coping and adapting to developmental changes, challenges, and opportunities using a patient education tool in family therapy. In D. Linville, K. Hertlein, and Associates, *The therapist's notebook for family health care: Homework, handouts, and activities for individuals, couples, and families coping with illness, loss, and disability* (pp. 31-39). Binghamton, NY: The Haworth Press.

Chapter 6

An Adaptive World Model for Meeting the Demands of Chronic Illness

W. David Robinson
Layne A. Prest
Jason S. Carroll

Type of Contribution: Intervention, Handout

Objective

For family members to learn the role each plays when one person in the family has a chronic illness, they must not neglect the role that the illness plays in the family. The objective of this chapter is to outline an intervention that shows family how to learn about and navigate these roles. Recent research has shown that: (1) helping families share their personal illness story, (2) family-experience genograms, (3) facilitating family reorganization with illness psychoeducation, and (4) shared experience building are all effective ways to address the affective demands of illness. Using these approaches, therapists are better able to assess additional areas of concern regarding where the patient and family members are in their adaptation to the illness, and to then facilitate growth through altered perceptions, expectations, experiences, and/or behaviors.

Rationale for Use

Chronic illness and disability place great affective demands on ill individuals and their family members (McDaniel, Hepworth, & Doherty, 1992; Shuman, 1996). Depending on the level of incapacitation as a result of the condition, patients and their family members frequently experience significant losses and must greatly alter their lifestyle and/or world view (Rolland, 1994). While family members often band together during a health crisis, chronic illness or disability can challenge the resilience of even the most committed family members. Depression, anxiety, frustration, anger, hopelessness, and helplessness are common feelings. As family members taper off in their expressions of concern and care-taking activities, the resulting isolation can make coping with illness even more difficult for the patient. This family system disengagement or disintegration is exacerbated when ill individuals, who already feel like a burden on the family, hold in their feelings and complaints (Robinson, Carroll, & Watson, 2005). Caregiving family members also suffer from feelings of isolation. They feel unable to share their burden of care-taking or concern due to fear of making things worse for the person who is ill or adding to the burden of other family members (McDaniel, Hepworth, & Doherty, 1997).

The emotional experience of chronic illness is complex and is further complicated by multiple experiences that exist within the family. No two individuals have the same experience with the illness. For example, it is a different experience as a daughter of a woman with breast cancer than as her husband. As a result, the foundation of therapeutic intervention should be a focus on these affective experiences that occur within the family. Helping family members create a shared meaning of the experience, while at the same time validating the lived experience of each person, can have profound results for family functioning. This illness-influenced experience of the family as a whole is distinct from that experienced by the majority of the other families with whom they associate. The "normal" experiences of life are limited or do not occur in the same way they used to because the illness limits family members' abilities to maintain everyday activities. Effects and side effects of medication and other treatments; physical, cognitive, and/or emotional limitations; and doctor's visits are a few examples of the constraints that make it difficult for the family to live a "normal" life.

As mentioned initially, an important issue to address with family members is the reciprocal link between illness and the family. Although this idea may seem like second nature for some therapists, it is foreign to others and the illness is generally seen as an individual's experience or as an outside entity that is (or should be) solely controlled by the medical profession. For this reason, patients and family members need to learn the role they play in the illness experience without forgetting the role the illness plays in their family. These issues and experiences can be explored in therapy through the use of several illness-experience focused interventions. These strategies foster a greater understanding of one another's experiences, a heightened sense of self-reflection, permission to constructively own and express emotions, and development of ways to handle them constructively. All of these changes foster a more positive adjustment among family members dealing with chronic illness and disability.

Instructions

These interventions are to be used to explore and treat the affective experiences of families who have a member with a chronic illness or disability. There are five steps: (1) family illness genogram, (2) sharing of personal illness story, (3) putting illness in its place, (4) psychoeduction, and (5) shared experience building. Supplies needed are white board or flip chart for completing the genogram and a copy of Handout 6.1 (located at the end of the chapter) for discussion about "Putting illness in its place."

Initial Stage of Therapy

Family illness genogram. Family therapists have long understood the importance of family history. Congruently, we have found that a useful way to begin therapy is by conducting an illness experience genogram. The important issues involved in constructing this type of genogram are: (a) understanding the organization of the family before and after the onset of illness; (b) inquiring into the family members' experiences with illness or other stressful events and how they dealt with them; (c) investigating family legacies that further explain how the family might deal with a stressful event; (d) including individuals outside the family who have been important during the illness; and (e) identifying changes in relationships that have occurred due to the illness (i.e., pulling away, reconnection).

Sharing personal illness stories. As another part of assessment and treatment, it is important for all family members to be given the opportunity to share their experiences with the illness from the beginning. One of the most important outcomes from sharing personal stories of illness is that family members are able to hear, usually for the first time, the complete story about the impact of the illness on other individuals in the family. These experiences help families develop greater empathy for one another. It is important for family members not to interrupt or correct the person sharing during this time. They should be asked simply to listen. Once the person finishes, the therapist can ask other family members about the individual's experience and have them identify issues of which they were not aware. This exercise is not designed to prove that one person has suffered more than another, but to bring perspective and empathy for the unique experiences due to the illness.

Treatment Stage of Therapy

Putting illness in its place: Old World versus New World. Another key therapeutic intervention is helping the family put the illness in its place. Families who get stuck focusing on the illness alone struggle because it begins to rule the family. Putting illness in its place is a way of containing the effects of the illness on the family. One way to do this is to help the family understand the dynamics of their life before the illness, as opposed to their new life with the illness—Old versus New World View.

Finding a balance between the old world of health versus the new world of illness can be difficult. Families are usually unprepared for the changes illness or disability bring, and often find that a new world has been created which can be compared to entering a new, uncharted land. Similar to immigrants in a new country, families begin the process of either accepting and creating a life in this new world or taking extreme measures to keep life how it used to be. Because illness inevitably changes life, families need to learn how to move forward and develop a life that includes the illness component (see Handout 6.1). Therapists can use Handout 6.1 as the organizational structure for a family discussion. In this discussion and through homework, the family can identify the key areas that they need to address to limit the impact of illness in their daily lives (see Handout 6.1).

Psychoeducation. Psychoeducation is an important way for therapists to help families understand key components and areas of the illness. This is an important part of therapy because family members often seek information about what is "normal." They tend to cope better to the extent that the therapist can realistically assist them in seeing their emotions and behavioral reactions as normal. A variety of information can be given to the families through short psychoeducational pieces during or after the therapy sessions. For therapists unfamiliar with particular illnesses, using Rolland's typology of illness (Rolland, 1994) can be very helpful. It addresses the key psychosocial issues inherent in different types of illness.

Creating a forum for shared experience building. Finally, the overarching goal of therapy for dealing with the affective demands of illness is to create the forum for shared experience building (Robinson, Carroll, & Watson, 2005). Families usually do not spontaneously engage in indepth interactions concerning illness. They may have discussed aspects of the illness, but not delved into the many important issues that are often addressed in therapy (e.g., sexual intimacy, anger, fairness, spiritual crises).

Shared experience building is based upon developing a shared experience of healing, not necessarily of illness. The key component is helping family members develop a shared experience in the healing process without devaluing individual experiences. This process begins to occur during the sharing of stories when family members identify similarities between what they experienced and what was shared. Through this exercise, family members are able to build greater connection with one another, develop greater empathy for one another, and learn how to cope more effectively with the illness.

Brief Vignette: The Young Diabetic

Fifteen-year-old Corey's stepmother, Phyllis, asked his physician for help after a period of a few months when Corey had become increasingly defiant and resistant about giving himself his injections and following the recommended dietary guidelines. He had first been diagnosed with juvenile onset (Type I) diabetes at ten years of age. From the beginning, he had been fairly compliant, and even proactive, in managing his disease. So it came as a surprise to Phyllis, and Corey's father, Dennis, when his attitude and behavior changed rather suddenly. Corey had begun hiding his medication and eating foods in quantities he knew had an exacerbating effect on his blood sugar level.

Family dynamics. When confronted by Phyllis about his behavior, Corey became defensive and angry. Phyllis would then complain to Corey's father, who would alternately excuse his behavior or angrily chastise him. In response, Corey often became silent or would tearfully blame Phyllis in some way. This was increasingly straining Dennis and Phyllis's relationship. Phyllis reported that the conflict was upsetting to the rest of the family as well. Corey and his thirteen-year-old sister Sara are Dennis's children from a previous marriage. The three of them had lived together for two years after Dennis and their mother's divorce, prior to Dennis and Phyllis meeting. A year-long courtship preceded their marriage. During this period, Phyllis and her three children (currently eight, ten, and thirteen) began to spend increasing amounts of time with Dennis and his family. They were married approximately one year ago.

With the seven members of the family coming and going at all hours of the day, theirs was a busy household. This contributed to difficulty with scheduling and consistency. Complicating the situation was the fact that Corey's mother, who lived in the same city but chose not to have custody of her children because of "emotional problems," was inconsistent in following the visitation schedule. Dennis worked construction, sometimes out of town, so by default it became Phyllis's job to take care of doctor's appointments, make sure Corey had his medical supplies and medicine, and that he followed through on medical recommendations given by the physician and dietician. Increasingly, Corey and Phyllis were having sometimes heated arguments about his behavior and "noncompliance." Corey complained to his father about Phyllis. Dennis was torn between wanting his son to take care of himself and supporting his wife, and not being perceived by his son as "being on her side." At times, Corey asked his biological mother about living with her instead. She would sometimes tell him he could if only his father and "that woman" would let him, but alternately not contact him nor follow through on promises to bring the topic up for discussion with Dennis. She would also avoid the topic or blame Corey for pressuring her to do something she felt she could not afford to do.

Dennis and Phyllis' combined incomes allowed the primary household to be more stable financially and even enjoy a higher standard of living than they could living separately, balancing these responsibilities with parenting and house maintenance was difficult. And as stated, the majority of this responsibility fell on Phyllis' shoulders.

Developmental changes, challenges, and opportunities. In the five years since Corey's diagnosis, there had been several significant changes: his parents' divorce, the custody decision and irregular visitation schedule, his father beginning the relationship with Phyllis, their courtship and marriage, the blending of the two families, Corey's transition into early and then middle adolescence (including the move into junior high and then high school), and the attendant increasing bids for autonomy and identity development.

Using the interventions. In the first session of therapy at which all family members who lived in the household were present, the therapist engaged them in a conversation by asking them to tell the story of their life together as a family. This involved some discussion of their unique family histories prior to Dennis and Phyllis' marriage, as well as the ongoing transition and adjustment to life as a family in their own right. The therapist began to reframe some of their struggles in terms of the developmental transitions, normalizing where possible some of their problems. During this discussion, the therapist also began constructing a family illness genogram. This intervention involved eliciting family members' perspectives on Corey's adjustment to the diagnosis, what they thought about his having diabetes, and family members' attempts to cope and go on with their lives. Although Corey was encouraged to tell his personal illness story (sharing how his life was before the illness, his reaction to the diagnosis, and struggles and strengths that have come since diagnosis), he stated he wasn't comfortable doing so in front of his younger siblings or Phyllis. Therefore, the conversation was shifted toward other issues of daily living. In a subsequent session with Corey and his father, Corey told his personal illness story. He was alternately sad, proud, angry and defiant, minimizing, and afraid as he talked about his experience. His father shared his own perspective, including fears and worries, frustration with Corey for not taking care of himself, and sadness and guilt that Corey had been diagnosed in the first place.

In a follow-up family session, Corey was supported by his father and the therapist to share parts of his illness story as he felt comfortable. As Corey did so, the members of the family seemed to listen carefully and supportively, adding their own similar or contrasting experiences. They all agreed that family life would be more peaceful if the illness wasn't so out of control and disruptive. The therapist suggested they "gang up on" the illness. As a result, a strategy session was held during which the family members were asked to collaborate in designing a "battle plan" to be used in putting the diabetes in its place. Separate discussions with Dennis and Phyllis addressed the coparenting issues, their different roles relative to their own and each others' children, and how to reduce the day-to-day parenting burden on Phyllis. During subsequent sessions, the family was assisted in the process of shared experience building. Consistent with the previous description, Corey and his family members were helped to talk about a variety of issues that had previously been affected by his illness, with a focus on minimizing the day-to-day impact. Just as important, they were guided in creating a shared experience around nonillness-related events in their lives. For example, Corey was encouraged to talk with his siblings about positive family memories they all shared but which were clearer in his mind than in theirs. Doing so helped Corey to be in an authoritative position, but he also helped enrich his younger siblings' memories and family identity. In a conjoint session, Dennis and Phyllis were prompted to reminisce about their courtship days, and build in some more romantic and marital subsystem-oriented activities and discussions at home. The result seemed to be that family members' perspectives on their family became more balanced, communication was more open and spontaneous, and power struggles around Corey's illness diminished in frequency and intensity.

Contraindications for Use

With any illness, it is important to assess the family members for emotional overload and schedule appointments accordingly. If the ill individual is too fatigued or required to endure too many medical tests and/or procedures, the therapist should discuss with the family the appropriate number and duration of each session. There is also nothing wrong with seeing individual family members or small groupings of the family so as to not overstress each member. Therapy should be seen as a supportive and helpful endeavor not just one more appointment that must be kept. Similarly, the emotions that are discussed are often overwhelming and sharing them can be difficult—especially if mutual trust has broken down within the family or in certain dyads. During the initial sessions of therapy, the general process for coping with and sharing feelings within the family should be assessed. If it is determined that these are particular problem areas (e.g., premorbid marital discord, parenting difficulties, premorbid psychiatric disorders), then preliminary work may need to take place before these interventions can be carried out.

Suggestions for Follow-Up

It is important during the weeks following the intervention that the family attends regular sessions to ensure the process of establishing emotional closeness does not revert back to preintervention state. During the follow-up sessions, it is important to assess each individual and family subsystem. If difficulties are observed during the family session, the therapist should meet with the parents to assess possible difficulties that might exist (e.g., marital, emotional, discipline, sibling relationships). Individual sessions with family members who are struggling with emotional engagement with the family may also be warranted. It is especially relevant to meet with the person with the illness to assess feelings of guilt and perception of burden.

References

Cohen, M. H. (1993). Diagnostic closure and the spread of uncertainty. *Issues in Comprehensive Pediatric Nursing, 16*(3), 135-146.

Gonzalez, S., Steinglass, P., & Reiss, D. (1989). Putting the illness in its place: Discussion groups for families with chronic medical illness. *Family Process, 28,* 69-87.

Knowal, J., Johnson, S., & Lee, A. (2003). Chronic illness in couples: A case for emotionally focused therapy. *Journal of Marital and Family Therapy, 29,* 299-310.

McDaniel, S. H., Hepworth, J., & Doherty, W. (1992). *Medical Family Therapy.* New York: Basic Books.

McDaniel, S. H., Hepworth, J., & Doherty, W. J. (1997). *The shared experience of illness: Stories of Patients, Families and their Therapists.* New York: Basic Books.

Moyers, B. (1993). *Healing and the mind.* New York: Doubleday.

Robinson, W. D., Carroll, J. S., & Watson, W. L. (2005). Shared experience building around the family crucible of cancer. *Families, Systems & Health, 23*(2), 131-147.

Robinson, W. D., & Smith, C. (1998). *Understanding hemophilia: A family process of adaptation.* Unpublished manuscript.

Rolland, J. (1994). *Families, illness, & disability: An integrative treatment model.* New York: Basic Books.

Shuman, R. (1996). *The psychology of chronic illness: The healing work of patients, therapists and families.* New York: Basic Books.

Steinglass, P. (1998). Multiple family discussion groups for patients with chronic medical illness. *Families, Systems and Health, 16*(1/2), 55-70.

Wright, L., Watson, W., & Bell, J. (1996). *Beliefs: The heart of healing in families and illness.* New York: Basic Books.

Readings and Resources for the Professional

McDaniel, S. H., Hepworth, J., & Doherty, W. J. (Eds.). (1997). *The Shared Experience of Illness: Stories of Patients, Families, and Their Therapists.* New York: Basic Books.

Robinson, W. D., Carroll, J. S., & Watson, W. L. (2005). Shared experience building around the family crucible of cancer. *Families, Systems, & Health, 23*(2), 131-147.

Rolland, J. (1994). *Families, Illness, and Disability: An Integrative Treatment Model.* New York: Basic Books.

Shuman, R. (1996). *The Psychology of Chronic Illness: The Healing Work of Patients, Therapists, and Families.* New York: Basic Books.

Wright, L., Watson, W., & Bell, J. (1996). *Beliefs: The Heart of Healing in Families and Illness.* New York: Basic Books.

Bibliotherapy Sources for the Client

Fennel, P. A. (2001). *The Chronic Illness Workbook: Strategies and Solutions for Taking Back Your Life.* Oakland, CA: New Harbinger.

Frank, A. W. (1991). *At the Will of the Body: Reflections on Illness.* New York: Mariner Books.

HANDOUT 6.1.
Old World versus New World Views

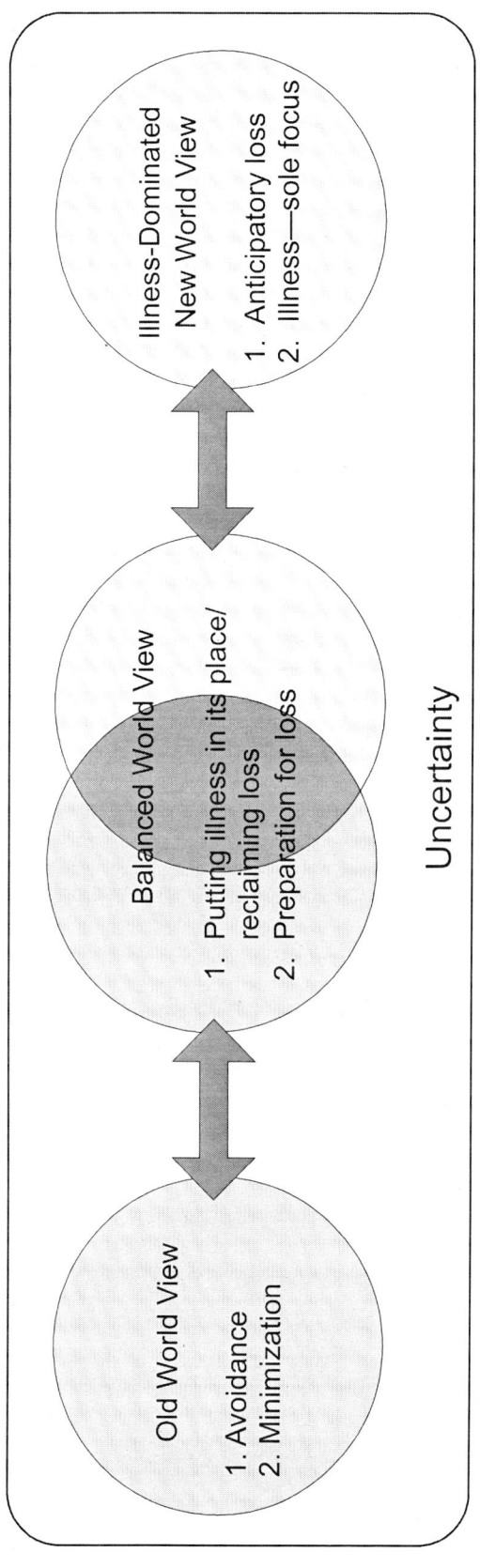

Robinson, W.D., Prest, L., & Carroll, J. (2007). An adaptive world model for meeting the demands of chronic illness. In D. Linville, K.M. Hertlein, and Associates, *The Therapist's notebook for family health care: Homework, handouts, and activities for individuals, couples, and families coping with illness, loss, and disability* (pp. 41-47). Binghamton, NY: The Haworth Press.

Chapter 7

Positive and Negative Feelings Boxes

Miriam Claire Godwin

Type of Contribution: Activity

Objective

This activity can be used with any family member coping with an illness, trauma, or disability of another family member. It can be used as an intervention in one session or throughout treatment.

Rationale for Use

Being a family member of a loved one who suffers from an illness, trauma, or disability can be difficult and is associated with many emotions, both positive and negative in nature. Family members may feel frustrated, angry, disappointed, helpless, or stressed, as well as feel joy about having the ill or disabled person in their lives. A wide range of emotions may surface because of the possible changes in roles associated with the illness or disability, such as the additional parental demands of caring for a child with a disability. Medical care for a family member with an illness or disability can pose a tremendous threat to healthy family functioning and can be associated with high financial and emotional demands. The duties of caring for a loved one in need can be associated with feelings of burn out and guilt at not being as effective a caregiver as deemed necessary.

The appropriate expression of all emotions is essential for healthy family and individual functioning. Communication in families is the cornerstone for cohesion and connectedness (Satir, 1972). Experiential theorists emphasize the importance of expressing emotions to support healthy family functioning and believe that the purpose of the family is to support the emotional growth of each member (Satir, 1972).

Although each family member is entitled to his or her emotions, he or she may not wish to always share the negative emotions experienced. However, the expression of these emotions is as important as the expression of positive emotions. Family members may claim that a lack of quality family time prevents them from openly expressing emotions on a daily basis, or that they do not feel comfortable enough with their family members to share negative thoughts or feelings in fear of hurting someone they love.

Family members may often direct their negative feelings toward the family member that has an illness or disability, rather than toward the illness or disability itself. The externalization of problems is an important element in Narrative Family Therapy. Bill O'Hanlon (1994, p. 28) encouraged therapists to, "believe, to the bottom of your soul, that people are not their problems." Narrative theorists use the paradigm that people are not the illness or disability, but rather a person is challenged by the demands of the illness or disability (Freedman & Combs, 1996). Narrative therapists use the externalization of illness or disability to support families in effectively coping with their challenges together.

This activity was designed to help clients manage the full range of emotions that can be associated with the illness/trauma/disability that afflicts their family. The purpose of this activity is to foster open family communication, explore appropriate means of expressing emotions, and to gain an understanding that the family member is separate from his or her illness or disability. In addition, negative emotions should be attributed to the illness or disability when appropriate.

Instructions

Supplies you will need for this activity include: two empty shoe boxes (per client), numerous old magazines, markers or paints/paint pens of various colors, glue, and scissors (child safe if used with young children). Optional materials include: fabrics, ribbons, buttons and plain paper.

The clinician should discuss with the clients the importance of appropriate expression of feelings, both positive and negative in nature. The clinician should then process with the clients how they currently express feelings and what feelings they choose not to express. The clinician should explore with the clients what prevents full expression of their emotions. The clients might share that they do not express feelings for various reasons, such as: not wanting to burden anyone with their feelings, not wanting to become vulnerable to others, or assuming others already know how they feel. The clinician should assess the client's motivation to change their challenges in communicating feelings and address their needs through further treatment.

The clinician should normalize for the client the experience of a having a wide range of emotions associated with family members. The clinician and clients should discuss how negative feelings are as important as positive feelings, as well as their right to feel and appropriately express both.

The clients should then choose one box to be their "Negative Feelings Box" and one box to be their "Positive Feelings Box." The clients should then decorate the outside and inside of the "Negative Feelings Box" with colors, pictures, and drawings that represent the negative feelings they have experienced associated with their family member's illness, trauma, or disability. One client, for example, could use paint to color the outside of his or her box black and the inside blue. The client might explain that on the outside negative feelings look dark and bad, but on the inside, negative feelings make you feel sad and "blue." The client might decorate the outside of the box with pictures of witches and ghosts because he or she thinks of these things as scary, just like the negative feelings.

The clients should then decorate the outside and inside of their "Positive Feelings Box" with colors, etc. that represent the positive feelings they have experienced associated with their family member that are not influenced by the illness, trauma, or disability. One client, for example, could use markers to color the outside of the box yellow because he or she thinks of yellow as a happy, or positive color. He or she could color the inside of the box green because he or she thinks of green as representing growth and he or she wants to use the positive feelings to grow or to prosper from the experiences with his or her family member's illness, trauma, or disability.

The clinician should instruct the clients to take the boxes home and write down each negative feeling they experience associated with their family member and/or their illness/trauma/disability. The clients should be instructed to place the feeling in the "Negative Feelings Box." The clinician should take the opportunity to encourage the clients to reframe negative thoughts directed toward an individual family member and instead direct them toward the illness/trauma/disability. The clinician should process with the clients how the illness/trauma/disability is external from their family member and negative feelings should be directed toward the illness/trauma/disability when appropriate.

The clinician should instruct the clients to follow the same procedure for the "Positive Feelings Box" each time they have a positive feeling about their family member that is challenged with the illness/trauma/disability. If the client expresses concern about his or her ability to think of positive or negative feelings, challenge him or her to write a least one feeling every day.

Each session after the creation of the boxes, the clinician should process with the clients what feelings they have been putting in the boxes and how they felt about the activity. The clinician could ask, "Did you have a positive or negative feeling about the activity?" "In what way was this activity helpful?" "In what way was this activity not helpful?" If the clients give examples of how the activity could have been more helpful, the clinician should offer to complete the activity again and regard the suggested changes.

During subsequent sessions the clinician should draw pictures of feelings with the clients, cut out pictures and words associated with the feelings experienced, and ask clients to include those feelings in the appropriate boxes. At this time, the feelings should be processed in a helpful way to the clients, supporting their expression of such feelings to other family members. The clients should be encouraged to share the contents of their feeling boxes at home, as well as in session. If the clients state they do not yet feel comfortable sharing certain feelings openly with others, the roadblocks to expression should be processed. Clients should always be encouraged to share both positive and negative feelings outside of sessions in an appropriate manner so that the family's communication can be as effective as possible for all members.

Brief Vignette

Lisa and Bert G. brought their oldest child, Bishop, to therapy with the presenting concern that she was having difficulty coping with her younger sister's illness. Bishop was a seven-year-old female and her six-year-old sister, Ann Parke, suffered from severe asthma and was often ill. Bishop claimed that she was having difficulty "getting along" with her sister and that she often became angry with her when she exhibited symptoms of her illness.

The therapist, Ila B., began processing with Bishop and her parents how they currently coped with Ann Parke's illness and the feelings they have associated with their family member. Ila explored with the family both positive and negative feelings and the importance of appropriately expressing both. Ila assessed the clients' present ability to openly communicate with one another and encouraged them to begin openly expressing feelings during the session and at home.

Ila provided Lisa, Bert, and Bishop with two shoe boxes each and various decorative materials. Ila worked with the family in discussing and decorating their "Positive Feelings Box" and "Negative Feelings Box." Bishop used paint to color the outside of her positive feelings box pink because she said, "pink makes me happy." Ila processed with Bishop the various emotions that can be associated with happy and when and how she expressed those feelings. Bishop painted the outside of her negative feeling box dark blue because she said, "dark blue is depressing, just like negative feelings."

Ila worked with the family members in planning where they would keep their boxes and how they would utilize them on a daily basis. Bishop decided to write her feelings on small pieces of paper and place them in her boxes during the session. Ila worked with Bishop in processing her feelings and how she expressed them in a way that would not be hurtful to her sister or other family members. Ila encouraged Bishop to separate the negative feelings that she had about her sister's illness and its' symptoms from the negative feelings she had about her sister. Ila explored with Bishop and her parents how illnesses are external to people and are not a part of a person, but rather something that challenges them.

Bishop was also encouraged to give her sister an opportunity to share the negative feelings she had about her illness, therefore providing them with an opportunity to connect on an emotional level. Bishop decided to give her positive feelings box to her sister as part of her birthday present to show her sister how much she really did care for and love her.

Suggestions for Follow-Up

The clinician should encourage the clients to share their positive and negative feelings boxes with their family members in session and at home. The clinician should process with the other family members their thoughts about the boxes and how they choose to appropriately express their emotions.

The "Positive Feelings Box" can be retitled "What I love about my _____" (i.e., brother, sister, daughter, etc.) and then given as a gift to the family member that is challenged by the illness/trauma/disability. The clinician could process with the receiving family member what it was like to receive such a gift and how he or she could do the same for other family members.

Contraindications for Use

This activity works best with children, but it can be used with clients of all ages, even adults. If a client is unable to create the boxes due to disability, the clinician could create the boxes under the client's directions.

References and Resources for the Professional

Freedman, J., & Combs, G. (1996). *Narrative therapy: The social construction of preferred realities.* New York: W.W. Norton & Company.
McDaniel, S. H., & Doherty, W. J. (Eds.) (2003). *The shared experience of illness: Stories of patients, families, and their therapists.* New York: Basic Books.
O'Hanlon, B. (1994). The third wave. *Family Therapy Networker, 18* (6), 28-29.
Rolland, J. S. (1994). *Families, illness, and disability: An integrative treatment model.* New York: Basic Books.
Satir, V. M. (1972). *Peoplemaking.* Palo Alto: Science and Behavior Books.

Bibliotherapy Sources for Clients

McKay, M., Davis, M., & Fanning, P. (1998). *Thoughts and feelings: Taking control of your moods and your life.* Oakland, CA: New Harbinger Publications.
Meyer, D., & Gallagher, D. (2005). *The sibling slam book: What it's really like to have a brother or sister with special needs.* Bethesda, MD: Woodbine House.
Meyer, D., & Pillo, C. (1997). Views *from our shoes: Growing up with a brother or sister with special needs.* Bethesda, MD: Woodbine House.

Chapter 8

Extraordinary Parts:
The Wife, Mother, and Survivor

Katherine M. Hertlein
Deanna Linville

Type of Contribution: Activity

Objective

The objective for this chapter is to use internal family systems theory (Schwartz, 1995) to better manage different parts of one's experience and personality in order to promote healing and emotional wellness for people living with chronic illness.

Rationale for Use

Biopsychosocial model. This chapter is primarily grounded in the biopsychosocial model. The biopsychosocial model emphasizes the interconnectedness among the physical, social, and psychological aspects of people. This same model underscores the field of medical family therapy and recognizes the interplay of physical and emotional well-being on a client's mental health (McDaniel, Hepworth, & Doherty, 1992). Specifically, medical family therapists consider how clients' physical symptoms inform their issues in therapy and vice versa.

Internal family systems theory. As a secondary framework, internal family systems therapy (IFS) helps the therapist and the client to focus on intrapsychic process in therapy (Schwartz, 1995). In the IFS approach, the therapist and client work with the many different "parts" of a client's system. The system parts include one's Self (the leadership part of the system) and other subparts or subpersonalities. The therapist can identify these parts by looking for polarizations within individuals or within systems. Some common polarized parts include: exiles (parts that have experienced trauma), managers (parts that keep control of the individual and run day-to-day life), and firefighters (groups of parts that attempt to control an individual's feelings) (Schwartz, 1995).

There are several goals outlined in IFS treatment: (1) to work toward balance in one's internal system, (2) to develop one's Self so that it will be able to effectively lead the system, (3) to have the other parts provide input but ultimately respect the Self's leadership and autonomy, and (4) to have all of the parts work together rather than live in isolated polarization. Overall, the therapist works to have the client's Self lead his or her decision making while considering input from all other parts and utilizing the benefits and talents of each part rather than discounting them.

Instructions

There are three distinct phases in using IFS with patients with chronic illness or disability: (1) identify polarizations in thoughts, attitudes, feelings, and behaviors, including those related to the illness, (2) pair up these polarizations with their accompanying parts (i.e., firefighter, manager, exile, etc.), and (3) use imagery to generate a symbol of the polarizations. When using imagery to generate a symbol of polarizations, one should also generate an image of the Self. Once this is developed, the therapist should encourage clients to use strategies for managing the disability and illness as a way to work toward better integration of the Self in other areas of life.

The first major task is to help clients identify and manage the personal and individual parts within their internal systems. Specifically related to illness and disability, the therapist encourages clients to consider parts in the individual system related to the illness/disability as these may be a mirror for how the parts are activated within one's system. Clients may report struggling with different roles (patient, mother, wife, etc.) and have difficulty switching between roles. Identification of multiple roles is one way the therapist can assess the different parts for the client. The therapist can then employ the specific IFS techniques by developing more questions around these multiple roles. In particular, the therapist should look for polarizations within the roles. Examples of questions might include (but are not limited to):

- "Are there any instances or times when you feel pulled from the patient role to another role (e.g., caregiving role)?"
- "Are there times when you feel that you are alternating from one end of the spectrum to another, perhaps from a self-sufficient recovering person to a sick and somewhat dependent person?"
- "Can you cite any instances when you have wanted to act in a certain manner and something has prevented you from saying what you really thought should be said? Or have there been any instances when you felt unable to act the way that you thought would have been best, perhaps with your physicians or support network? Describe those instances."

Following the IFS model, the therapist should continue by making an assessment of the extent to which the client is aware of his or her experience of the parts. In a couple or family relationship, the therapist can also ask questions about how aware each of the family members is of his or her individual parts as well as the parts of the other family members. The client(s) and therapist then work to develop an agreement around how the framework will be employed within their sessions. In this intervention, imagery is identified as the primary way to use the framework, but a collaborative agreement between the therapist and client may result in a slight variation. For example, therapists and clients may determine that using art rather than imagery can also be powerful in conducting this intervention.

Once the therapist and client are able to identify the roles, the second major task is for the therapist and client to attach IFS language regarding parts to the identified parts. For example, a desire to control feelings such as loss, anger, fear, and hurt might be activating one's firefighters. The therapist should introduce this language to the client(s) and work toward helping the client to integrate the language into his or her self-understanding (for greater detail on IFS therapy, see Schwartz, 1995).

The third distinct task in this intervention is learning to utilize imagery. Imagery is a powerful technique in getting clients to understand and possibly incorporate alternative perspectives into their awareness. Imagery is an important and powerful aspect of IFS treatment. The imagery in this activity is related to symbolism and most closely follows the work of Assagioli (1969). In such treatment, clients may be asked to think about a symbol that represents an object or event.

Clients may then be encouraged to focus on this symbol, paying particular attention to the details of the symbol. For example, the therapist should instruct the client to pay attention to the colors in the symbol, shape, and/or other physical properties of the image. A symbol of one's illness might be an image of a hospital or a physician, whereas a representation of wellness might be an image of outdoor activity.

After the images are generated and discussed, the therapist encourages the client to imagine the integration of the firefighters, exiles, and managers into the Self. This can be accomplished by having the client tell a story or journal about the symbols and working together for a unified self. In cases of illness, the therapist should ask the client to focus on a story that involves feelings toward illness, family dynamics related to the illness, etc. Once the client can see and accept this alternate reality, the therapist and client generate ways to implement Self-leading in the client's life.

Brief Vignette

Colleen, thirty-four, initially called for couples counseling. At the time of intake, she had been married for six years. She reported that she was having difficulty dealing with her husband's close relationship with a female friend of his and that she and her husband were fighting frequently. At the first session, Colleen's husband, Wayne, elected not to attend the session. Colleen reported that Wayne had moved out the weekend just before the first session, renting a townhouse at the other end of town. The couple had a three-year-old daughter, Alesha. Wayne was still communicating with Colleen regarding opportunities when he could see Alesha, but was otherwise not responding to Colleen's attempts to communicate with him either by phone or e-mail.

The course of therapy, then, moved from couple sessions to individual treatment for Colleen. In addition to the stressors of her relationship, she expressed sadness in relation to her husband's recent lack of support regarding her recovery from Non-Hodgkin's Lymphoma. She was diagnosed with this condition just prior to her wedding six years ago. Colleen reported that Wayne was a great support to her when she was initially diagnosed. Three years after her diagnosis, her cancer went into remission. From the inception of her diagnosis until just recently, Wayne attended all of her doctor appointments, was vigilant in terms of keeping her healthy, and attended the annual local cancer walk, cheering her on. Besides possibly losing her relationship, Colleen also faced the loss of a significant social support related to her health care. She reported that she recently went to her doctor to evaluate the state of her remission and that this was the first doctor appointment in the course of her illness that Wayne had missed. In addition to the recent separation, Wayne's connection with his female friend, and their increased conflict, Colleen was distraught at the possibility of losing this support system.

Over the course of the first few sessions, Colleen indicated that she was experiencing significant stress from the ongoing conflict of roles that she maintained. Although she reported that she had some anger at Wayne, she indicated that she was reluctant to disclose this because she was fearful that her anger would push Wayne further away from her. She was also struggling with her role as a parent because she was fearful about her personal health and whether the cancer would come out of remission. These fears had significant implications for the well-being of her daughter. Colleen reported that she "caught" herself wanting to discuss some of these issues with Wayne but did not want to intrude on his life by "demanding" his support.

After noticing how Colleen was engaging in a pattern of censoring herself, the therapist asked Colleen to identify conflicting thoughts and attitudes she often experienced. Colleen described the following polarized thoughts and feelings:

1. I should be extremely nice to get him back—I am very angry with him.
2. I am saddened by his lack of support—I don't need someone who won't be supportive anyway.
3. I want to use Alesha to entice him to come home—I know it is wrong to use Alesha as a pawn.

The therapist wrote these polarized statements opposite one another on a whiteboard in the therapy room. Once these statements were represented, the therapist and Colleen worked to assign parts-related labels on each of these polarizations. Manager parts included (1) the feelings that she had to be overly nice to Wayne as a way to get him back, and (2) the thoughts of using Alesha to get Wayne back. Colleen used caretaking toward Wayne and being controlling in regard to her daughter to manage painful feelings of rejection. An example of her exiles would be the angry fearful parts related to her husband leaving and thoughts about being alone to deal with her health issues. Once these feelings were activated, her firefighters came in to rescue her so she would not have to experience the negative feelings. Behaviors used by the firefighters to keep the exiles in hiding was her passive-aggressive behavior toward her husband, trying to be nice so that he would return to her, but all the while building up resentment and not being true to herself.

Related to chronic illness, emotions such as fear, anger, and sadness were particularly pronounced in Colleen as a reaction from her Non-Hodgkin's Lymphoma diagnosis. Colleen indicated that in both instances, she felt as if she was experiencing a loss of control over her own life and the most recent events in her relationship left her with similar feelings. The therapist and Colleen discussed the firefighter parts in her system which controlled or extinguished the feelings that she was uncomfortable managing.

Per IFS treatment, the therapist began with working on the protective parts first. The therapist allowed Colleen to discuss her fears related to allowing her anger to be expressed toward her husband and also to allowing her anger to be expressed in session. Working with Colleen to help her bring down the curtain of protection around her behavior was critical in being able to reach her managers, firefighters, and exiles.

The therapist then asked Colleen to generate images of her firefighters, starting with the firefighter that was preventing her from experiencing the anger related to her husband's close relationship with a female friend. Colleen described picturing a large blanket over a tightly wound and knotted ball of rope. This process of generating images and describing these images was repeated for the following parts and feelings: exiles, managers, feeling loss of control, sadness related to her current separation from her husband, her feelings of inadequacy as a wife (partially prompted by her diagnosis), and anger at Wayne for withdrawing his support related to her illness. The therapist specifically instructed Colleen to examine the images she had related to feelings about her illness (fear, shame, loss of control) and compare them with the images she generated regarding her present situation. Colleen reported that she imagined the current operations of her managers, exiles, and firefighters to be the same that she experienced after being diagnosed, but since her separation, the imagery became more pronounced.

The therapist instructed Colleen over the week to write two short stories. The first short story was to be about how, after her diagnosis, her parts were able to integrate and allow her to Self to lead. Colleen described how she imagined the support from co-workers, her family, and particularly Wayne as instrumental in minimizing the function of the firefighters. Around these individuals, she felt comfortable to be vulnerable with her feelings, thereby reducing the demand on the firefighters. Further, she indicated that the amount of social support she received allowed her mangers to relax and experience the hurt that she was feeling. In her second story, she was instructed to describe the images taking pieces of themselves and putting them in a melting pot to blend the parts together and integrate them into one large part. In this way, each of the parts retained its own individuality while still contributing to the Self leader. This imagery was consistent with demonstrating respect for the parts while maintaining balance by not allowing the parts to overwhelm the Self.

The therapist encouraged Colleen to apply the techniques she had employed in managing her parts at the time of diagnosis to the current situation. Using her Self to lead, Colleen reported that she felt that it was important that she express her anger and disappointment to Wayne, but in a way that was appropriate, nonblaming, and assertive. Afterward, she indicated that she felt positive about the experience and that she was generating respect for herself. She worked harder between sessions to be more genuine and reduce instances of passive-aggressive behavior. At the close of therapy, Wayne had moved back home and was attempting to work on his relationship with Colleen.

Suggestions for Follow-Up

Although this vignette depicts the treatment of an individual patient in therapy, the same steps can be employed with couples and families in treatment. For example, if Wayne had been present for couples therapy, the therapist may have worked on each of their parts together and learned how each part could interact with the parts from the other person.

Contraindications for Use

This intervention, although effective in this case in bringing the couple together, should not be interpreted as a method of attempting couples therapy through individual treatment. As literature in the field of couples therapy finds, couples therapy with only one partner attending treatment is not as effective as conjoint therapy (Nichols & Schwartz, 1998). Furthermore, the goals of treatment in this case were not to work toward reestablishing the couple relationship, but rather to work with the individual client to develop an integrated sense of self and make her decisions based on her personal goals and leadership of Self rather than polarized parts. The maintenance of the couple relationship was incidental. In addition, in IFS the therapist is also advised to be aware whether they are working with the Self or one of the parts. Working with the Self is ideal, but in some cases parts are heavily protecting the Self, and the success of the treatment depends on the access to the Self.

References

Assagioli, R. (1969). Symbols of transpersonal experience. *Journal of Transpersonal Psychology, 1*, 33-45.
McDaniel, S., Hepworth, J., & Doherty, W. J. (1992). *Medical family therapy: A biopsychosocial approach to families with health problems.* New York: Basic Books.
Nichols, M. P., & Schwartz, R. C. (1998). *Family therapy: Concepts and methods.* Boston: Allyn & Bacon.
Schwartz, R. (1995). *Internal family systems therapy.* New York: Guilford.

Readings and Resources for the Professional

Breunlin, D., Schwartz, R., & Kune-Karrer, B. (1992). *Metaframeworks: Transcending the models of family therapy.* New York: Guilford.
Schwartz, R. (1995). *Internal family systems therapy.* New York: Guilford.
Singer, J. L. (2005). *Imagery in psychotherapy.* Washington, DC: APA.

Bibliotherapy Resources for Clients

Boss, P. (2000). *Ambiguous loss.* Massachusetts: Harvard University Press.

Deutsch, M. W., & Cangemi, G. (1998). *Are you tired again? I understand: An activities book to help children understand and live with a person who has a chronic illness or disability.* Los Angeles: Western Psychological Services.

Fincannon, J., & Bruss, K. (2002). Couples Confronting Cancer. American Cancer Society. Atlanta, Georgia.

Chapter 9

The Healthy Families Project

Lisa Lavelle

Type of Contribution: Multiple Family Discussion Group

Objective

The Multiple Family Discussion Group (MFDG) (Steinglass, 1988) model has been successfully used to address various medical conditions including schizophrenia, alcoholism, and cancer. The MFDG examines the psychosocial functioning of families with an ill family member. The group enables families to experience the myriad ways family relationships impact an illness and how an illness impacts family relationships. It challenges the idea of the illness as the central organizing principal for families in all phases of the family life cycle. The initial model was structured and has most effectively been applied to white middle-class families. This chapter will examine the ways in which the model has been adjusted to meet the needs of low-income families of color with a chronic illness.

Rationale for Use

Recruitment for the MFDG has historically been one of the most difficult aspects of this model. The primary issues involved with recruitment difficulty in this low-income Harlem community of color are time commitment and a history of mistrust with the medical system. First, the illness takes on the role of an unwanted house guest that refuses to leave. Families are forced to make space and time for the illness. Time is taken away from the day-to-day tasks of attending school activities, going to work, and the demands of a single-parent household. For many families the thought of carving out time for one more activity feels simply impossible. Time becomes scarce and even more difficult to negotiate as a chronic illness enters family life. Second, historical family beliefs and experiences are negatively loaded in this domain. The Tuskegee Syphilis Study set a historical precedent.

In the six session Steinglass model (Steinglass, 1998), several families meet once per week for two hours at the same day and time every week for a total of six weeks. Two clinicians serve as facilitators to engage families in discussions related to illness and its impact on family life. The definition of family used to recruit participants assumes that family means a nuclear model of family living under the same roof sharing day-to-day experiences, which is true of many white middle-class families. The Steinglass model employs the *family bumper sticker* by asking families to create a phrase or motto that captures the essence of who they are in terms of their beliefs and values. In its use of *family identity,* the Steinglass model makes no direct reference to an exploration of family culture or ethnicity.

While conducting a two-phase needs assessment comprised of a one-to-one patient/family member questionnaire and family focus groups, we learned about the challenges, effects, and changes in daily routines as a result of living with a chronic illness. Families talked about the dilemma of juggling the roles of caregiver and patient. Most critical, we learned that in most of these families it was more the rule than the exception that there was *more than one person in the family with an illness*. This was our first indicator that the Steinglass model of "one illness per family" would fall short in meeting the needs of low-income families of color with chronic illnesses. In assessing the data collected from the questionnaire, focus groups, our knowledge of family systems and low-income families of color, we came to realize that various components of the Steinglass model did not readily lend themselves to the east Harlem community. Specifically, the variables of the definition of family, one illness per family, family bumper sticker, and the requirement to include culture in any conversation of family identity. These concepts were modified to reflect cultural awareness and cultural sensitivity.

The narrow Steinglass definition of family does not readily lend itself to working with families of color whose composition, more often than not, expands beyond the boundaries of who lives together under the same roof; it would have eliminated a high number of families in east Harlem. We expanded the definition of family in our work to include kinship networks, which are commonplace among families of color, especially African Americans and Latinos. As Boyd-Franklin states, "the emotional significance of relationships is not determined solely by the immediacy of blood ties. In fact, 'family' is an extended system of blood related kin and people who are informally adopted into this system," (Boyd-Franklin, 1989, p. 38). More often than not, family members reside in close proximity to one another or in the same neighborhood which ultimately allows for daily interaction around day-to-day tasks. "Indeed some members of the 'extended' or nonhousehold family are as intimately involved in family matters as are 'nuclear' or household members. This may be particularly true in a crisis such as a chronic illness," (Holder et al., 1998, p. 4).

In poor communities such as east Harlem, the model of 'one illness per family' is simply not applicable. Poor or no health care, ethnicity and social-class marginalization, and lack of access to services often result in low-income families of color having more than one family member with one or more chronic illnesses. The role of ill family member and caregiver may fall upon the same person or vary interchangeably among family members. A single mother may care for her adolescent son with asthma who in turn may care for her.

The idea of a *bumper sticker* lacks meaning for low-income families of color, as a bumper sticker implies one has a car or access to one. Many families who participated in the Healthy Families Project do not have resources to afford a car and due to their environment rely solely on subways, buses, taxis, or other public transportation. Adapting the model to make it more relevant to low-income families of color, the *bumper sticker* was replaced by *family song title*. Music has historically been a part of African-American, Afro-Caribbean, and Latino cultures. Singing in churches, song as a part of ethnic pride, and song for survival as used during slavery, are one of the cornerstones of ethnic and racial heritage for people of color. More specifically for African Americans, call and response songs were used during slavery as a method of communication and safety as slaves were denied access to a common language.

One cannot work with families of color, engage them in a conversation about family identity, without also addressing issues of culture and ethnicity. An examination of family identity was expanded to include: What stories of pride and shame do you have about your culture/ethnicity? What does it mean to be a family in your culture/ethnicity? What are the beliefs about illness in your culture/ethnicity?

The issue of culture is easy to ignore when talking about whites and is almost often raised with non-white populations. Culture is a *constant,* important variable regardless of race, class, or ethnicity. This idea must not be overlooked when working with any population, including whites. In order to be meaningful, a discussion of family identity *must* include a conversation about culture.

Instructions

Session 1—Patient Perspective

Session 1 focuses on the experience of the patient. The goals are to first, identify illness-related issues, concerns, and stressors as these relate to patient and family. Second, the facilitators encourage family members to talk to individuals other than their own family about the illness experience in an effort to highlight elements of similarity and difference among families as it relates to illness management and its impact on family relationships. This is done using the *group within a group model* or "fishbowl technique." The fishbowl technique divides the group into patients and caregivers such that group members are in observation of one another. In a small, inner circle, patients discuss their feelings and experiences in relation to having an illness within their specific family. Caregivers from all families sit in a larger, outer circle to listen and observe this process. Then the dynamic shifts so that the caregivers discuss their experiences of an illness in their specific family and the patients listen and observe.

Session 2—Caregiver Perspective

The format of Session 2 is similar to Session 1, with the focus now being the experience of the caregivers/family members. The goals of this session are as follows: (1) to identify illness-related issues and perspectives via the caregiver experience, (2) to highlight similarities and differences among families around these issues, and (3) to connect and share around like experiences, ideas, and feelings as it relates to the illness lifecycle. Using the fishbowl technique, caregivers/family members are asked to meet with a facilitator in a smaller subgroup discussing the experience of being a family member of someone with an illness.

Session 3—Family Development

Session 3 examines family beliefs about the illness. The goal of this session is to give families a framework for understanding how the illness has affected their sense of identity as a family. Using a workshop format, families begin to think about how to make needed and necessary accommodations for the illness while not allowing the illness to overwhelm their lives and a sense of who they are as a family. To help engage families in this process, a flip chart with the categories *before* and *now* is used by the facilitator to write down ideas, phrases, and activities that characterized family life during the respective time. Families are then invited to think about themselves in terms of what makes them unique, special, or different from other families. Each family is asked a series of questions which serve as a catalyst to get families to see themselves through a non-illness perspective and to get them to think about the real meaning of who they are. What are you most proud of about your family? What makes your family unique? What would someone be surprised to learn about your family? The concept of the *family song* is introduced and families are asked to create a song title that reflects the essence of who they are in terms of family, coupled with their dilemma of "honoring the illness while putting the illness in its place" (Steinglass, 1998 p. 67).

Session 4—Art Collages "Family Life Before the Illness" and "Family Life Now"

Each family will then work together to create a collage of what family life was like *before* the illness and what family life is like *now*. The goal of this session is to demonstrate visually to the group how each family sees itself *before* and *now* with the illness.

Session 5—Presentation of Collage

The collages are mounted on the wall and facilitators lead a discussion with one family at a time about their *before* and *now* collages. Families are asked what they hope family life will look like one year from now. Observing families can help other families examine family themes, challenge family beliefs about the future, and problem solve. At the last session, each family is asked to bring a symbol that will signify where they see themselves next year.

Session 6—Next Year's Family

Using the object brought in by each family coupled with their family motto to help them achieve the dual goal of "honoring the illness while putting the illness in its place," facilitators work with each family to create a meaningful ritual using their illness reminder.

To mark the end of the six sessions MFDG families participate in a ritual. This includes certificates of completion as in a graduation and summary reflections from facilitators and families highlighting shifts in each family made during the MFDG.

Brief Vignette

One example of the impact of the Healthy Families Project is of a three-generation family of African-American women consisting of mother, daughter, and granddaughter. Mother had been diagnosed with asthma and diabetes and her daughter had been diagnosed with asthma. The granddaughter had no reported illness. Mother had a history of poor medical management of her diabetes. Medical care had been characterized by frequent visits to the emergency room and hospitalizations as a result of not taking her insulin. Mother and daughter argued continually about the illness to the point where a classic role reversal had taken place; Mother had become the daughter and daughter had become the parent. Mother and daughter had the experience that talking about the illness made things worse in their relationship. Illness conversations had gone underground, creating distance and alienation between mother and daughter. After the six-week session intervention, mother and daughter reported improved communication between each other, especially in regards to illness dialogue. ER visits were replaced by appointments with a primary care physician. The role reversal between mother and daughter resumed normal family functioning because the daughter no longer needed to play the role of mother in the family and mother started managing her insulin. The family utilized support from families sharing the same illness, validation, and problem solving as created by the Healthy Families Project.

Suggestions for Follow-Up

Research has shown that the MFDG works successfully to address the impact of a chronic illness on family relationships and how those relationships then impact the illness. More work has been done applying this model to white middle-class families with "one illness per family." Its use in poor urban areas with families of color has required changing various aspects of the model to make it more culturally sensitive. What continues to be challenging with the model is the recruitment phase, especially for low-income people of color.

Further development of this model should include participation in MFDGs as a required aspect of medical protocol. In the same fashion that a doctor would recommend a person with diabetes to a nutritionist, patients struggling with chronic illness should be referred to MFDGs. In order for this concept to be effective and become a standard part of medical treatment, physicians must widen the medical lens to see the family as the patient, and not just the individual with the illness. Illness has a profound impact on families and families impact an illness. Recognition of this idea is critical to the future implementation of the MFDG.

Contraindications for Use

This approach may not be effective for patients with a dual diagnosis of a serious mental illness and a chronic illness. The MFDG model is best applied to single health/mental health issues, especially with regard to its psychoeducational component. In addition, couples for whom there is active domestic violence may not be a good fit as the MFDG does not lend itself to the in-depth exploration of psychological and safety issues.

References

Boyd-Franklin, N. (1989). *Black families in therapy: A Multi-systems approach.* New York: Guilford Press.

Holder, B., Turner-Musa, J., Kimmel, P., Alleyne, S., Kobrin, S., & Simmens, S., et al. (1998). Engagement of African American Families in Research on Chronic Illness: A Multisystem Recruitment Approach. *Family Process 37,* 127-151.

Steinglass, P. (1988). Multiple Family Discussion Groups for Patients with Chronic Medical Illness. *Family Process, 16,* 55-70.

Readings and Resources for the Professional

Gonzales, S., & Steinglass, P. (2002). Application of multifamily groups in chronic medical disorders. *Multiple family groups in the treatment of severe psychiatric disorders.* New York: Guilford Press.

Gormley, M. (1999). The role of fertility control in socio-economic development. *Journal of the History Students of San Francisco University, Volume VIII.* San Francisco State University.

Imber-Black, E., & Roberts, J. (1993). *Rituals for our times: Celebrating, healing, and changing our lives and our relationships.* New York: W.W. Norton & Co.

Jones, J. H. (1993). *BadBlood: The Tuskegee syphilis experiment.* New York: Free Press.

McFarlane, W. R. (2002). *Multiple family groups in the treatment of severe psychiatric disorders.* New York: Guilford Press.

Rolland, J. (1994). *Families, illness and disability: An integrative treatment model.* New York: Basic Books.

Steinglass, P. (1988). Multiple family discussion groups for patients with chronic medical illness. *Family Process, 16,* 55-70.

Bibliotherapy Resources for Clients

Imber-Black, E. (1998). *The secret life of families.* New York: Bantam Books.

Morris, D. (2000). *Illness and culture in the postmodern age.* Berkeley and Los Angeles California: University of California Press.

Videotape for Clients

BD Diabetes Center (Producer). (2005). *Diabetes: A Team Effort* [Videotape]. (Available from BD Diabetes Center, Morristown, NJ 07962.)

SECTION II:
INTERVENTIONS FOR WORKING WITH CHILDREN AND ILLNESS

Chapter 10

Fun with Bubbles: Relieving Childhood Pain and Physical Symptoms

Olivia Chiang
Jeri Hepworth
Susan McDaniel

Type of Contribution: Intervention/Homework

Objective

Bodily symptoms in children can be terrifying to children and to their family members. This playful "bubble" intervention provides a way for a child and his or her family members to help manage somatic complaints, such as pain, through knowledge and diaphragmatic breathing. When children feel their bodies are out of control, this intervention is an active approach that can lessen fear and anxiety and increase their sense of agency (McDaniel, Hepworth, & Doherty, 1992). It gives a sense of control to the child and his or her family, and it provides an easy and efficient method of teaching diaphragmatic breathing in a manner that is developmentally appropriate for children. The task of blowing bubbles provides feedback and a sense of fun. As an activity for the entire family, blowing bubbles can reinforce the child's ability to relieve symptoms, while increasing family play and connectedness.

Rationale for Use

Children with medical illnesses and consequent anxiety and/or depression report a wide variety of bodily symptoms: pain, nausea, diaphoresis, tingling, numbness, temperature changes, dyspnea, and heart palpitations. With any symptom, children look first to their parents for help. When faced with these concerns, parents can panic as well and feel helpless and out of control. Sometimes these feelings lead to frantic calls to physicians or visits to Emergency Departments.

Diaphragmatic breathing is a helpful technique for breaking the cycle of increasing pain and fear in response to physiologic symptoms (Benson, Beary, & Carol, 1974; Lehrer, Carr, Sargunaraj, & Woolfolk, 1994; National Institute of Health Technology Assessment Panel on Integration of Behavioral and Relaxation Approaches into the Treatment of Chronic Pain and Insomnia, 1996). Adults usually can understand that deep breathing helps relax tight muscles and decreases shallow breathing or palpitations. It is more difficult for children to intuitively understand that some of their symptoms are responses to fear, and can be decreased with slower breaths and relaxation.

Blowing bubbles is a way to ensure deep breathing. It is not necessary to understand the process or even understand that blowing bubbles is deep breathing. It is a way of turning attention to something other than the pain or fear, and slowing breath to disrupt the pain-fear-hyperventilation cycle. As the child's breath is slowed with the bubble exercise, parents' fears are also quickly reduced.

This exercise is informed by medical family therapy (McDaniel, Hepworth, & Doherty, 1992). Medical family therapists work with families struggling with illness or disability. Chronic illness can often take a central role in the family, resulting in disrupted roles and coping styles. Particularly for childhood illness, the family can feel helpless in managing symptoms and consequent impact. Goals of medical family therapy are to increase the family's sense of agency and connectedness with one another to respond to the illness and care for all family members. Several other theoretical constructs support this family intervention.

David Reiss, Sandra Gonzalez, and Norman Kramer (1986) describe how a family's paradigm for coordination is an important factor in its ability to handle illness and relationships with the health care system. Coordination is the family's level of readiness to experience themselves as a single unity especially when faced with stress. This family based exercise helps put parents back in charge of helping to comfort a sick child.

A second relevant theory is the family adjustment and adaptation response model (McCubbin & Patterson, 1982), which combines family stress theory and family systems theory. This model considers how families manage the demands of chronic illnesses through coping patterns, resources, and beliefs. The Bubbles exercise helps organize somatic symptoms into a dynamic experience affected by physical and emotional interactions. Children and families learn the relationship between fears and concerns and their somatic problems. The exercise offers a fun coping strategy to manage that interaction.

Finally, the Family FIRO Model (Doherty, Colangelo, & Hovander, 1991) offers three dimensions of family interactions—inclusion, control, and intimacy. Illness can exclude family members from one another, as families learn to depend on outside sources for relief, thus impairing connectedness with one another. This intervention explicitly involves the entire family, not just the sick child. In fact, siblings often benefit from this task as they can help cue the intervention when they notice a sibling needs help. This also helps with control. The child, siblings, and parents can all initiate the exercise. The exercise paves the way for close personal exchanges amongst the family, which are fun and meaningful. The powerful impact of the feared symptoms is reduced for all family members.

Instructions

The Bubbles intervention is appropriate for children who are also under the care of medical providers who have determined that diaphragmatic breathing is not harmful to their medical condition. As this intervention requires blowing bubbles, it is appropriate for children ages three and up. However, two-year-olds can enjoy trying to blow bubbles with their families even when they are unable to do so successfully. Materials needed include an easel pad, a set of crayons/markers, jars of bubbles, and bubble wands. (Alternatively, a dish of bubbles can be made with water and dish detergent.)

The therapist explains that many things can happen to the body when a person experiences pain. This acknowledges that everyone gets scared when he or she is in pain and helps establish the link between the mind and the body. The therapist then draws a large outline of a body onto the easel pad. With younger children, the therapist can identify the picture as the child. The therapist asks the child to imagine what happens to his or her body when he or she is in pain. If the child has difficulty, the therapist can ask family members to help give a clue or an actual somatic complaint. Once the child offers a symptom, the therapist asks the child to draw the symptom onto the body. Each family member can take turns identifying a symptom and drawing the symptom. Examples include shortness of breath, muscle tightness, headaches/stomachaches, palpitations, negative thoughts, and feeling anxious or scared.

After the body drawing is completed, the therapist summarizes what happens to our bodies when we are in pain. The therapist asks what easy thing can be done to help a person feel better. Many suggestions are helpful, but the discussion targets breathing as an activity that can lessen the symptoms or help them go away altogether. With a very short explanation, the therapist describes how breathing changes when people are in pain, scared, sad, or angry. Discussion with the family highlights how people tend to either hyperventilate or hold their breath. Each family member can be asked how they tend to respond, which normalizes how breathing changes for everyone when under stress. For older children or parents, the therapist explains that both ways of breathing lower the body's oxygen level, which increases the painful and frightening symptoms.

The therapist then passes out the bubble solution and wands to each family member. The family will start experimenting with the bubbles. The therapist encourages them to try to blow when they are holding their breath, or when they have very short breaths. They will see that this results in few or tiny bubbles. Many or large bubbles will only occur with sustained breathing. The therapist will help the child and parents identify that big or many bubbles mean "healthy breathing." The exercise typically includes silly behavior, and therapists can note how laughing also can diminish pain and fear.

Homework should continue the sense of play. Parents and children can practice before bed, sometimes with actual bubbles, and sometimes by pretending to blow bubbles. Eventually children and parents notice when the child's body starts to get upset because of pain and find that children can blow real or imaginary bubbles right away and disrupt the cycle. To keep this intervention useful and fun, parents should be encouraged to use real bubbles at home, even if pretend bubbles are all that are necessary to alleviate an acute reaction. In addition, the body drawing is given to the family to take home. The family is instructed to post the drawing where it can be easily seen and the parents and/or the child can reference the symptoms when they occur. The parents can point out the child's current symptoms with the ones on the drawing. Accordingly, bubble blowing is then prompted as a way to aid in managing the symptoms. The therapist can refer to the drawing at home at subsequent sessions to follow up on the intervention. Ongoing communication and collaboration with the family physician, pediatrician, or nurse practitioner is important to the comprehensive care of the child.

Variation

Some families and children may also enjoy blowing bubbles in water. In the bath, or in a large pot of water, children can put their mouth under water and blow bubbles by "sounding like an engine." They can be encouraged to keep blowing and making noise for longer periods before taking a breath of air. They can discuss how this breathing and blowing helps take good oxygen from the air and send it around the body where it is needed. Blowing old air into the water makes room for the new air that the body needs.

Brief Vignette

Julio, an eight-year-old boy with chronic pain and von Willebrand's disease, also suffered from depression and a significant amount of anxiety. Von Willebrand's disease is a lifelong bleeding disorder in which a protein in the body's blood system is missing or does not work well. The missing or malfunctioning protein, Factor VIII, helps blood to clot. Thus, symptoms include frequent nosebleeds, bruising, and heavy bleeding after surgery or injury. This disease is similar to hemophilia, a more severe bleeding disorder. Julio's symptoms included frequent nosebleeds and bruising.

Julio's family had recently moved from Puerto Rico for medical care when they were told that nothing more could be done for him in his hometown. They left a close knit extended family and were now a family of four: Julio's parents, his brother, and Julio. Julio's parents brought him to the pediatrician or emergency room on a weekly basis because Julio was so concerned about his pain that he would become agitated and vomit. Julio's depressive and anxious symptoms and medical visits resulted in significant school absences and unsuccessful performance. He would often cry in school and home. Julio's pediatrician was becoming concerned at the frequency of his symptoms and believed there to be a significant psychosocial component of the problem, so he made a referral to a family therapist working in the pediatric clinic. By the time of referral, Julio had become afraid to sleep in his own bed or even go to the bathroom by himself.

Julio's parents attended without him for the first therapy session and described their distress about his symptoms, depression, and withdrawal. They saw each separate symptom as indicative of a serious medical problem and despaired over how much time they had spent searching for medical diagnoses. They disclosed their fear that Julio had cancer and would likely lose his kidney function and require dialysis. They had two family members who had required dialysis and subsequently died, so were particularly fearful about Julio's prognosis. His parents strongly identified their desire to help Julio but felt helpless and unsure about how to do so.

Julio was apprehensive at the second session but quickly warmed up to explaining his pain and frustration. He reported he would often go to bed at night with a symptom, such as pain. Upon waking in the morning, he would feel worse and tell his mother. His mother described how she would rub his back or give him some medicine but neither would have any benefit. She reported that Julio often then felt nauseous and threw up. His parents would bring Julio to the pediatrician's office where the pediatrician would consider additional possible diagnoses and order new tests. Instead of feeling reassured, his parents were fearful Julio might have a new disease. The cycle repeated itself almost weekly.

Pain was acknowledged as a big problem for Julio. The bubble intervention was suggested as a way to help reduce Julio's pain, with his parents and younger brother's help. Julio and his family were very interested in the idea. The rationale and picture was completed and Julio was especially vocal about all the symptoms that would go through his body when he was in pain. "Being scared" about pain and "feeling helpless" were feelings that were validated with Julio and his family. They appreciated the description about how limited oxygen in the body contributed to all of his symptoms. Julio and his family enjoyed the bubble blowing exercise and agreed to practice it as homework. They were also reminded that deep breathing is a tool to be used in addition to the pain management techniques suggested by his pediatrician. The pediatrician, whenever he saw Julio or his family, supported the therapy, reassured Julio and his family, and encouraged them to continue working on the "bubbles" homework assignment.

At the therapy session one week later, Julio and his parents reported that they felt happier and more in control. Julio had been able to use bubbles on his own and his parents had helped him at other times. Julio reported a small decrease in pain. Julio's brother also reported he was less fearful when Julio was in pain and felt he could participate in the family intervention. His parents were pleased they had an additional way to help Julio and his brother. With this immediate change, the family seemed more comfortable about continuing therapy and considering additional ways to increase structure and support for Julio. By the end of therapy, Julio and his family reported improved sense of control and ability to manage. Julio was functioning well and had returned to school where he again was a successful student. Finally, Julio and his parents greatly reduced their visits to the pediatrician and emergency room. The pediatrician was very pleased with the progress of Julio and his family.

Suggestions for Follow-Up

At later sessions, families can be encouraged to persist if they didn't practice enough. The therapist can also suggest that deep breathing is effective for managing anger as well. The therapist can note that being angry, depressed, anxious, in pain, or sick may have the same effect on breathing, and all these situations may respond to the breathing/bubbles exercise.

As demonstrated with the clinical case, this exercise can set the stage for families' acceptance of additional pain and anxiety management strategies, and ongoing family therapy. Subsequent sessions can help children and families anticipate acute responses and recognize the links between somatic symptoms and consequent anxiety and mood.

Contraindications for Use

Close collaboration with medical professionals is crucial to ensure that this exercise is helpful and not harmful. This exercise may not be helpful for symptoms not typically related to anxiety, but still may provide some comfort, reassurance, and a sense of play for children and families.

The largest concern with this intervention is the misperception that if one can reduce symptoms through breathing, then the patient must be manufacturing or "faking" the symptoms. Children and families need to be reassured that the symptoms are real, that pain is a real response to fear, and that a child is not pretending to feel pain or somatic symptoms. Families can be informed that mind-body medicine is a new frontier (Astin, Shapiro, Eisenberg, & Forys, 2003), and there is much that physicians and therapists are learning. Each family can be a part of this new understanding of health. As they learn specific ways to manage their own pain, they help us learn more for other families in the future.

References

Astin, J., Shapiro, S., Eisenberg, D., & Forys, K. (2003). Mind-body medicine: State of the science, implications for practice. *Journal of the American Board of Family Practice, 16,* 131-147.

Benson, H., Beary, J., & Carol, M. (1974). The relaxation response. *Psychiatry, 37,* 37-46.

Doherty, W. J., Colangelo, N., & Hovander, D. (1991). Priority setting in family change and clinical practice: The family FIRO model. *Family Process, 30,* 227-240.

Lehrer, P. M., Carr, R., Sargunaraj, D., & Woolfolk, R. L. (1994). Stress management techniques: Are they all equivalent, or do they have specific effects? *Biofeedback and Self Regulation, 19,* 353-401.

McCubbin, H. I., & Patterson, J. M. (1982). Family adaptation to crisis. In H. I. McCubbin, A. Cauble, & J. M. Patterson (Eds.), *Family stress, coping, and social support* (pp. 26-47). Springfield, IL: Charles C Thomas.

McDaniel, S., Hepworth, J., & Doherty, W. (1992). *Medical family therapy: A biopsychosocial approach to families with health problems.* New York: Basic Books.

National Institute of Health Technology Assessment Panel on Integration of Behavioral and Relaxation Approaches into the Treatment of Chronic Pain and Insomnia. (1996). Integration of behavioral and relaxation approaches into the treatment of chronic pain and insomnia. *Journal of the American Medical Association, 276*(4), 313-318.

Reiss, D., Gonzalez, S., & Kramer, N. (1986). Family process, chronic illness, and death: On the weakness of strong bonds. *Archives of General Psychiatry, 43,* 795-804.

Readings and Resources for the Professional

Gatchel, R. J., & Turk, D. C. (1996). *Psychological approaches to pain management: A practitioner's handbook.* New York: Guilford Press.

Gimpel, G., & Holland, M. (2003). *Emotional and behavioral problems of young children: Effective interventions in the preschool and kindergarten years.* New York: Guilford Press.

Bibliotherapy Sources for Clients

Caudill, M. (1995). *Managing pain before it manages you.* New York: Guilford Press.

Davis, M., Robbins Eshelman, E., & McKay, M. (2000). *The relaxation and stress reduction workbook.* USA: New Harbinger Publications, Inc.

Goleman, D., & Gurin, J. (1993). *Mind-body medicine.* Yonkers, NY: Consumer Reports Books.

Chapter 11

The Superhero in All of Us

Deanna Linville
Michelle R. Ward

Type of Contribution: Activity/Homework Assignment

Objective

Anxiety has become a common presenting problem for young children in family therapy, particularly those who are experiencing loss, illness, and disability. The purpose of this activity is to provide children with some security about their own strengths, empowering their self-perceptions and eventually reducing their symptoms of anxiety and worry. The therapist and client create a personal "superhero" for the child in the therapy session. This superhero is unique in that it identifies strengths that the child considers important to overcome difficult obstacles. The power of this intervention is that the therapist relates these "superpowers" to the already existing strengths intrinsic to the child's personality. Once completed, the superhero reflects the child's "superpowers." By identifying the child's strengths as "superpowers," this activity boosts the child's self-concept and fosters an ability to cope during difficult times. After the child and family review the child's superpowers, the family takes the superhero home to be mounted in a visible place. The presence of this superhero in the child's everyday world serves as a reminder of the strengths that will help him or her cope with life's struggles.

Rationale for Use

Oftentimes the fear of the unknown involved in dealing with illness and disability can produce significant anxiety in young children, as their ability to process and verbalize difficult emotions is not fully developed. In this activity, the therapist and child create a "superhero" to help externalize the child's strengths in a fun and creative way. Each superhero is individualized to the client's unique personal strengths, as well as to the child's perception of what attributes are considered powerful. This activity externalizes the child's strength through a combination of art and expressive play therapy techniques.

Several theoretical frameworks influence this activity. First, this activity is influenced by the use of externalization in narrative family therapy (White & Epston, 1990). Narrative therapy helps therapists to work with families to experience shifts in the problem context. By externalizing problematic behaviors for families, the problems can be attributed to external factors rather than internal characteristics within the individual or family (White & Epston, 1990). This

---

This activity was created by Sarah S. Briggs, LPC, RPT-S.

also allows clients to develop an alternative story separate from the problem-saturated story with which they have been plagued.

The second theoretical framework that influences this activity is play therapy. Play is viewed as the most effective means for children to communicate and process their experiences. Through expressive and art play therapy, children are able to externalize what is happening internally in an organized manner. The therapist observes the process of play, as well as the content, and aims to provide a safe environment and develop a warm and accepting relationship for the child. In addition, the therapist works to help the child understand his or her experiences and link that understanding with feelings (Gil, 1991).

The third theoretical framework that influences this activity is the biopsychosocial model. The biopsychosocial model takes into account the interaction between family behavior and characteristics of the illness and how this mutual interaction can have a positive or negative influence on the course of the chronic illness (Rolland, 1994, p. 6). Biological, social, and psychological aspects of people are viewed as important in the assessment and treatment phases of treatment.

Instructions

This activity takes place is session with the child and therapist. To begin this activity, the therapist will need to have the following supplies available in session: a roll of butcher paper, a pencil, and various art supplies, including markers, crayons, glue, glitter glue, stickers, yarn, and/or paint. The therapist presents the idea of "creating a superhero" with the child at the beginning of session. The therapist then unrolls a sheet of paper as long as the child is tall. The therapist instructs the child to lay down on the piece of butcher paper so that all body parts are resting on the paper. The therapist then traces the child's body with a pencil, creating a life-size outline of the child on the paper. Once the child's outline is completed, the therapist will ask the child to use the provided art supplies to create an image of a superhero while prompting the child to brainstorm about the strengths of his or her favorite superhero. As the conversation develops, the therapist asks the child about the superhero's powers, incorporating these powers into the child's outline by writing them on the paper near the body part that the superpower would be found. For example, if the child identifies "superhuman strength" as one of the superhero's powers, then the therapist might write, "Strong Muscles" next to the arms and legs of the child's outline. If the child states that his or her superhero can fly, the child and therapist may create a "cape" for the superhero and identify the superpower near the cape as "The Power to Fly." Other superhero strengths that are commonly mentioned include "Moves Fast," "Strong Voice," "Fast Feet/Fast Runner," "Strong Ears/Listening," "Powerful Sight/Hearing," and "Able to Rescue/Save People." A strength that should always be included on the child's list of strengths, even if at the therapist's suggestion, is the strength of being very clever or having a "Strong Brain." This strength is one that children can identify with because it is a reality-based strength that involves little magical powers. Children tend to identify with their superhero's "strong brain" and are often able to cite examples of times when they use their own strong brain superpowers.

This activity can vary in the amount of time necessary to complete the superhero. Some children complete their superhero in one session, and other children use more than one session to complete their work. If working primarily with younger children, the therapist should adjust the language of the superhero's powers to reflect the level of verbal skills of the child.

Brief Vignette

The Smith family came to therapy due to the anxiety that their eight-year-old son, Mark, was having at bedtime when he said good night to his parents. He became fearful of the dark and concerned that intruders would enter the home. The behaviors and anxiety began soon after Mark's mother had been diagnosed with a rare form of cancer and had begun undergoing chemotherapy. Because Mark was having difficulty being alone in the dark, the family superhero activity fit well with this family, as he could hang his superhero in his room and feel less alone and more secure and powerful against the feared intruders.

Mark was very engaged in the superhero activity and was able to identify many superhero powers that were integrated into his superhero figure, including "super smart," "strong muscles," "fast runner," and "not afraid of the dark." Mark invited his family into the session to introduce them to his superhero and describe all of the superpowers that he possessed. Mark's family was asked to hang his superhero wherever Mark felt it would be best, in a place where he could see it from his bed.

The family returned the next week reporting that the superhero had a powerful affect on Mark's ability to separate from his parents at night. He reported feeling much "stronger" at bedtime and less alone. Although his fears about intruders were still present, his fear that he would come to harm was greatly reduced. His parents incorporated a discussion about his superpowers into their nighttime routine, so that it became a part of the family's bedtime structure. Mark had a significant reduction in anxiety symptoms and was able to sleep on his own without exhibiting a fear response when his parents said good night.

Suggestions for Follow-Up

After the creation of the superhero, the therapist can ask several important process questions in relation to the activity's completion. These questions will also serve as a way to solidify the language used around the superhero at home, as the therapist models strength-based comments about the child's work. The therapist can ask such questions as, "What was it like to create your superhero?" "Which of these superpowers do you recognize in yourself?" and "Which superpower feels most helpful?" These questions ask the child and the family to comment on the child's strengths and self-empowerment. This is a positive, externalizing way that the therapist, and thus the child and family, frames what they may not have recognized in the past, thus externalizing the problem even further.

Contraindications for Use

This activity may not be appropriate with families who have not come to terms with the illness and therefore are not willing to accept that their child might be experiencing problems due to their fears about the illness. In addition, the child's feelings of anxiety should be normalized by both the family and therapist recognizing such feelings as a normal response to a parent being diagnosed with cancer. This activity is not meant to suggest that the child needs to feel less anxious but is intended to empower the child to manage his or her anxiety in a productive and playful manner.

References

Gil, E. (1991). *The healing power of play.* New York: Guilford.
Rolland, J. (1994). *Families, illness, & disability.* New York: Basic Books.
White, M., & Epston, D. (1990). *Narrative means to therapeutic ends.* New York: Guilford.

Readings and Resources for the Professional

Gil, E. (1991). *The healing power of play.* New York: Guilford.
Leff, P. T., & Walizer, E. H. (1992). *Building the healing partnership: Parents, professionals, & children with chronic illnesses and disabilities.* Cambridge, MA: Brookline.
Rolland, J. (1994). *Families, illness, & disability.* New York: Basic Books.
Sapolsky, R. M. (2000). *Why zebras don't get ulcers: An updated guide to stress, stress-related diseases, and coping.* New York: W.H. Freeman.
White, M., & Epston, D. (1990). *Narrative means to therapeutic ends.* New York: Guilford.

Bibliotherapy Resources for Clients

Barrett Singer, A. T. (1999). *Coping with your child's chronic illness.* San Francisco: Robert D. Reed.
Bluebond-Langner, M. (1996). *In the shadow of illness: parents and siblings of the chronically ill child.* Princeton, NJ: Princeton University Press.
Clark, C. D. (2003). *In sickness and in play: Children coping with chronic illness.* New Brunswick, NJ: Rutgers University Press.

Chapter 12

The Angry Feelings Toolbox

Michelle R. Ward
Deanna Linville

Type of Contribution: Activity/Homework Assignment

Objective

Anger is a common stage of grief and loss, even for children. Many children who are coping with illness, death, or disability experience a natural stage of overwhelming anger about such difficult situations. For young children in family therapy, this activity may be useful in helping families help children deal with their difficult emotions. The purpose of this activity is to provide children with a system that they can use at home, with the help of their family, to develop healthy coping skills when feeling angry. The therapist and client create a personalized anger-management rating system and various verbal and physical techniques that are used by the child as a safe outlet for angry feelings. This intervention gives families hands-on solutions to helping their child manage his or her feelings in a healthier way.

Rationale for Use

Children respond to loss, illness, or disability in many ways. Anger is a potential stage in the grieving process. In this activity, the therapist and child create an anger-management system to help children cope with their anger in a healthy and productive manner. Each anger management "toolbox" is individualized for the specific child, so that the child chooses which techniques to use and when. This allows children to determine which coping skills are helpful or not helpful, giving them control of how they help themselves.

Several theoretical frameworks influence this activity. First, this activity is influenced by the use of cognitive-behavioral therapy as it attempts to recognize certain thoughts and behaviors and then modify them. Emotions are included in assessment and treatment phases, and cognitions are considered to be the intervening variable between a stimulus and a response. Two main goals of cognitive-behavioral therapy are for the client to become aware of the cognitive processes that contribute to maladaptive behaviors or disturbed mood, and for the therapist to help the client build skills necessary for successful interpersonal interactions (Lynn & Garske, 1985).

The second theoretical framework that influences this activity is play therapy, which assumes that a child can best communicate and process his or her emotions through play (Gil, 1991). Through expressive and art play therapy, children are able to externalize their internal world in an organized manner. One goal of play therapy is to help bring relief of clinical symptoms while removing impediments to the child's continuing development. Children are able to release emotions in a healthy and productive manner through a process that is natural for them.

Lastly, this activity is influenced by solution-focused family therapy insofar as it focuses on what has worked and not worked in the past and how clients can be empowered to find a solution within themselves to solve their own problem (Lipchik, 2002; O'Hanlon & Weiner-Davis, 1989). Assumptions guiding solution-focused therapists include the following: (1) every client is unique, (2) clients have the inherent strength and resources to help themselves, and (3) change is constant and inevitable; a small change can lead to bigger changes (Lipchik, 2002).

Instructions

The start of this activity takes place in a family session, where the therapist has introduced the question, "What do you do when you get angry?" This session is an important launching pad for the anger management system. This question can begin a process of increased understanding about the family's current use of coping skills, including whether their current "toolbox" feels helpful or not helpful, useful or not useful, and hurtful or not hurtful. Once the therapist has explored with the family what is or is not working, the idea of creating a useful "toolbox" can be introduced. At this time, the therapist can describe the anger management activity to the family.

The actual expressive art portions of this activity initially take place with the child and therapist. The activity takes place in three parts, which can be separated into two or more sessions. To begin the first part of this activity, the therapist will introduce the child to the use of a verbal rating scale to measure his or her level of angry emotions. The therapist will teach the child to rate his or her level of anger on a scale of zero to ten. Once the child has mastered and practiced this new skill, the therapist and child can create an "anger thermometer" together. To create this thermometer, the therapist will need to have the following supplies available in session: a sheet of poster board, a pencil, and various art supplies including markers, glue, foam cutouts and/or glitter glue. With a pencil, the therapist draws a large thermometer on the poster board delineating the numbers from zero to ten along one side of the thermometer, with zero being at the bottom of the thermometer and ten at the top of the thermometer. As the child works on personalizing his or her thermometer by decorating it with the art supplies, the therapist describes how a thermometer works and discusses with the child how the thermometer might relate to angry feelings. This concept can be initiated by asking the child, "Do you know what a thermometer does?" The therapist can guide the discussion in a way that captures the idea that a thermometer measures heat. As a thermometer measures heat (i.e., angry feelings), it gets redder and redder as it gets hotter. When the thermometer fills with red, it blows! This concept is a visual representative of the angry emotions. Children can begin to visualize their anger getting higher and higher, up to the top of the thermometer, as they color the "red" of their angry feelings on their poster board. Once the thermometer has been personalized and has been filled with the red of the angry feelings, the child can then begin to learn about the various items that he or she will use to make the thermometer a helpful part of managing angry feelings. The supplies needed for this part of the activity include: a shoebox, paper, pens/pencils, small plastic bags, a stretchy play animal or sticky ball, a small pillow, and bubble wrap (the type with large bubbles works best), cut into 8" × 10" sheets. These supplies are used to teach the child a variety of new anger management techniques in session. As the therapist teaches the techniques to the child, the child is then asked to practice what he or she has learned in session. The therapist begins each introduction by asking the child to conjure up something that he or she has felt angry about in the recent past. The child is then asked to let his or her angry feelings be felt in the moment, during the session. Once the child begins to experience the angry feelings, the therapist can introduce the techniques so the child can determine how helpful or not helpful he or she manages the angry feelings while using it. Ideally, the child should recreate the angry feelings enough to build up some level of physical energy but not so much that he or she is overcome by emotion. The anger management techniques are listed in order of least to greatest physical exertion required to complete task:

- Using Words: The therapist prompts the child to state loudly what he or she is feeling angry about. The therapist encourages the child to do so until the angry energy dissipates. When using this activity at home, the child is told to go outside or to a private place (such as his or her room or the basement or garage) to use the loud, angry voice. The therapist clarifies for the child that the loud, angry voice is used to get out the angry feelings and is not to be directed at another person or family member.
- Pillow: The therapist asks the child to yell his or her angry feelings into a pillow. Encourage the child to yell as loudly and as long as he or she needs until the angry feelings are managed.
- Scribbling/Drawing: The therapist asks the child to scribble his or her angry feelings onto a piece of paper. Or, depending on age and motor skill abilities, the child could be asked to "draw" his or her anger, if that seems to fit better. Some children enjoy the visual creation of their "anger," while others seem to feel better with the physical act of scribbling, which works to exert their angry energy. If children are able to do so, ask them to say what they feel angry about as they scribble or draw.
- Paper Ripping: The therapist gives the child a sheet of paper. Once the child has activated his or her angry feelings, he or she is instructed to tear the sheet of paper up into tiny, little bits. Once the child has torn the paper into however many pieces he or she needs to, the child is asked to put all of the pieces into a plastic bag, tie it up tightly, and throw the bag of angry paper shreds in the trash. If children are able to do so, ask them to state their angry feelings as they shred the paper.
- Bubble Wrap: The therapist puts a sheet of bubble wrap on the floor in front of the child. The therapist asks the child to "stomp out" all of the angry energy onto the bubble wrap until the angry energy has been released. If children are able to do so, ask them to state their angry feelings as they pop all of the bubbles with their feet, stomping as hard as they can on the bubble wrap.
- Safe Throwing: The therapist gives the child a stretchy animal or sticky ball (either can be purchased from play therapy supply catalogs) and asks him or her to practice throwing the sticky item at a blank wall, using as much angry energy as he or she can to throw it as hard as possible against the wall. The therapist encourages the child to throw the item over and over again until all of the angry energy has been released. It is clarified for the child that these items are only to be thrown on a wall that the family has predetermined as okay for this purpose. It is also made clear that the item is only to be thrown at the wall and not at anything other than the wall.

We have found that children respond to these activities in a very positive way, as they are fun, creative, and physical. We have also found that children are energized by the therapist's participation in the activity. For example, in the use of the bubble wrap exercise, we always put a sheet of bubble wrap down for the therapist, too, and jump alongside our clients on the first try. Then we ask the child to try on his or her own as practice. As the child sees us using our physical energy to stomp the bubbles, rip up the paper, or throw the sticky ball, it models for him or her the use of fun coping skills to manage difficult feelings. It sometimes serves as a great stress reliever for the therapist, too!

Once the technique or techniques have been practiced, the child can then invite his or her family into session to "teach" the parents how the child uses the newly learned anger-management skill. With the family in the room, the child decides which techniques feel most helpful at what level of anger. In this part of the activity, the child is asked to assign a technique to an anger level on his or her anger thermometer. The therapist uses the previously decorated anger thermometer to write the name of the technique next to the corresponding level of anger that the use of the technique will feel most helpful. The ratings can be given a range, so that the child can choose four or five of the techniques. An example of this could be:

Anger Level	Corresponding Technique
0-3	Pillow
4-6	Scribbling
7-8	Bubble Wrap
9-10	Safe Throwing

The family is then asked to create a visible place at home where the thermometer can be hung (the back of a basement or pantry door is often a favorite spot). When the child is at home and experiences angry feelings, he or she can use the anger thermometer to rate the level of anger. Then the child can choose the technique from his or her tool box based on his or her anger level. If techniques require supplies to be readily on hand, it is helpful for families to keep each technique nearby in a separate shoebox labeled with the rating scale (i.e., Box 1 labeled as "0-3," Box 2 labeled as "4-6," and so on). Within each box, supplies should be kept stocked and ready for children to use as they are experiencing their angry feelings.

Brief Vignette

The Clark family sought family therapy due to extreme outbursts of anger by daughter, Jessica, age eight, who had been diagnosed with Diabetes I six months ago. During these episodes, Jessica became enraged, often screaming at her parents and sometimes hitting them or biting her siblings. The family was seeking help in controlling Jessica's anger in a safe and healthy way. Jessica and her family were engaged in having a conversation about how the family was currently expressing anger. Jessica was able to identify the ways that her body sometimes feels when she has angry emotions. Some of her physical experiences of anger included her muscles tightening, her fists and jaw clenching, her face getting red, her voice getting loud, and an uncontrollable impulse to lash out. Jessica's anger was reframed using the thermometer analogy. The therapist normalized Jessica's physical responses to anger and described her loss-of-control feelings as "blowing up." This family session laid the foundation for a play therapy session with Jessica individually where she could create her anger thermometer.

Jessica was very interested in the decorating and creating of her thermometer. She suggested that it be titled, "Jessica's Anger Thermometer." She responded positively to the idea of the thermometer measuring her angry feelings to prevent it from "blowing" over the top. Jessica was also interested in and excited about the use of the physical techniques, especially the sticky balls and the bubble wrap. She was energized as she learned and practiced her newfound skills, and as she taught her family each of the techniques in her toolbox, she appeared to have great pride in her family's *positive* attention about her anger feelings. The family left the final session with hope and purpose about helping Jessica cope with her difficult feelings. The message they took home with them (along with their box of start-up supplies) was that it is okay and normal for Jessica to feel her angry feelings, as long as she expresses them in a safe and productive way.

The next week, the Clark family reported that Jessica had great success with the physical techniques but that the verbal techniques seemed less helpful. During the session, Jessica was able to choose all physical techniques and do away with the less helpful verbal techniques. This reassignment of techniques fit for Jessica because of the strong physical response she had when experiencing angry feelings. Once Jessica was able to manage her angry feelings in a more productive way, Jessica and her family were able to explore what was behind the angry feelings in family therapy. Over time, Jessica's angry feelings became better understood. With the initial management of her physical expressions of anger, Jessica and her family eventually improved their ability to verbally express their angry feelings. Jessica's extreme physical responses to anger eventually lessened as she learned to practice her verbal skills in family therapy sessions with her family.

Suggestions for Follow-Up

After the client has successfully used his or her coping skills for dealing with anger successfully for two months, it may be useful to use the same intervention with other emotions often associated with managing a chronic illness, such as sadness or anxiety. If family members or other supports are involved in the client's therapy, you may wish to describe how the family can facilitate shared emotional expression through developing a family toolbox with family coping skills inside.

Contraindications for Use

This activity may not be appropriate with children who are not able to verbally rate their level of anger on a scale of one to ten. It may also be contraindicated for children who have been diagnosed with attachment disorder or conduct disorder and have used their aggressiveness to control or manipulate their environment and those around them. Finally, the success of this intervention depends on the willingness of the child's family to support the use of the child's chosen coping skills and therefore, may be inappropriate with a family that is unsupportive of the therapy process or is too rigid to allow new strategies or behaviors.

References

Gil, E. (1991). *The healing power of play.* New York: Guilford.
Lipchik, E. (2002). *Beyond technique in solution focused therapy.* New York: Guilford.
Lynn, S., & Garske, J. (Eds.) (1985). *Contemporary psychotherapies: Models and methods.* Columbus, Ohio: Charles E. Merrill Publishing Co.
O'Hanlon, W., & Weiner-Davis, M. (1989). *In search for solutions.* Ontario, Canada: Penguin Books.

Readings and Resources for the Professional

Imber-Black, E., Roberts, J., & Whiting, R. (Eds.) (1988). *Rituals in families and family therapy.* New York: W.W. Norton.
Lipchik, E. (2002). *Beyond technique in solution focused therapy.* New York: Guilford.
McGoldrick, M., & Walsh, F. (2004). *Living Beyond Loss.* New York: W.W. Norton & Company.
Sapolsky, R. M. (2000). *Why zebras don't get ulcers: An updated guide to stress, stress-related diseases, and coping.* New York: W.H. Freeman.

Bibliotherapy Resources for Clients

Barrett Singer, A. T. (1999). *Coping with your child's chronic illness.* San Francisco: Robert D. Reed.

Bluebond-Langner, M. (1996). *In the shadow of illness: parents and siblings of the chronically ill child.* Princeton, NJ: Princeton University Press.

Clark, C. D. (2003). *In sickness and in play: Children coping with chronic illness.* New Brunswick, NJ: Rutgers University Press.

Mazur, M. L., Banks, P., & Keegan, A. (1995). *The dinosaur tamer: And other stories for children with diabetes.* Alexandria, VA: American Diabetes Association.

Sheppard, D., & Jones, T. (2004). *Life with diabetes: Lacie the lizard's adventure.* USA: Critters, Inc.

Chapter 13

Why Is My Kid Doing This and What Can I Do? Facilitating Family Problem Solving Using Scatterplots

Theodore A. Hoch

Type of Contribution: Homework, Handout

Objective

Parents of any child are faced with challenges as the child and family go through typical stages of development. Families of children with developmental disabilities are often faced with unique, complex challenges. These children often experience medical difficulties ranging from acute and life threatening to chronic and multiply handicapping. Parents carry out medical, behavioral, educational, and analytic functions as they care for these children, often with very little training or prior experience in these domains. Developmental delays these children exhibit can include delayed or completely missed developmental milestones, with sitting unassisted, pulling to stand, and first words coming much later than for others, or not at all. Behavioral problems can occur when medical and developmental differences converge and the child's world becomes more complex. These problems can include feeding problems, disordered sleep, self-injury, aggression, property destruction, self-stimulation, enuresis, encopresis, vomiting, rumination, and others—and can themselves have medical consequences. Parents of typically developing children sometimes feel overtaxed. Families of children with developmental disabilities can feel completely bewildered.

The wide array of alternative and controversial therapies proffered to treat or cure developmental disabilities complicates matters. Often promoted online or in publications that do not have rigorous empirical standards, therapies such as chelation therapy to cure autism or megavitamins to cure mental retardation are touted to desperate parents who purchase the therapies, but who are not given methods of assessing whether the therapy is having any effect. One certain effect of some of these therapies is lost money, lost time, and lost opportunities for more effective, empirically supported therapies.

This assignment is intended to help families of children with developmental disabilities identify patterns and factors contributing to behavioral or health related problems such children may exhibit. The tool discussed is called a scatterplot. Once patterns are identified, families can sometimes make changes on their own, and sometimes in consultation with a medical professional, to remedy the difficulties. The family and professional then use the scatterplot to measure the effectiveness of those changes and determine future changes. Alternatively, the scatterplot can help measure effectiveness (or lack thereof) of controversial therapies, providing parents a more objective method of evaluating results and of determining whether to continue expending time, effort, and money.

Rationale for Use

Children with developmental disabilities often present with complex, multiple-determined problems. Systemic therapists, and behavior analysts in particular, understand that this often means that what appears to be one kind of problem may actually indicate a variety of factors producing the identified problem, and so multiple factors may need to be assessed and addressed. Consider, for example, a growing child with cerebral palsy and a seizure disorder who often appears lethargic and behaves in an inattentive and irritable manner at school and at home. The lethargy, inattentiveness, and irritability may be related to dosing schedule of the child's antiepileptic drugs; poor fit between the child's growing body and the child's custom-molded wheelchair; schedule of curriculum activities at school in relation to the medication dosing schedule and changes in alertness and arousal the medication may produce at various points in the drug's half-life; and nature of demands and expectations placed on the child by teacher and parents at various times in the midst of all of this. To simply reinforce the child's behavior when the child behaves in a more alert, compliant, pleasant manner may not address all relevant factors in this situation. Behavior analysts and other systemic therapists understand that working with such a child and family would require collaboration with and among multiple professionals, and that this collaboration must be sufficiently informed by those with the child most often to permit effective decision making and evaluation of those decisions.

A scatterplot is a simple method of documenting when problems occur. It involves making a grid and plotting when the problem happens, shortly after it happens. Aggregating several or more of these marks can permit parents and consulting professionals to see patterns in when the problems happen, and directs them to questions about possible relationships between the problem and other events that occur in time (Touchette, MacDonald, & Langer, 1985). For example, noticing that irritability often begins around 11:30 am, 3:00 pm, and 5:30 pm for a child who does not speak or feed himself may suggest that providing a meal or snack earlier may help alleviate the irritability. Should the parents and teacher change meal and snack times and subsequently see fewer or no instances of irritability plotted, the intervention has been successful. Should they, however, see just as many (or more) instances of irritability plotted, the intervention has not been successful, and another change is needed.

Instructions

Instructions for developing and plotting on the scatterplot are straightforward. Interpreting the scatterplot and determining what changes to make is sometimes less straightforward, and is often helped by jotting notes when entries are made on the scatterplot. Evaluating effectiveness of the changes made, however, is also straightforward. Fewer entries on the scatterplot means a decrease in frequency of the problem, unchanged frequency of entries means unchanged problem frequency, and increased entries means increased problem frequency. In addition to its utility in helping assess and remedy behavioral and health-related difficulties for children with disabilities, the scatterplot may also be used to identify potentially contributing factors for a wide variety of physical or relational phenomena experienced by individuals, couples, or families.

1. Help the client to operationally define the problem. Rather than asking the client to plot each instance of lethargy or irritability on the chart, guide the client through stating and writing down exactly what she or he sees and hears the person doing when the lethargy or

irritability is happening. This should be a concrete listing of what the target person does and any person who reads the definition should be able to state with certainty whether the defined problem is or is not happening at that moment. This statement is the operational definition.
2. Instruct the client to make a grid, or make one with the client. This is easily done in Microsoft Word using the Table feature, or in Microsoft Excel by highlighting cells within a spreadsheet and adding borders using the Format Cells feature. Once the grid is made, enter time of day (which can be in sixty, thirty, or fifteen minute increments) in the first vertical column, day of week in the row second from the bottom, and date in the cells making up the bottom row.
3. Type the operational definition somewhere on the page so it and grid appear in the same place.
4. Instruct the client to shade in the cell that corresponds to the time, day, and date that the problem has happened, whenever the problem happens.
5. In some cases, it is also helpful to ask the client to make a note on the back of the scatterplot whenever a cell is shaded in, describing the circumstances under which the problem occurred (e.g., where, in whose presence, what happened next, etc.).
6. Instruct the client to bring the scatterplot to each session.
7. Review the scatterplot with the client at each session. Examine any recurrence of the problem in terms of time of day, day of week, etc., in which the problem tends to occur. Discuss with the client what's different about those times as opposed to when the problem didn't occur. Discuss possible changes that can be made, and determine with the client how those changes will be made, and by whom. Two good frameworks from which to ask questions at this point are Bailey & Pyles' (1989) behavioral diagnostics interview, and Vollmer & Matson's (1996) *Questions About Behavioral Function*. The former considers a wide range of possible environmental, medical, logistical, and other variables that might contribute to the problem, whereas the latter considers immediate antecedents and consequences that may have contributed to the problem.
8. Continue reviewing the scatterplot with the client at each session, seeking additional consultation from other professionals (i.e., teacher, physician, psychiatrist, etc.) as suggested by the scatterplot.

Brief Vignette

Martin is a seven-year-old boy who lives with his parents and younger sibling. He is diagnosed with autistic disorder, severe mental retardation, and a generalized seizure disorder. Martin does not speak, but has been using a picture exchange system for several years, and is beginning to use American Sign Language. His seizure frequency has been greatly reduced after numerous medication trials, although he still experiences several seizures per week. Martin's parents sought help for his self-injurious behavior, tantrums, and periodic food refusal. They reported that these three behaviors tended to occur together and occurred on most days, occasionally with a day or two passing between instances. The therapist helped Martin's parents operationally define each of these behaviors. "Tantrum" was defined as Martin yelling, screaming, crying, or whimpering loud enough to be heard from at least ten feet away, lasting for longer than one minute, when no obvious event had triggered the behavior. "Self-injury" was defined as Martin pounding his abdomen with his fist or slapping it with his open hand, or banging his head against any nearby surface. "Food refusal" was defined as Martin consuming one-fourth or less of an age-appropriate sized meal, when no snacking had taken place for at least two hours before the meal.

Once the problems were operationally defined, the therapist helped Martin's parents make a scatterplot in Microsoft Excel, and placed the operational definitions on the scatterplot. She instructed Martin's parents to use one color per defined behavior, to shade in the cells that corresponded to when the problems occur, to indicate on the grid when seizures occured, and to bring the scatterplot to the next session.

While reviewing the scatterplot at the next session, the therapist noted that several seizures had occurred during the week, and that the self-injury and tantrums tended to occur together. She also noted a period in which no problems were noted. When queried about this, Martin's parents reported that nothing had been done differently on those days, although Martin did have a rather large bowel movement at the beginning of the first day. The therapist asked Martin's parents to also plot his frequency of bowel movements on the scatterplot, and bring it to the next session (see Handout 13.1).

The next review of the scatterplot indicated infrequent bowel movements, with problems occurring more frequently on days during which bowel movements did not occur and less frequently on days with bowel movements. The therapist contacted Martin's physician and discussed the data with him. From this conversation, Martin's parents and the therapist learned that it was possible that Martin's antiepileptic drug regimen was producing constipation, which could account for the infrequent bowel movements, but also contribute to food refusal, self-injury, tantrums, and impaired seizure control. As a result of this consultation, the physician added a bowel regimen. After several days of implementing the bowel regimen, Martin's parents saw that he had regular bowel movements, exhibited fewer instances of tantrums, self-injury, and food refusal, and appeared to have better seizure control.

Suggestions for Follow-Up

Not only is the scatterplot used to determine whether patterns exist with regard to when and if problems occur, and not only to guide questioning about circumstances of problems' occurrence to help determine necessary changes. The scatterplot is also an essential tool to assess effectiveness of those changes, and determine other changes that the family can make. In the vignette provided, initial review and discussion of the scatterplot did not produce a solution, but instead led to another question. When the additional information was provided, another question was posed, and collaboration with another treating professional brought about an intervention, but also another question: would it work? Subsequent recording on the scatterplot indicated there was, indeed, improvement.

This is not always the case. Sometimes additional factors need to be considered as previous factors are ruled out, and sometimes partial remedies are encountered as the additional factors are addressed. The scatterplot can be an important tool in determining whether improvement, partial improvement, or no improvement has occurred, as a result of the changes made by the family and consulting professionals.

Contraindications for Use

The scatterplot can be used by any parent, teacher, or professional who is interested in determining if there are relationships between when problems and other events happen. It can also be used to determine whether there are relationships between when things go well and when other things happen. The reader is cautioned, however, that although such relationships can be made clearer or be suggested by a scatterplot, that sometimes such relationships do not exist, or that sometimes such relationships only become clearer after further analysis is conducted (Kahng, Iwata, Fischer, Page, Treadwell, Williams, & Smith, 1998; O'Neill, Horner, Albin, Sprague, Storey, & Newton, 1997). Parents should always consult with prescribing medical professionals before changing medications, dosing schedules, or dosages; or with their child's physician or a pharmacist before using or changing over the counter medication with a child for whom other medications have been prescribed.

References

Bailey, J. S., & Pyles, D. A. M. (1989). Behavioral diagnostics. In E. Cipani (Ed.), *The treatment of severe behavior disorders: Behavior analysis approaches.* Washington, DC: American Association on Mental Retardation, pp. 85-107.

Kahng, S. W., Iwata, B. A., Fischer, S. M., Page, T. J., Treadwell, K. R. H., Williams, D. E., & Smith, R. G. (1998). Temporal distributions of problem behavior based on scatter plot analysis. *Journal of Applied Behavior Analysis, 34,* 593-604.

O'Neill, R. E., Horner, R. H., Albin, R. W., Sprague, J. R., Storey, K., & Newton, J. S. (1997). *Functional assessment and program development for behavior problems.* Pacific Grove, CA: Brooks/Cole.

Touchette, P. E., MacDonald, R. F., & Langer, S. N. (1985). A scatter plot for identifying stimulus control of problem behavior. *Journal of Applied Behavior Analysis, 18,* 343-351.

Vollmer, T. R., & Matson, J. L. (1996). *Questions about behavioral function.* Baton Rouge, LA: Disability Consultants, LLC.

Readings and Resources for the Professional

Ansbaugh, R., & Peck, S. (1998) Treatment of sleep problems in a toddler: A replication of the faded bedtime with response cost protocol. *Journal of Applied Behavior Analysis, 31,* 127-129.

Bosma, A., & Mulick, A. (1990). Ecobehavioral assessment using transparent scatterplots. *Behavioral Residential Treatment, 5,* 137-140.

Iwata, B. A., Kahng, S. W., Wallace, M. D., & Lindberg, J. S. (2000). The functional analysis model of behavioral assessment. In J. Austin and J. E. Carr (Eds.), *Handbook of applied behavior analysis* (pp. 61-89). Reno, NV: Context Press.

Kahng, S. W., Iwata, B. A., Fischer, S. M., Page, T. J., Treadwell, K. R. H., Williams, D. E., & Smith, R.G. (1998). Temporal distributions of problem behavior based on scatter plot analysis. *Journal of Applied Behavior Analysis, 34,* 593-604.

O'Neill, R. E., Horner, R. H., Albin, R. W., Sprague, J. R., Storey, K., & Newton, J. S. (1997). *Functional assessment and program development for behavior problems.* Pacific Grove, CA: Brooks/Cole.

Symons, F. J., McDonald, L. M., & Wehby, J. H. (1998). Functional assessment and teacher collected data. *Education and Treatment of Children, 21,* 135-159.

Touchette, P. E., MacDonald, R. F., & Langer, S. N. (1985). A scatter plot for identifying stimulus control of problem behavior. *Journal of Applied Behavior Analysis, 18,* 343-351.

Vollmer, T. R., & Matson, J. L. (1996). *Questions about behavioral function.* Baton Rouge, LA: Disability Consultants, LLC.

Bibliotherapy Sources for the Client

Bailey, J. S. & Pyles, D. A. M. (1989). Behavioral diagnostics. In E. Cipani (Ed.), *The treatment of severe behavior disorders: Behavior analysis approaches* (pp. 85-107). Washington, DC: American Association on Mental Retardation.

Batshaw, M. L., & Perret, Y. M. (Eds.) (1992). *Children with disabilities: A medical primer* (3rd ed). Baltimore, MD: Paul H. Brookes.

Jacobson, J. W., Foxx, R. M., & Mulick, J. A. (Eds.) (2005). *Controversial therapies for developmental disabilities: Fads, fashion, and science in professional practice.* Hillsdale, NJ: Lawrence Erlbaum Associates.

Positive Strategies. (2004). Scatter Plot [Recording form]. Valhalla, NY: Westchester Institute for Human Development. Available from http://www.wihd.org/pbs.

Special Connections. (2005). What is a scatter plot and how do you use it? Lawrence, KS: University of Kansas. Available from http://www.specialconnections.ku.edu.

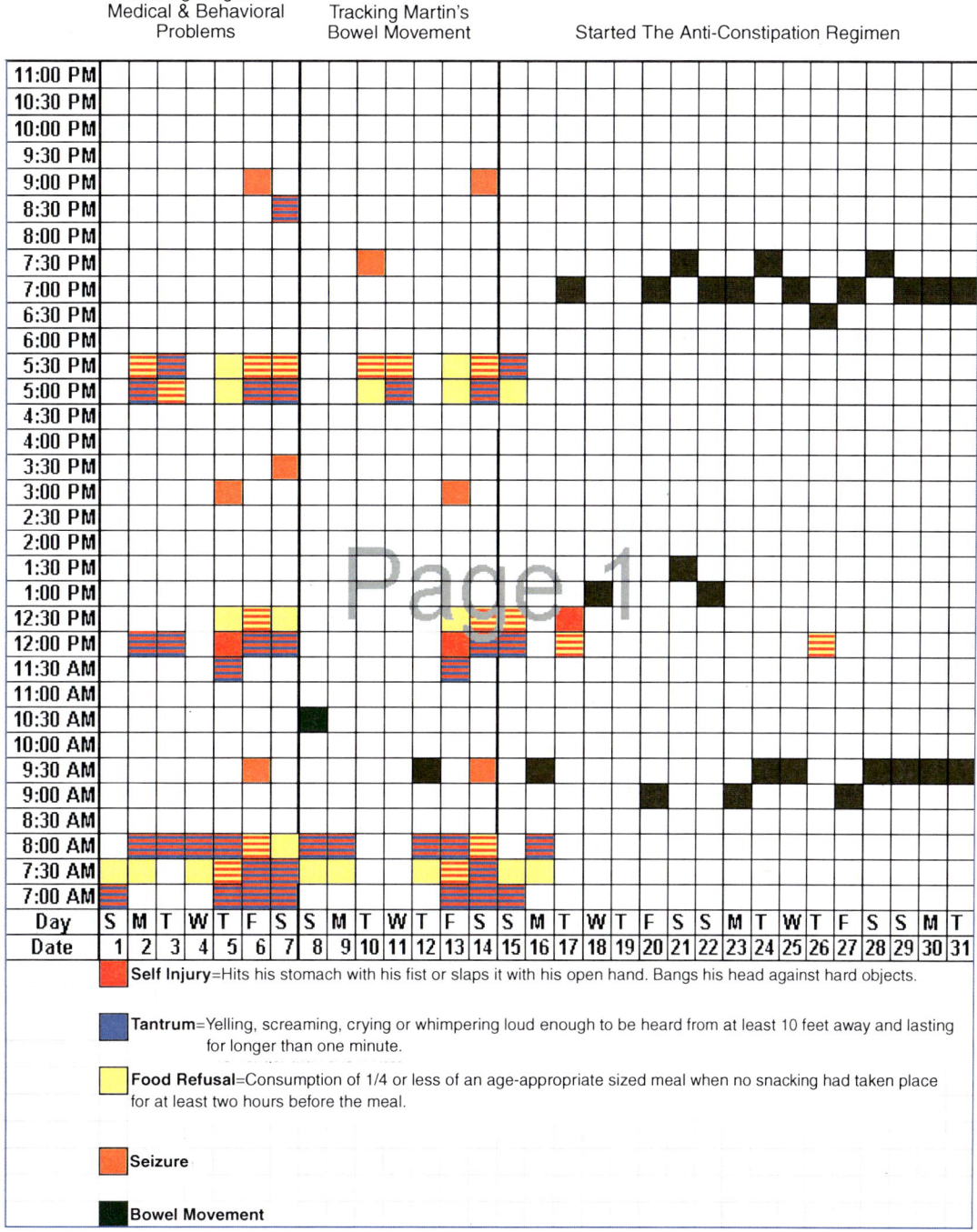

Hoch, T. (2007). Why is my kid doing this and what can I do? Facilitating family problem solving using scatterplots. In D. Linville, K.M. Hertlein, and Associates, *The therapist's notebook for family health care: Homework, handouts, and activities for individuals, couples, and families coping with illness, loss, and disability* (pp. 83–89). Binghamton, NY: The Haworth Press.

Chapter 14

The ANGELS
(*A* Neighbor *G*iving *E*ncouragement, *L*ove, and *S*upport): A Collaborative Project for Teens with Diabetes

Tai J. Mendenhall
William J. Doherty

Type of Contribution: Activity, Handout

Objective

Community-based participatory research (CBPR) represents an action research approach that emphasizes close collaboration among clinical providers and community participants (patients and families). Our primary objective in writing this account is to highlight a novel intervention that is oriented to adolescents with diabetes and was designed and implemented through CBPR. This partnership involved the active engagement of medical and mental health providers, situated in a large academic hospital, with teenage patients and their families.

Rationale for Use

Diabetes is one of the most widespread chronic diseases in the United States, with current estimates exceeding 18 million. More than 2,000 new cases of the disease are diagnosed each day, and it represents the seventh most common presenting problem in family medicine (American Diabetes Association, 2005). Globally, an estimated 194 million people live with diabetes, and this is expected to rise to over 333 million by 2025 (International Diabetes Federation, 2005). Over 6 percent of the U.S. population is directly affected, and racial/ethnic minorities are disproportionately affected (Centers for Disease Control and Prevention, 2000; National Institute of Diabetes and Digestive and Kidney Diseases, 2004).

In synchrony with these alarming trends across the general population, diabetes in children and adolescents is also rising. Type 1 diabetes is now the third most common chronic illness in youth, and Type 2 diabetes (once thought to occur almost exclusively in adults) is consistently correlated with pandemic increases in childhood and adolescent obesity and physical inactivity (Fagot-Campagna, Burrows, & Williamson, 1999; Hampson et al., 2004). These trends cut across all ethnic/racial categories, and follow adult patterns with Native American, Hispanic, and African-American youth being the hardest hit (Glaser & Jones, 1998; Hale & Danney, 1998; Onyemere, Lipton, Baumann, Silverman, & Brodsky, 1998).

Adolescents as a group maintain the worst glycemic control when compared to any other age group (Anderson, Ho, Brackett, & Laffel, 1999; Anderson & Laffel, 1996; Gage et al., 2004). Although some declines in metabolic control are attributable to normal physiological changes that occur during teenage years, much is linked to declines in both overall self-care and disease management (Diabetes Control and Complications Research Group, 1994; Gage et al., 2004). This represents a significant concern in health care, because poor diabetes management during adolescence is strongly associated with the onset and progression of a variety of short- and long-term physical complications (Couper, Fotheringham, Taylor, & Sawyer, 1999; Hampson et al., 2001).

It is also important to note that adolescents with diabetes are significantly more likely than their non-diabetic counterparts to experience a variety of psychiatric and adjustment problems. Low self-esteem, depression, eating disorders, and unhealthy eating attitudes and behaviors are all more prevalent in teens who have diabetes and are even worse in diabetic adolescents whose metabolic control is poor (Jacobson et al., 1997; Kovacs, Goldston, Obrosky, & Bonar, 1997; Wysocki, Hough, Ward, & Green, 1992). Children and adolescents with diabetes are also more likely to evidence higher rates of school absences and lower rates of academic achievement (Holmes, Dunlap, Chen, & Cornwell, 1992; Ryan, Longstreet, & Morrow, 1985).

While the majority of interventions for treating diabetes show modest improvements across a variety of outcomes, extensive methodological and systemic reviews maintain that these improvements are often not sustained over time (Delamater et al., 2001; Gage et al., 2004; Hampson et al., 2001). Diabetes is a disease that does not go away, and attention to effective disease management should similarly endure. As providers, clinical researchers, patients, and families struggle with this issue, they must uncover new ways to design and implement programs that are sustainable within their communities. One such program is the ANGELS (*A Neighbor Giving Encouragement, Love, and Support*). Guided by a community-based participatory research approach, this initiative encompasses an active participation and co-ownership by professionals and lay persons alike and is supported by human and tangible resources that are not connected to temporary external funding sources (Mendenhall & Doherty, 2005).

Community-based participatory research (CBPR) is an action research approach that emphasizes close collaboration among researchers and community participants who are directly affected by an issue to generate knowledge and solve local problems. Hierarchical differences are flattened through this partnership and all participants work together to create knowledge and effect change (Agency for Healthcare Research and Quality, 2004; Lewin, 1946; Mendenhall & Doherty, 2005). Because CBPR focuses on a problem within a specific site or community, the "local" problem is addressed directly and in context (Caballero, 1999; Hambridge, 2000). Several key assumptions permeate these projects (Bradbury & Reason, 2003; Mendenhall & Doherty, 2005). Themes include: (1) a democratic partnership between all project members (i.e., clinical researchers, community participants) as collaborators through every stage of knowledge and intervention development, (2) a deep investment in change that carries with it an element of challenging the status quo and improving the lives of members in a community or practice, (3) a cyclical process in which a problem is identified, solutions to address it are developed within the context of the community's existing resources, interventions are implemented, outcomes are evaluated according to what is essential in the eyes of participants, and interventions are modified in accord with new information as necessary, (4) project members' humility and flexibility to accommodate changes as necessary across any part of a project, and (5) recognition that CBPR can be a slow and messy process, especially during its initial phases.

The Citizen Health Care Model

Handout 14.1 outlines the main principles of Citizen Health Care. The model is a systematic way to access a resource that is largely untapped in our contemporary health care system: the knowledge, lived experience, wisdom, and energy of individuals, families, and communities who face challenging health care issues in their everyday lives. This is different from the conventional way of perceiving an activated patient who becomes a responsible agent for his or her own health. The notion of "citizen" refers to people becoming activated along with their neighbors and others who face similar health challenges in order to make a difference for a community. Ordinary citizens become assets in heath care as they work as coproducers of health for themselves and their communities. They no longer assume passive roles whereby they are simply consumers of services and look out only for their own health and that of their immediate loved ones.

Instructions

Since 1999, we have done twelve projects in Citizen Health Care and the larger Families and Democracy Project in which this work is positioned (Doherty & Carroll, 2002; Mendenhall & Doherty, 2003; Mendenhall & Doherty, 2005). These efforts have spanned across a diverse range of communities and problem areas and are guided by the following action strategies:

1. Get buy-in from key professional leaders and administrators.

These are the gatekeepers who must support the initiation of a project based on its potential to meet one of the goals of the health care setting. However, we have found it best to request little or no budget aside from a small amount of staff time, in order to allow the project enough incubation time before being expected to justify its outcomes.

2. Identify a health issue that is of great concern to both professionals and members of a specific community (clinic, neighborhood, cultural group in a geographical location).

Stated differently, the issue must be one that a community of citizens actually cares about, not just something that we think they should care about, and the professionals initiating the project must have enough passion for the issue to sustain their efforts over time.

3. Identify potential community leaders with personal experience with the health issue, whom have relationships with the professional team.

These leaders should generally be ordinary members of the community who in some way have mastered the health issue in their own lives and who have a desire to give back to their community. "Positional" leaders who head community agencies are generally not the best group to engage at this stage, because they bring with them institutional priorities and constraints.

4. Invite a small group of community leaders (three to four people) to meet several times with the professional team to explore the issue and see if there is a consensus to proceed with a larger community project.

These are preliminary discussions to see if a Citizen Health Care project is feasible and to begin creating a professional/citizen leadership group.

5. This group decides on how to invite a larger group of community leaders (ten to fifteen) to begin the process of generating the project.

One invitational strategy we have used is for providers to nominate patients and family members who have lived expertise with a health issue and who appear to have leadership potential.

6. Over the next six months of biweekly meetings, implement the following steps of community organizing:

- Explore the community and citizen dimensions of the issue in depth
- Create a name and mission
- Have one-to-one interviews with a range of stakeholders
- Generate potential action initiatives, processing them in terms of the Citizen Health Care Model and their feasibility with existing community resources
- Decide on a specific action initiative and implement it

7. Employ the following key Citizen Health Care processes:

Democratic planning and decision making at every step. This requires training of the professionals who bring a disciplined process model and a vision of collective action that does not lapse back into the conventional provider/consumer model, but who do not control the outcome or action steps the group decides to take.

Mutual teaching and learning among community members. Action initiatives consistent with the model first call upon the lived experience of community members, with the support of professionals, rather than recruiting community members to support a professionally created initiative.

Creating ways to fold new learnings back into the community. All learnings can become "community property" if there is a way for them to be passed on. Currently we have vehicles for professionals to become "learning communities," but few vehicles outside of Internet chat rooms for patients and families to become learning communities.

Identifying and developing leaders. The heart of community organizing is finding and nurturing people who have leadership ability but who are not necessarily heads of organizations with turfs to protect.

Using professional expertise selectively—"on tap," not "on top." In this manner, all knowledge is public knowledge, democratically held and shared when it can be useful. Professionals bring unique knowledge and experience as well as access to current research to Citizen Health Care initiatives. But everyone else around the table also brings unique knowledge and expertise. Because of the powerful draw of the provider/consumer way of operating, professionals must learn to share their unique expertise when it fits the moment, and to be quiet when someone else can just as readily speak to the issue. A community organizing axiom applies here: Never say what someone in the community could say, and never do what someone else in the community could do.

Forging a sense of larger purpose beyond helping immediate participants. Keep the Big, Hairy, Audacious Goal (BHAG) in mind as you act in a local community. Citizen Health Care is not just about people helping people—it is about social change toward more activated citizens in the health care system and larger culture. This understanding inspires members of the Citizen Health Care project about the larger significance of their work. It also attracts media and other prominent community members to seek to understand, publicize, and disseminate Citizen Health Care projects.

Brief Vignette: The ANGELS

The ANGELS initiative, described here and adapted from Mendenhall & Doherty (2005), represents the application, guiding principles, and strategies of the Citizen Health Care Model to adolescent diabetes.

Providers in the pediatric department of a large academic hospital had been long frustrated with their adolescent patients diagnosed with diabetes. Although many teens adhered (on their own or at their parents' insistence) to prescribed regimens of physical activity, diet, blood sugar monitoring, and insulin administration, a large proportion of patients were managing their disease quite poorly. Repeated efforts across conventional interventions were not working—from teaching community classes about diabetes and self-care, to hosting diabetes-related fairs and public forums, to the consistent provision of warnings during standard care visits about a variety of long-term consequences associated with poor metabolic control. Adolescent patients continued to evidence unhealthy physiological indicators (e.g., hemoglobin A1c and body mass index) and little apparent motivation to change. Parents complained about being "nags" to teenagers who wanted to be left alone. Patients complained about adults, both parents and providers, who would not "get off their backs" or allow them to have the same freedom and spontaneity as their peers. Providers felt triangulated into family conflicts, oftentimes in the exam room, without any clear direction other than recite the same old information and cautionary warnings.

Initial conversations between the director of pediatrics and the first author, a marriage and family therapist (MFT), ensued to identify new ideas for this old and increasing problem. Having recently been involved in the development of a CBPR initiative oriented to adults called "Partners in Diabetes" (Mendenhall & Doherty, 2003), the MFT suggested that a community-based participatory research approach be applied to this problem to move efforts beyond the conventional top-down services. Unfamiliar with flat-hierarchy interventions involving active patient and family participation in partnership with providers but maintaining an investment to address the problem with an openness to try new solutions, the director mobilized other providers to meet, learn about CBPR, and decide whether and how to proceed.

Early meetings between the first author and providers addressed how to engage patients as collaborators in the design of supplemental services to standard care. This would tap a variety of resources previously untapped, including patients' and families' lived experience and wisdom of living with diabetes on a day-to-day basis. The Citizen Health Care Model was introduced as a guiding framework for this work. Through the lens of this model, the first author explained how providers are viewed as citizens with knowledge and skills who work actively with other citizens who also possess important knowledge and skills. He explained how participants in this work self-consciously and explicitly avoid conventional provider/consumer dynamics by recognizing and valuing all members' respective contributions to a common mission. Families are active producers and co-creators of action and change, and thus do not function in a conventional consumer/patient role.

Six families were invited to meet with providers and discuss ideas regarding the building of a citizenship initiative that would benefit adolescents and parents struggling with diabetes. The stage was set to work collaboratively, and a great deal of attention was spent discussing and understanding how these efforts would not follow the conventional top-down sequences of a provider-led approach. Adolescents and parents were enthusiastic about creating something new through CBPR, with the larger vision of developing a model of care by and for its citizens with all participants functioning as stakeholders in the process. The group collaboratively identified key areas of concern and developed solutions within the contexts of the hospital and surrounding community's resources. As adolescents, parents, and providers met over the following months, an exciting new program was named by the group and began to take root.

Through the ANGELS (*A Neighbor Giving Encouragement, Love, and Support*) adolescents and their parents with lived experience with diabetes (called "support partners") are connected with other families (called "members") struggling with the illness. These efforts begin at the time of diagnosis, which occurs almost universally in the context of emergency hospitalization. It is during this time that the initiative's teens maintained that they wanted the ANGELS to connect with members, because the motivation to adopt healthy lifestyles is the highest at a time of crisis. Support partners and members meet in a variety of combinations (e.g., adolescents with adolescents, parents with parents, families with families), and continue to meet off hospital grounds (or via telephone, e-mail, internet discussion boards) after initial hospitalization. Sometimes members simply need a pep talk; other times ongoing support is offered for several months.

Adolescents and parents in the ANGELS program worked democratically with providers throughout every stage of the program's development, beginning with the initial brainstorming regarding the program's mission, naming process, training design, public-visibility efforts, and continuing through implementation and ongoing problem solving and maintenance. Although functioning under the auspices of an official hospital volunteer program, the ANGELS training reflected citizens' viewpoints regarding how to best prepare for the role of a support partner, going far beyond basic provider-designed training about generic volunteer, health, or diabetes-related topics. Intentionally relying on existing community resources, the ANGELS program has maintained its democratic character and ensured its long-term viability as a resource within its community. Initial efforts are now in process for training a new generation of support partners, many of whom were former members connected with this program during their own crisis and early struggles with diabetes. Support partners' sense of personal ownership in the ANGELS continues to be reflected in this progression as they assume responsibility for components of this training and long-term vision.

Contraindications for Use

It is important to emphasize that community-based participatory research is often slow and messy work. Stops and starts, trials and errors, and repeated sequences of problem solving and going back to the drawing board are commonplace. This is important to understand from the beginning and to normalize to participants before and during the initial processes and sequences of this work. If a professional is situated in an organization that is not sensitive to this, extending efforts to engage community members through CBPR could be risky. Without a champion of influence in the institution (e.g., a clinic administrator or department head), it is remarkably difficult to successfully create the space, keep up the morale, and accommodate the requisite time to create these types of projects. Relatedly, until a project is grounded in an institution's culture and practices (e.g., incorporated into standard care protocols and design), these initiatives are quite vulnerable to shifts in the organizational context.

It is also important to note that external funding at the outset can be a trap. With grants come timelines and predefined deliverables that can sabotage the CBPR process of collaboratively exploring and addressing a problem through the development of new knowledge and novel interventions. Funding can be useful for capacity building to learn the model or for expanding the scope of citizen projects once they are developed, but it should not be elemental in a project's initiation or early phases.

Suggestions for Follow-Up

Two of the most common questions that interested colleagues have asked us about this work relate to time: (1) How much time does it take to be involved in a Citizen Health Care project?

and (2) How long does a Citizen Health Care project take to create and implement? To begin, this work does not require a large amount of professionals' time in the short run (an estimated six to eight hours per month). Community-based participatory research projects are owned and operated by the communities in which they are positioned, and much of the work is done by the patients and families who are directly involved (i.e., professionals do not do all of the work). However, Citizen Health Care projects entail a considerable amount of time to establish, and thereby require a sustained commitment, usually several years.

The pull of the traditional provider/consumer model is very strong on all sides, and democratic decision making requires eternal vigilance. Professionals are socialized to be experts vis-à-vis patients, and patients are socialized to be directed by their providers. This type of work requires that all involved learn a different way of relating with one another, and this is oftentimes easier said than done. Patients and families will often turn to providers to answer questions that arise or outline solutions to problems that are identified, and providers are often quick to respond. Providers will often make decisions without the active collaboration of patients and families, and patients and families are often more comfortable being told what to do or expect. Consistently referring to the Citizen Health Care Model, running problems and questions through the model's guiding principles, and regular attention to keeping one another in check is essential.

For MFTs, physicians, and other providers, it is important to understand that this kind of work requires considerable mentorship. There are no quick training programs to teach professionals the public skills of engaging other citizens in community organizing projects with flattened hierarchies. We are now creating a Citizen Health Care Program in which professionals can participate in face-to-face training and long-distance mentoring as they create a new project, and through these efforts we hope to advance the scope and practice of this work.

Conclusion

Many observers believe that the United States health care system needs a fundamental redesign if we are to have a healthier population and avoid exhausting our economic resources (Future of Family Medicine Project, 2004; Institute of Medicine, 2001). We believe that work guided by the Citizen Health Care Model is beginning to answer this call. Initiatives like the ANGELS are adopting new forms of democratic partnership between citizen professionals, patients, and their families. The driving mission of these initiatives is to create a democratic model of health care that unleashes the capacity and energy of ordinary citizens as producers of health for themselves and their communities. For providers, this work is about an identity transformation as a citizen professional, not just learning a new set of skills. It is about seeing one's self as a contributor to a much larger mosaic of knowledge and skills in partnership with others—patients, families, and other professionals—and about pursuing goals much larger than treating one patient or family at a time.

References

Agency for Healthcare Research and Quality. (2004). *Community-based participatory research: Assessing the Evidence.* Rockville, MD: AHRC.

American Diabetes Association. (2005). *Diabetes statistics for Native Americans.* Retrieved on January 30, 2006, from http://www.diabetes.org/diabetes-statistics.jsp.

Anderson, B., Ho, J., Brackett, J., & Laffel, L. (1999). An office-based intervention to maintain parent-adolescent teamwork in diabetes management: Impact on parent involvement, family conflict, and subsequent glycemic control. *Diabetes Care, 22,* 713-721.

Anderson, B., & Laffel, I. (1996). Behavioral and family aspects of the treatment of children and adolescents with IDDM. In D. Porte, R. Sherwin, & H. Rifkin (Eds.), *Ellenberg and Rifkin's Diabetes Mellitus* (5th ed., pp. 811-825). Stamford, CT: Appleton & Lange.

Bradbury, H., & Reason, P. (2003). Action research: An opportunity for revitalizing research purpose and practices. *Qualitative Social Work, 2,* 155-175.

Caballero, B. (1999). Obesity prevention in American Indian school children: Pathways. *American Journal of Clinical Nutrition, 69,* 745S-824S.

Centers for Disease Control and Prevention. (2000). *Diabetes surveillance report.* Retrieved January 30, 2006, from http://www.cdc.gov/diabetes/statistics/surv199/chap2/contents.htm.

Couper, J., Fotheringham, M., Taylor, J., & Sawyer, M. (1999). Failure to maintain the benefits of home-based intervention in adolescents with poorly controlled Type 1 Diabetes. *Diabetes Care, 22,* 1933-1937.

Delamater, A., Jacobson, A., Anderson, B., Cox, D., Fisher, L., Lustman, P., et al. (2001). Psychosocial therapies in diabetes. *Diabetes Care, 24,* 1286-1292.

Diabetes Control and Complications Research Group. (1994). Effect of intensive diabetes treatment on the development and progression of long-term complications in adolescents with insulin-dependent diabetes mellitus. *Journal of Pediatrics, 125,* 177-188.

Doherty, W. J., & Carroll, J. S. (2002). The families and democracy model. *Family Process, 41,* 579-589.

Fagot-Campagna, A., Burrows, N., & Williamson, D. (1999). The public health epidemiology of type 2 diabetes in children and adolescents: A case study of American Indian adolescents in the Southwestern United States. *Clinica Chimica Acta, 289,* 81-95.

Future of Family Medicine Project. (2004). The future of family medicine: A collaborative project of the family medicine community. *Annals of Family Medicine, 2,* S3-S32.

Gage, H., Hampson, S., Skinner, T., Hart, J., Storey, L., Foxcroft, D., et al. (2004). Educational and psychosocial programmes for adolescents with diabetes: Approaches, outcomes and cost-effectiveness. *Patient Education and Counseling, 53,* 333-346.

Glaser, N., & Jones, K. (1998). Non-insulin-dependent diabetes mellitus in Mexican-American children. *Western Journal of Medicine, 168,* 11-16.

Hale, D., & Danney, K. (1998). Non-insulin dependent diabetes in Hispanic youth. *Diabetes, 47*(suppl 1), A82.

Hambridge, K. (2000). Action research. *Professional Nurse, 15,* 598-601.

Hampson, S., Foxcroft, D., Skinner, T., Kimber, A., Hart, J., Cradock, S., et al. (2004). Behavioral interventions for adolescents with type 1 diabetes: How effective are they? *Diabetes Care, 23,* 1416-1422.

Hampson, S., Skinner, T., Hart, J., Storey, L., Gage, H., Foxcroft, D., et al. (2001). Effects of educational and psychosocial interventions for adolescents with diabetes mellitus: A systemic review. *Health Technology Assessment, 5,* Number 10.

Holmes, C., Dunlap, W., Chen, R., & Cornwell, J. (1992). Gender differences in the learning status of diabetic children. *Journal of Consulting and Clinical Psychology, 60,* 698-704.

Institute of Medicine (2001). Crossing the quality chasm: A new health system for the 21st century. Washington, DC: Author.

International Diabetes Federation. (2005). *World Diabetes Day 2005: Diabetes and foot Care.* Retrieved January 30, 2006, from http://www.idf.org/home/index.cfm?node=1294.

Jacobson, A., Hauser, S., Willett, J., Wolfsdorf, J., Herman, L., & de Groot, M. (1997). Psychological adjustment to IDDM: 10 year follow-up of an onset cohort of child and adolescent patients. *Diabetes Care, 20,* 811-818.

Kovacs, M., Goldston, D., Obrosky, D., & Bonar, L. (1997). Psychiatric disorders in youths with IDDM: Rates and risk factors. *Diabetes Care, 20,* 36-44.

Lewin, K. (1946). Action research and minority problems. *Journal of Social Issues, 2,* 34-46.

Mendenhall, T., & Doherty, W. (2003). Partners in diabetes: A collaborative, democratic initiative in primary care. *Families, Systems & Health, 21,* 329-335.

Mendenhall, T., & Doherty, W. (2005). Action research methods in family therapy. In F. Piercy and D. Sprenkle (Eds.), *Research Methods in Family Therapy* (2nd ed., pp. 100-117). New York: Guilford Press.

National Institute of Diabetes and Digestive and Kidney Diseases. (2004). *National diabetes statistics.* Retrieved January 30, 2006, from http://diabetes.niddk.nih.gov/dm/pubs/statistics/#10.

Onyemere, K., Lipton, R., Baumann, E., Silverman, B., & Brodsky, I. (1998). Onset features of insulin-treated atypical type 1 and early onset type 2 diabetes in African American and US Latino children. *Diabetes, 47*(supp 1), A25.

Ryan, C., Longstreet, C., & Morrow, L. (1985). The effects of diabetes mellitus on the school attendance and school achievement of adolescents. *Child Care, Health & Development, 11,* 229-240.

Scott, C., Smith, J., Cradock, M., & Pihoker, C. (1997). Characteristics of youth-onset noninsulin-dependent diabetes mellitus and insulin-dependent diabetes mellitus at diagnosis. *Pediatrics, 100,* 84-91.

Wysocki, T., Hough, B., Ward, K., & Green, L. (1992). Diabetes mellitus in the transition to adulthood: Adjustment, self-care, and health status. *Journal of Developmental and Behavioral Pediatrics, 13,* 194-201.

Readings and Resources for the Professional

Agency for Healthcare Research and Quality. (2004). C*ommunity-based participatory research: Assessing the Evidence.* Rockville, MD: AHRC.

Bruce, T., & McKane, S. (Eds.). (2000). *Community-based public health: A partnership model.* Washington, DC: American Public Health Association.

Doherty, W. J., & Carroll, J. S. (2002). The families and democracy model. *Family Process, 41,* 579-589.

Gage, H., Hampson, S., Skinner, T., Hart, J., Storey, L., Foxcroft, D., et al. (2004). Educational and psychosocial programmes for adolescents with diabetes: Approaches, outcomes and cost-effectiveness. *Patient Education and Counseling, 53,* 333-346.

Hagey, R. (1997). The use and abuse of participatory action research. ChronicDiseases in Canada. Retrieved on January 30, 2006, from http://www.phac-aspc.gc.ca/publicat/cdic-mcc/18-1/a_e.html.

Hampshire, A., Blair, M., Crown, N., Avery, A., & Williams, I. (1999). Action research: A useful method of promoting change in primary care. *Family Practice, 16,* 305-311.

Hampson, S., Skinner, T., Hart, J., Storey, L., Gage, H., Foxcroft, D., et al. (2001). Effects of educational and psychosocial interventions for adolescents with diabetes mellitus: A systemic review. *Health Technology Assessment, 5,* Number 10.

Macaulay, A., Commanda, L., Freeman, W., Gibson, N., McCabe, M., Robbines, C., et al. (1999). Participatory research maximises community and lay involvement. *British Medical Journal, 319,* 774-778.

Mendenhall, T., & Doherty, W. (2003). Partners in diabetes: A collaborative, democratic initiative in primary care. *Families, Systems & Health, 21,* 329-335.

Mendenhall, T., & Doherty, W. (2005). Action research methods in family therapy. In F. Piercy and D. Sprenkle (Eds.), *Research Methods in Family Therapy* (2nd ed., pp. 100-117). New York: Guilford Press.

Minkler, M., & Wallerstein, N. (Eds.). (2003). *Community based participatory research for health.* San Francisco, CA: Jossey-Bass.

Smith, S., Willms, D., & Johnson, N. (Eds). (1997). *Nurtured by knowledge: Learning to do participatory action-research.* New York: The Apex Press.

Bibliotherapy and Resources for Clients

American Diabetes Association. (2005). *The American Diabetes Association Complete Guide to Diabetes (4th ed.).* Alexandria, VA: American Diabetes Association.

American Diabetes Association. (2006). The American Diabetes Association Home Page. Retrieved on January 30, 2006, from http://www.diabetes.org/home.jsp.

Bradbury, H., & Reason, P. (2003). Action research: An opportunity for revitalizing research purpose and practices. *Qualitative Social Work, 2,* 155-175.

Macaulay, A., Commanda, L., Freeman, W., Gibson, N., McCabe, M., Robbines, C., et al. (1999). Participatory research maximises community and lay involvement. *British Medical Journal, 319,* 774-778.

Mendenhall, T., & Doherty, W. (2003). Partners in diabetes: A collaborative, democratic initiative in primary care. *Families, Systems & Health, 21,* 329-335.

Minkler, M., & Wallerstein, N. (Eds.). (2003). *Community based participatory research for health.* San Francisco, CA: Jossey-Bass.

Wysocki, T. (2004). *Ten keys to helping your child grow up with diabetes* (2nd ed.). Alexandria, VA: American Diabetes Association.

HANDOUT 14.1.
Citizen Health-Care Model: Core Principles

1. The greatest untapped resource for improving health care is the knowledge, wisdom, and energy of individuals, families, and communities who face challenging health issues in their everyday lives.

2. People must be engaged as coproducers of health care for themselves and their communities, not just as patients or consumers of services.

3. Professionals can play a catalytic role in fostering citizen initiatives when they develop their public skills as citizen professionals in groups with flattened hierarchies.

4. If you begin with an established program, you will not end up with an initiative that is "owned and operated" by citizens. But a citizen initiative might create or adopt a program as one of its activities.

5. Local communities must retrieve their own historical, cultural, and religious traditions of health and healing, and bring these into dialogue with contemporary medical systems.

6. Citizen health initiatives should have a bold vision (a BHAG—a big, hairy, audacious goal) while working pragmatically on focused, specific projects.

Mendenhall, T.J., & Doherty, W.J. (2007). The ANGELS (*A N*eighbor *G*iving *E*ncouragement, *L*ove, and *S*upport): A collaborative project for teens with diabetes. In D. Linville, K.M. Hertlein, and Associates, *The therapist's notebook for family health care: Homework, handouts, and activities for individuals, couples, and families coping with illness, loss, and disability* (pp. 91-101). Binghamton, NY: The Haworth Press.

Chapter 15

Facilitated Mirroring: Building Perspective in Clients with Asperger's Syndrome

Nan Gray Lester

Type of Contribution: Intervention

Introduction

Odd, quirky, uniquely intelligent, rigid, "difficult," and terminally uncomfortable in their own skin—these are some of the adjectives routinely used in describing individuals with Asperger's Syndrome (AS). In my experience as an advocate, university educator, psychological consultant, and parent of a child with Asperger's Syndrome, a clear understanding of this emerging diagnosis is best realized by making a personal connection to someone known. When lecturing on the subject, I often begin with a painful description of "that kid from school," the weirdo with no friends, who tripped over his own feet, wore the same ill-fitting clothes day after day, and seemed to connect only with the science teacher. Unstructured times such as recess, lunch, and study hall proved a social nightmare for this poor soul, while his attempts to make social connections often involved inappropriate bursts into conversations of others, only to be met with odd stares and fits of giggles. The opening of his locker promised an avalanche of homework brilliantly completed but never turned in. His annoying, even repulsive, habits ran the gamut from jiggling knees, endless rocking and knuckle-crunching, to chewing the sleeves of his well-worn shirt into sopping shreds. My description never fails to bring flickers of recognition in the eyes of my audience members, which is why I resort to such obvious generalizations. My next questions are, "What became of this child?" "Did he or she find a way to channel his or her talents into a meaningful career?" "What about relationships?"

Given that one in 250 to 500 people meets the diagnostic criteria for Asperger's Syndrome (Myles, 2002), there is a good chance that most clinicians have encountered clients affected by AS in their clinical practice. Because of the genetic predisposition for developing the disorder (Volkmar, 2000), it is highly likely that work with this client will involve multiple family members within his or her family system who meet the criteria for AS, or were raised by, or with, someone on the spectrum.

The limited space of this chapter does not allow for an extensive clinical overview of this perplexing, pervasive developmental disability, nor does it allow me to reflect anecdotally on the many reasons why I love working with children and adults affected by Asperger's Syndrome: the talent, intelligence, humor, sensitivity, honesty, loyalty, insightfulness . . . the list goes on.

Within this brief framework, my goal is to present clinicians working with this population with a method that I have found to be effective in building self-awareness and positive relationships. Over the past two years, I have developed the intradiagnostic-intergenerational peer mentoring model and have successfully implemented it in a group therapy setting.

Objective

Functional perspective of self and others is often the greatest barrier to success for individuals affected by Asperger's Syndrome. Facilitated Mirroring is a method of building self-awareness through a triangulated process involving others with AS and a neurotypical translator (the therapist). The method involves a systematic, literal breakdown of life experiences as described by one individual with Asperger's Syndrome, and, in turn, reflected upon by others with AS. It is the therapist's role to contain and facilitate the mirroring process and to provide the framework for teaching self-awareness and self-regulation through a contextual understanding of the diagnosis. It is a rigorous exercise for the clients that combines a visceral experience with an intellectual one. Ideally, this merges the disjointed perceptions, reactivity, and literal adherence associated with AS into a revelatory and empowering process that is aided by others with the same challenges.

Rationale for Use

Traditional psychotherapy techniques are generally ineffective for individuals with AS (Jacobson, 2003). There are many reasons for this, and I have included books in my bibliography that go into much greater detail, particularly with regard to Theory of Mind. However, I have observed that traditional therapies fail on two levels: (1) a lack of understanding on the part of the clinician regarding the complexities of the diagnosis, and (2) a clinician's failure to adhere to literal meaning in all things said and done, no matter how trivial they may seem.

Before I describe the Facilitated Mirroring process, there are two misconceptions regarding AS that I feel must be addressed. Unfortunately, the first misconception is also a current descriptive within DSM IV-TR diagnostic criteria. The idea that individuals affected by AS lack empathy is semantically inappropriate. At best, a lack of empathy can be described as a casual disregard for the feelings of others or, at its most extreme, descriptive of sociopathology. What people with Asperger's Syndrome lack is perspective, not empathy. Perspective is defined as having a mental view of aspects of a subject as they relate to one another, an understanding of the relative importance of things. This distinction will become more apparent as I explain the Facilitated Mirroring intervention technique and how it relates specifically to the hallmark features of Asperger's Syndrome.

Second, Asperger's Syndrome is not mild autism. There is nothing mild about having a pervasive developmental disability with lifespan implications. Over the course of my work, I have witnessed tremendous strides in childhood diagnosis and corresponding educational and psychosocial services regarding Asperger's Syndrome. However, my current focus has turned toward adults, the majority of whom have never received educational or social support services of any type. In fact, obtaining a diagnosis is highly problematic for adults, with services all but nonexistent for a condition that is still considered a "childhood disorder" and therefore confined to pediatric and behavioral/developmental domains. Adding further complexity to the diagnostic picture is the prevalence of comorbid psychiatric conditions. It is estimated that greater than 60 percent of individuals with AS meet the criteria for other Axis I diagnoses (Myles, 2002), including anxiety, depression, ADHD, bipolar disorder, and less frequently, schizophrenia. I continually speculate with my adult clients as to the origin of these comorbid conditions. Perhaps they are symptomatic of living life as an undiagnosed autistic, with all of the residual trauma that implies.

The most important aspect of Facilitated Mirroring is the inclusion of more than one individual with AS in the process. Authentic validation of the difficulties encountered living with Asperger's Syndrome is a core rationale for the use of Facilitated Mirroring. The difficulties of coping with what I refer to as the "Key Three" (Key III) deficits defining the disorder—executive function, sensory integration, and social—cognitive are most effectively validated by another person with the same functional challenges.

The analogy to any support group model is obvious; however, as with "all things Asperger's" the process is more complex. The desired outcome in Facilitated Mirroring is building perspective of self and others while developing an understanding of the how the disorder affects one's behavior and how one is perceived by others. The role of the facilitator is crucial but not central to the process. The model of Facilitated Mirroring is that of an inverted triangle, with the neurotypical facilitator (you) at the bottom (see Figure 15.1). Part of the experience for the client(s) is that they outnumber the neurotypicals in the equation, perhaps for the first time in their lives. My clients report that this is deeply liberating.

Instructions

The group can be comprised solely of individuals with Asperger's Syndrome or include family members. The essential feature is that more than one individual in the group must have Asperger's Syndrome. I begin each Facilitated Mirroring group therapy session with a diagnostic explanation of the Key III characteristics of AS categorized as executive function, sensory integration, and social-cognitive deficits.

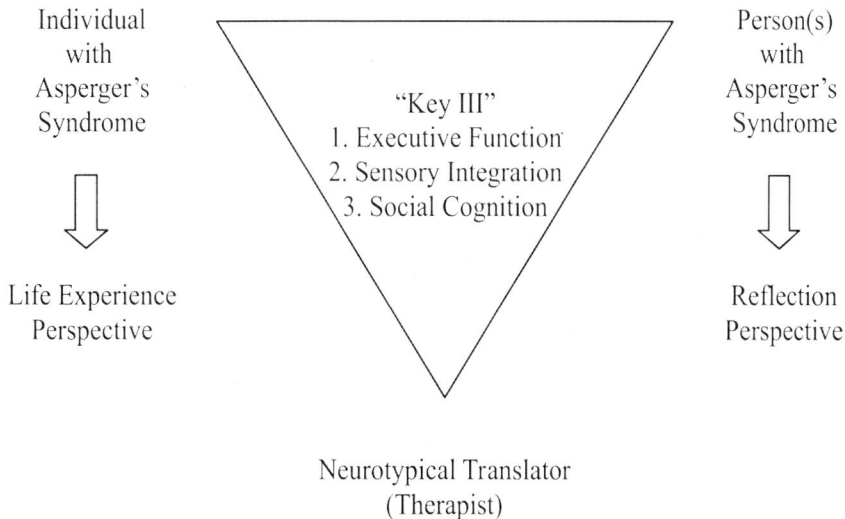

FIGURE 15.1. Facilitated Mirroring Model. *Source:* From Lester, N.G. (2007). Facilitated Mirroring: Building Perspective in Clients with Asperger's Syndrome. In D. Linville, K.M. Hertlein, and Associates, *The Therapist's Notebook for Family Health Care: Homework, Handouts, and Activities for Individuals, Couples, and Families Coping with Illness, Loss, and Disability.* Binghamton, NY: The Haworth Press.

Executive Function Challenges—Broadly defined as a frontal lobe deficit that impairs mental flexibility and central coherence. Difficulties in this area may include:

- Multitasking, shifting focus, and prioritizing
- Determining relevance in thought/action/objects and the perspective of others
- Narrow, perseverating interests
- Difficulty following instructions, particularly those involving sequence and chronology
- Lapses in word finding and thought continuity
- Inflexible adherence to literal language
- Difficulty with generalizing information
- Resistance to change, fixed routines, and extreme difficulty coping with transitions.

Sensory Integration Dysfunction (SID)—Challenges of the central and peripheral nervous system in receiving and processing sensory information. These generally present as *hyper-* or *hypo*sensitivity of the sensory processing system, including:

- Tactile: Over- or under-reactive to tactile stimuli (fabrics, foods), low or high pain tolerance
- Visual: Light sensitivity, diminished ocular control
- Auditory: Difficulty with auditory information processing, decoding sounds, and hypersensitivity to auditory input
- Gustatory and Olfactory: Hyper- or hyposensitivity and reactivity regarding odors and taste
- Vestibular and Proprioceptive: Difficulties with posture, balance, joint stability, muscle strength and tone, motor planning and control, perception of depth and movement, and bilateral coordination

Social-Cognitive Deficit—Social cognition is often referred to as theory of mind (ToM); however, I have experienced difficulty in communicating this abstract concept to my clients with Asperger's Syndrome. I have had more success with the term social-cognitive deficit. Many of my clients report this as the most challenging aspect of living with AS. Difficulties in this area may include:

- Limited understanding of the perspectives, emotions, intentions, motivations, behaviors, and reactions of others
- Impaired ability to read and provide nonverbal communication
- Impaired interpersonal communication skills, including reciprocity, topic content and relevance, conversational shifts and transitions
- Literal communication and atypical (pragmatic, pedantic) language
- Difficulty understanding and modeling appropriate social behavior
- Impaired understanding of interpersonal contexts and expectations
- Rigid expectations of others, strict adherence to rules, hypervigilance

Teaching the Key III to clients is an exciting feature of Facilitated Mirroring. Intellectually understanding the aspects of the disability and how it manifests in their daily lives is a revelatory and perspective-building exercise for people with AS.

Focusing on a client's deficits goes against the principals of most strength-based psychotherapeutic modalities, however, it is important to remember that this process is not based on a normative model. These are the experiences of intelligent individuals who are fully aware that they are coping with the difficulties of living with a pervasive developmental disability. They are looking for information and strategies on how to navigate more comfortably and successfully in the world. With Facilitated Mirroring, you will come to realize that despite the focus on diagnostics, teaching to the Key III is strength-based. It capitalizes on clients' intelligence and analytic ability while helping them gain perspective on behavior. Self-regulation cannot be achieved without building self-awareness and perspective.

After introducing the Key III, the next step for the therapist is to clarify the topical focus of the session. Interpersonal relationships, childhood experiences, and employment issues resemble the topics introduced within any group therapy structure. Within the model of Facilitated Mirroring, however, they are explored within the context of the disability and how it affects function. Topics may be predetermined by the therapist, agreed upon by the group at the end of the previous session, or established as a result of an impending or emerging issue on the part of one of the group members. If the latter is the case, I instruct my clients to contact me ahead of time so that I am prepared to establish the topic within the relevant frame of reference. In my experience, I do not advise an open-ended format or a call for topical ideas, as the options may overwhelm and dominate the group energy from the onset.

The framework for group sharing must be highly structured for the perspective building objectives of Facilitated Mirroring to occur. After introducing a topic, I will invite someone to share a relevant incident or experience. It is important that this individual be describing an event and not an idea. The group then begins a round-robin sequence. Each member is asked to make observations on what Key III elements may be relevant in the story, his or her perceptions of how the fellow group member may have felt, and how he or she believes the incident may have been perceived by others. This exercise is an intellectualization of diagnostic references combined with perspective building observations, a process that you will find the group amazingly intrigued by and comfortable with over time.

The job of the therapist is to facilitate and help interpret meaningful reflections between the individual sharing the experience and the other members of the group. Whether or not others can interject out of sequence or there is cross-sharing is a matter of a therapist's individual comfort level with the group dynamic. I personally welcome deep discussion, but also keep a tight rein on the length of time that any one participant is allowed to share. Remember the communication difficulties inherent in the diagnosis of Asperger's Syndrome. Once you become more familiar with the disorder and how it manifests, you will become more comfortable with the blunt style you may need to develop to meet the needs of your group.

There are many continuing themes in working with people with Asperger's Syndrome. The two that I recognize as causing the deepest emotional scarring over time is the fear of making mistakes, particularly at work, school, or in social situations, and the subsequent humiliation of a public "meltdown" over the incident. The AS meltdown is described as having a near blackout quality. This experience, combined with the Key III diagnostic complications at play during the incident, often leave the individual with limited perspective on what actually occurred. These events are rarely, if ever, honestly apprised after the fact by a neurotypical interpreter. In my experience, people with Asperger's Syndrome have a tremendous need to process these incidents.

This is another important part of Facilitated Mirroring. You are working with people who often describe their life experience as feeling like an alien in their own culture. In fact, many of my clients report feeling more comfortable functioning in foreign countries, where it is already assumed that their behavior may be atypical. In processing these incidents, there is no room for nuance or subtlety; literal interpretation is absolutely critical. The triad model of Facilitated Mirroring is essential to the process. The perspective and validation offered by another individual with the same neurological challenges is tremendously supportive for the client.

Brief Vignette

Anne is a forty-one-year-old unmarried woman with Asperger's Syndrome, who is an undergraduate student studying human services. Although the university she attends is relatively large, the program is a smaller, cohort model that places tremendous emphasis on teamwork and respectful relationships among group members. Anne shared a story in group where the topic was "social confusion." A recent class assignment in her school program required breaking up into self-organized groups to develop a project and make a presentation. Joining informally organized groups causes Anne a tremendous amount of anxiety, and she was not primed for the assignment, as it had not been indicated on the syllabus. The crowded, poorly lit, and acoustically vibrant classroom, which had been a difficult environment for her all term, became even noisier and chaotic as people moved their chairs to connect into groups with their preferred classmates. Anne felt overwhelmed and disoriented. By the time she had mustered the courage to ask to join a team that included anyone she felt comfortable with, there was no space for her. She finally found a group to join, but she wasn't familiar with any of the members. She was still dragging her chair across the room when the instructor began giving the directions.

From the beginning, Anne had difficulty understanding the instructions of the project. She was reluctant to ask for more information from the instructor, whom she perceived as "brusque." The group decided not to meet again before the presentation, and to conduct all further communication by e-mail. Anne was too nervous to provide input on the decision, yet she felt terrified by its ramifications. All of the students in the group were much younger than Anne and very comfortable with technology; she had difficulty communicating by e-mail, because she was intimidated by the technology and unsure of her ability to communicate her ideas with clarity. The other students seemed impatient and even unwilling to help her; she felt intimidated.

On the day of the presentation her anxiety was high, but she had completed her portion of the work and felt good about its content. Shortly after beginning her presentation, she sensed a hushed and hostile silence around her. A member of her group called out to her in a voice loud enough for all to hear to "watch out for political correctness!" Anne turned to her, startled. She had heard this term repeatedly in her studies, but it had never been defined for her and she had never fully grasped its meaning. At this point her mind went blank, and she panicked. The same group member came over and told her "don't say negro!" while presenting her categorical statistics. Anne tried desperately to track where she was in the presentation, fighting her instinct to start from the beginning. She decided to pick up at the word that was apparently the issue, and tried the word "black" this time in describing her statistics. Both negro and black had been acceptable terms where she grew up. Anne sensed a growing discomfort in the crowded room, but forced herself to complete her presentation. As soon as she finished, a member of her group stepped up to the podium and profusely apologized for Anne's "offensive" remarks.

Anne was deeply humiliated and horrified, but had no idea what was so offensive about what she said or done. She wanted to bolt from the room, but forced herself to go up to the group and ask what she had done wrong. They looked at her incredulously, and told her that the politically correct terminology is "African American!" Anne had thought this term referred to people who had recently immigrated to the United States from Africa. At this point, the instructor came forward and said she wanted to meet with the whole group after class to discuss what had happened. At the very least, the instructor explained, the group needed to meet with the higher faculty and make a formal apology over e-mail to the entire cohort. In the end, none of this actually took place, as the incident occurred during the last days of the term. Anne never understood or felt closure about the incident.

Anne reported feeling extremely depressed and anxious after this experience. She even seriously considered suicide. Her roommate talked her out of it and, upon Anne's request, supported Anne by accompanying her to the first class the following term. Anne was extremely nervous about facing her fellow students and the faculty upon her return to school. One of the African-American students who had taken the most offense approached her and they talked. Anne explained her limited understanding of "politically correct" terminology and apologized. They embraced, and even ended up going to lunch together. This meant a tremendous amount to Anne, even though she still didn't fully understand everything that had occurred.

The group members had no difficulty using the Facilitated Mirroring process to relate to this incident. As a group they readily identified the Key III elements at play in Anne's experience. In order to concisely illustrate their comprehension, I'll focus on what, to a neurotypical observer, may seem to be a minute aspect of the incident, but to individuals with AS would be a functional nightmare within the context of the Key III.

The group understood how Anne felt when faced with the unstructured group selection process (executive function and social cognitive). In visceral terms, they deeply empathized with the process Anne went through as she dragged her chair across the noisy, crowded room to join the group (sensory overload) of students she did not know or feel comfortable with (social cognitive). They described the panic she must have experienced as the instructor began giving the directions while Anne was still enroute across the noisy room (executive function, sensory). This seemingly trivial sequence of the larger story occurred within a matter of minutes, but the implications of the Key III for the individual with AS are glaring.

After providing a Key III assessment of the incident, including the group members' perspective on Anne's emotions, the group shared similar experiences. Anne's confusion over the term "political correctness" and her misunderstanding of the African-American ethnic label offer an outstanding illustration of the ensuing social predicaments associated with adherence to literal meaning. Each client was able to attribute a similar experience including the emotional devastation that occurred as a result of their faux pas. Outcomes of stories such as these range from embarrassment, to social exclusion, to criminal arrest.

Suggestions for Follow-Up

Each session should end with a discussion of solution-focused strategies. In the presented case, Anne was given much positive feedback for the support she sought from her roommate regarding her anxiety, depression, and suicidal thoughts. It is advisable to check in with the individual after he or she relates the dominant story used in the Facilitated Mirroring process. It is my recommendation that this "check in" take place informally within the group at the close of the session, and be followed up by a private conversation with the individual. The individual may benefit from further processing of the incident discussed, or by a continued discussion about perspective building and self-regulation strategies.

Contraindications for Use

After starting my group, I found it necessary to develop a policy of inclusion based on client profile. As mentioned earlier, the prevalence of comorbid psychiatric conditions is extremely high for individuals with Asperger's Syndrome. I have experienced difficulty maintaining the focus of the group when it is being affected by individuals who are not following medical treatment for mood disorders. Another area of difficulty arises when including others who are lower functioning on the autism spectrum or have pervasive developmental disabilities not otherwise specified (PDD-NOS). A lower level of cognitive function may interfere with the ability of such individuals to participate.

Currently, I am using this method solely with an adult population with an age range of nineteen to eighty-seven years old. All of the members have, or are actively seeking, a medical diagnosis of Asperger's Syndrome. In the near future, I will be introducing the use of Facilitated Mirroring with an adolescent population in a middle and high school setting. Use in a family therapy context is appropriate only if multiple members are recognized as having Asperger's Syndrome.

References

Jacobson, P. (2003). *Asperger Syndrome and psychotherapy: Understanding Asperger perspectives.* New York: Jessica Kingsley.

Myles, B. S. (2002, October). *Asperger Syndrome: The Diagnostic Process.* Lecture presented at the second annual Asperger Advocacy Coalition Conference, Eugene, Oregon.

Volkmar, F. R. (2000). Diagnostic issues in Asperger Syndrome. In A. Klin, F. R. Volkmar, & S. S. Sparrow (Eds.), *Asperger Syndrome* (pp. 25-71). New York: Guilford.

Readings and Resources for the Professional

Attwood, T. (1998). *A guide for parents and professionals.* New York: Jessica Kingsley.

Grandin, T. (1995). *Thinking in pictures and other reports of my life with Autism.* Doubleday: New York.

Gutstein, S. E., & Sheeley, R. K. (2002). *Relationship development intervention for children and adults: Social and emotional development activities for Asperger Syndrome, Autism & PDD.* New York: Jessica Kingsley.

Klin, A., Volkmar, F. R., & Sparrow S. S. (Eds.) (2000). *Asperger Syndrome.* New York: Guilford.

Smith-Myles, B., & Southwick, J. (2005). *Asperger Syndrome and difficult moments: Practical solutions for tantrums, rage, and meltdowns.* Shawnee Mission, KS: Autism Asperger.

Willey, L. H., & Attwood, T. (1999). *Pretending to be normal: Living with Asperger Syndrome.* New York: Jessica Kingsley.

Recommended Web Sites and Resources

Asperger Information: http://www.aspergerinformation.org.

Asperger Syndrome Coalition of the U.S.: http://www.asperger.org.

ASPIRES/Asperger Syndrome Partners and Individual Resources, Encouragement & Support: http://justgathertogether.com/aspires.html.

Autism/Asperger Publishing Company: http://www.asperger.net.

Autism Society of America: http://www.autism–society.org.

IDEA Practices/Professional Development Resources: http://www.ideapractices.org.

Online Asperger Syndrome Information and Support (OASIS): http://udel.edu/bkirby/asperger/messageboards.html.

SECTION III:
ILLNESS-SPECIFIC INTERVENTIONS FOR FAMILIES

Chapter 16

Adaptation of the Family Systems Illness Model for HIV/AIDS Patients and Their Partners

G. Bowden Templeton
Shayne R. Anderson
Stephanie R. Burwell

Type of Contribution: Handout

Objective

This handout provides information for therapists dealing with issues that may arise in treating the psychosocial aspects of HIV/AIDS in the context of gay relationships. The handout may be used as a psychoeducational tool that can be easily adapted to individual, couple, or family therapy sessions. The handout illustrates the multiple challenges faced by patients and their loved ones as they confront HIV/AIDS and is relevant for all stages of therapy.

Rationale for Use

HIV presents a unique set of challenges to patients, their partners, and health care providers. Stigma, discrimination, isolation, grief, loss, role strain, fear, distrust, and uncertainty are commonly experienced by patients and partners who must adapt to and cope with this disease. In addition, gay couples may not be aware of the unique legalities involved in their interactions with the financial, judicial, and medical systems. Illness adjustment and coping efforts are further complicated by cultural norms and sexual orientation. For these reasons, it is important for therapists to be informed of the many issues gay couples face as they cope with and manage HIV/AIDS. With this information, clinicians will also be better prepared to actively collaborate with other health care providers.

While patients and their loved ones once considered a diagnosis of HIV/AIDS to be a death sentence, this is no longer the case. With the advent of antiretroviral treatments, patients are now living longer and what was once a terminal disease is now considered a chronic illness. As such, couples face prolonged exposure to a host of psychosocial stressors. The convergence of these factors creates a tremendous need for the development of resources that can be used to educate patients and providers about the issues that may arise across the illness trajectory.

The experiences of patients and their partners will vary at different stages in the life cycle of an illness. One particularly useful way to conceptualize illness and the demands it places on family systems at different stages has been proposed by Rolland's Family Systems-Illness Model (1994, 2003). This model takes into account interactions between the type of illness, the individual, family, and illness life cycles, and the social context. According to this model, illnesses can be categorized along four dimensions (onset, course, outcome, and incapacitation) and transition through specific developmental time phases (crisis, chronic, and terminal). Thus, AIDS is viewed as an illness with a gradual onset, progressive course, fatal outcome, and severe incapacitation. Further, AIDS places different demands on a couple at various phases of the illness.

This typology has important implications for therapists working with gay couples where one partner has AIDS. A diagnosis of AIDS is clearly a crisis that brings with it countless unanswered questions and concerns. Yet, the gradual onset of its associated symptoms may be respite in the midst of crisis because it allows time for couples to address other important and stressful issues that emerge. With medical management of the illness underway, a patient may focus on dealing with the shock and grief associated with diagnosis. The couple may have time to explore the possibility that the diagnosis reveals infidelity and betrayal or a substance abuse problem. It may allow time for the couple to contact extended family and reveal undisclosed lifestyle choices. Each of these represents unique opportunities for therapists to help navigate difficult conversations between partners and among extended family members.

The chronic phase of AIDS also brings with it extensive exposure to unique stressors that will challenge even the most committed couples. As the initial shock of diagnosis wears off, stigma may begin to take its toll. Patients may be unwilling to leave their homes and socialize with other people. Patients may be reluctant to attend appointments with their physician for fear of being seen entering an infectious disease clinic. Partners also face the long-term implications of managing the day-to-day tasks of living with a partner who has a chronic illness. Shared household responsibilities may now become one person's burden. Further, a partner may be increasingly anxious about whether or not he has been infected. Concern related to lack of financial support and uncertainty about medical treatments increases. Couples in this phase of the illness need to be flexible and open to change. They also need information and extensive ongoing support.

The terminal phase of illness is characterized as a period of mourning and bereavement in which the inevitability of death is apparent. In the terminal phase of illness, the infected patient may find himself in and out of hospitals and dealing with increasing symptom-related discomfort. He may experience increased apprehension about the course of the illness and impending death. The partner may find himself giving injections and changing bedpans, while continuing to provide emotional support for his partner. The couple may struggle with the implications of being in a relationship not legally recognized by most states and the reality that a partner is not allowed to participate in treatment planning or even visit the patient in the hospital.

The social context in which HIV/AIDS exist also constitutes a significant stress on the couple. Gay patients whose cultural or religious background scorns homosexuality face additional difficulties because their family and social network may not be supportive or they may be outcast. At best, if a patient is willing to share his illness narrative with family members, he runs considerable risk that he will lose their support. Issues of poverty and substance use are also significantly related to HIV/AIDS and complicate access to treatment and support services.

Instructions

This handout provides an overview of the issues that gay couples face when one partner is being treated for HIV/AIDS. It is adapted from the Family Systems-Illness Model (Rolland, 1994, 2003). The handout is organized by stage of the illness (crisis, chronic, terminal) and details many of the unique and often unexpected issues that a gay couple may confront during the course of treatment. Clinicians are encouraged to have the handout readily available to reference during treatment planning and in subsequent therapy sessions. Some clinicians may choose to share copies of the handout with their clients. By having quick access to this information, clinicians will be better prepared to meet the needs of gay couples at every stage of the illness. In addition, the nature of the organization and content of the handout makes it readily adaptable to individual and family therapy sessions as well.

Brief Vignette

Joe and Dave were referred for couple's therapy by a local agency serving HIV/AIDS patients and their families. Agency staff was concerned that the stress placed on the relationship as a result of Joe's HIV-positive status was more than the couple could manage without additional support and resources. At their first therapy appointment, Joe and Dave described the history of their relationship. They had been committed to each other for more than twenty years and owned a home together. Each shared equally in day-to-day tasks and both had full-time jobs. They described themselves as happy and comfortable until Joe's illness changed their lives dramatically.

Over the course of the next few therapy sessions, more details emerged about their relationship and the strain it was experiencing. Joe described feeling depressed and using alcohol as a coping mechanism. Conversations that were once friendly and engaging for the couple now became argumentative and antagonistic. They bickered constantly. In addition to his HIV-positive status, Joe also coped with diabetes, encephalopathy, liver disease, and a recent hernia. His medical conditions required significant attention and care and Dave became the primary caregiver.

Dave is Hispanic and worked in a warehouse. He closely guarded his sexual orientation by choosing to share this information with only a few very close friends. Dave was not out to family, primarily due to his cultural belief that men should be strong and provide for the family, certainly not be gay. This concern that his family and co-workers would not approve of his lifestyle resulted in Dave spending most of his time alone with Joe. He was isolated and as the stress of caring for his sick partner increased, Dave realized that he needed additional support.

After a three-month period in which the couple discontinued treatment, Dave contacted the clinic to say that Joe had died suddenly and that he wanted to resume therapy. Over the course of several months, he reported feelings and difficulties he had experienced with his partner's illness and subsequent death. He described having survivor guilt and talked about feeling torn between the responsibility of caring for his aging parents and his dying partner. He felt like he had no time or energy to care for himself. His thought process became quite negative and resulted in having little capacity to see that the care he provided was substantial.

Dave also expressed a great deal of pain around the injustices he experienced during his partner's illness and death. On several occasions, he had not been allowed to visit Joe in the hospital or participate in treatment decisions. Because Joe and Dave did not have wills or power of attorney, property that they owned jointly was left to Joe's family rather than Dave. As a result Dave found himself in the awkward position of owning his home with his partner's father, a man who did not approve of their lifestyle and relationship.

Suggestions for Follow-Up

The issues that couples face in dealing with HIV/AIDS are monumental and can only be addressed over time. This handout can facilitate open communication among partners and family members as they share their experiences with how the illness has impacted their lives.

Contraindications for Use

Therapists must always be sensitive to the emotional states and needs of their clients. Patients and their partners may feel overwhelmed at certain times or by certain material and, therefore, careful attention should be paid to gently timing when and how these topics are brought up in therapy.

Professional Readings and Resources

Campbell, T. (1999). AIDS-related death: A review of how bereaved gay men are affected. *Counseling Psychology Quarterly, 12*(3), 245-252.

Grossman, G. (1996). Psychotherapy with HIV-infected gay men. In P. M. Kato & T. Mann (Eds.), *Handbook of diversity issues in health psychology* (pp. 237-260). New York: Plenum.

Kurdek, L. A. (2005). What do we know about gay and lesbian couples? *Current Direction in Psychological Science, 14*(5), 251-254.

McDaniel, S. H., Hepworth, J., & Doherty, W. J. (1992). *Medical family therapy: A biopsychosocial approach to families with health problems.* New York: Basic Books. Particular attention should be paid to Chapter 8 and Chapter 10.

Oram, D., Bartholomew, K., & Landolt, M. A. (2004). Coping with multiple AIDS-related loss among gay men. *Journal of Gay & Lesbian Social Service, 16*(2), 59-72.

Rolland, J. S. (1994). *Families, illness, and disability: An integrative treatment model.* New York: Basic Books.

Rolland, J. S. (2003). Mastering family challenges in serious illness and disability. In F. Walsh (Ed.), *Normal family processes* (3rd ed., pp. 460-489). New York: Guilford Press.

Springer, C. A., & Lease, S. H. (2000). The impact of multiple AIDS-related bereavement in the gay male population. *Journal of Counseling and Development, 78,* 297-304.

Resources for Clients

Bartlett, J. G., & Finkbeiner, A. K. (2001). *The guide to living with HIV infection: Developed at John Hopkins AIDS clinic* (5th ed.). Baltimore: John Hopkins University Press.

Lambda Legal Defense and Education Fund (1998). Life planning: Legal documents and protections for lesbians and gay men. Retrieved November 14, 2005, from http://www.lambdalegal.org/sections/library/lifeplanning.pdf.

Shernoff, M. (Ed.). (1997). *Gay widowers: Life after the death of a partner.* Binghamton, NY: The Haworth Press.

HANDOUT 16.1.
Adaptation of the Family Systems Illness Model for HIV/AIDS Patients and Their Partners

Stage	Patient	Partner
Crisis	• **Diagnosis:** Explore initial feelings of shock and grief related to diagnosis.	• **Diagnosis:** Explore initial feelings of shock and grief related to the patient's diagnosis.
	• **Disclosure:** Diagnosis may necessitate disclosing to family and friends otherwise unknown lifestyle choices. Explore who to tell, when, and how. Role play the disclosure process.	• **Inadequate information:** Partner may not have adequate information about the illness leading to fear and uncertainty. Provide information and referrals for partners. Collaborate with health care professionals.
	• **Stigma:** Process feelings related to stigma. Educate that family, friends, and neighbors may shun the patient and partner. Explore ways in which stigma may impact their lives on a day-to-day basis and develop plans for managing those situations. Work to heal these relationships.	• **Betrayal:** Partner may feel angry or confused if the illness is a result of an affair or drug use. Facilitate conversations between the partners to heal differences.
	• **Fear of contagion:** Educate family and friends about the transmission process and related medical issues.	• **Fear of infection:** Provide referral for testing and facilitate discussions to work through the possibility of infection.
	• **Loss of social support:** Work to establish or extend networks of social support. Provide referrals to services that are supportive and designed to meet specific needs.	• **Support system:** Partner may not be "out" and thus lack the support system of family and friends to process the diagnosis. Facilitate discussions about coming out and expanding the support system.
	• **Legal and financial issues:** Patients may not be aware of the implications of being in a same-sex relationship as it relates to living together agreements, powers of attorney, wills, living wills, revocable trusts, and funeral arrangements. Explore needs and provide appropriate referrals.	• **Dealing with issues related to obtaining medical information from health care professionals:** Assist partners in planning for legal issues early in the illness as this may serve to prevent or minimize frustration. Encourage and make referrals to attorneys who are knowledgeable of medical, legal, and financial issues as they relate to same-sex couples.
Chronic	• **Coping with emotions:** Allow for expression and normalization of feelings related to sadness, loss, confusion, loneliness, and suicidal ideation.	• **Social support:** Explore sources of support available to the partner. Assist in developing plans that ensure continued social interaction and leisure activities.
	• **Exposure to trauma and fear:** Address feelings related to recurring illness episodes and the impending loss of hopes and dreams.	• **Role shifts and strain:** Explore feelings related to changes in roles assumed in the relationship. Partners may find themselves providing more and more care to the patient, creating instability and imbalance.

Templeton, G.B., Anderson, S.R., & Burwell, S.R. (2007). Adaptation of the family systems illness model for HIV/AIDS patients and their families. In D. Linville, K.M. Hertlein, and Associates, *The Therapist's notebook for family health care: Homework, handouts, and activities for individuals, couples, and families coping with illness, loss, and disability* (pp. 113-118). Binghamton, NY: The Haworth Press.

HANDOUT 16.1 (continued)

Stage	Patient	Partner
	• **Physical decline:** Patient's physical abilities diminish and activities of daily living become much more challenging. Explore feelings related to being a burden on those providing care. Assist in finding new ways to make meaningful contributions to family life. • **Normalcy in daily routine:** May experience the loss of a sense of predictability and control in their lives. • **Isolation:** Patients may spend increasing amounts of time in isolation. Assist in finding ways to engage in social interaction. Provide appropriate referral to support groups. • **Sexuality:** Explore new and safe opportunities for sexual expression. • **Guilt related to infecting others:** Explore feelings of fears and guilt related to the possibility of having infected others. Challenge irrational fears and develop strategies to work with rational fears.	• **Social rejection/isolation:** Partner may fear social rejection, loss of a job, and/or housing as a result of being associated with a person with HIV/AIDS. They may decide to conceal the illness from family and friends. • **Caregiver fatigue and burnout:** Explore feelings of being overwhelmed and burned out by the responsibilities of providing day-to-day care for the ill partner. Consider home health or other services to alleviate caregiver burden. • **Lack of financial and emotional support:** Explore stress related to inadequate financial and emotional support. • **Sexual relationship:** Partner may experience a loss over a lack of sexual involvement with their partner. • **Fear of HIV/AIDS testing:** Partners may be reluctant to be tested for fear of learning that they are seropositive. Be prepared to make appropriate referrals for testing when the partner is ready.
Terminal	• **Coming to terms with the inevitability of death:** Assist patients in processing feelings related to impending death. Facilitate contact with a religious or spiritual leader. Explore patient's beliefs about homosexuality as they relate to death. • **Fear of what lies ahead:** Explore beliefs about life after death. Educate about end of life and dying. Collaborate with palliative care providers. • **Symptomology:** Patients may experience an exacerbation of illness-related symptoms resulting in numerous hospitalizations or may utilize hospice care.	• **Caregiving responsibilities change:** Partners may provide intensive, front-line medical care including keeping track of medications, giving injections, inserting catheters, or cleaning wounds. • **Feelings of loss and grief:** Explore feelings associated with the impending loss of the patient. • **Feelings of helplessness:** Ensure that partners are in contact with appropriate support networks charged with caring for the caregiver. • **Treatment decisions:** Partners may find themselves limited by legal issues in the role they can play in making treatment decisions. Explore and actively pursue legal means through which partners can be involved. Provide appropriate referrals. • **Estate planning:** Partners may experience frustration with the legal challenges associated with executing the will of a patient in a same sex-couple.

Templeton, G.B., Anderson, S.R., & Burwell, S.R. (2007). Adaptation of the family systems illness model for HIV/AIDS patients and their families. In D. Linville, K.M. Hertlein, and Associates, *The Therapist's notebook for family health care: Homework, handouts, and activities for individuals, couples, and families coping with illness, loss, and disability* (pp. 113-118). Binghamton, NY: The Haworth Press.

Chapter 17

Quilting As a Meaning-Making Intervention for HIV/AIDS

Shoshana D. Kerewsky

Type of Contribution: Activity

Objective

This activity uses personal and collaborative quilting as a way for people with HIV/AIDS and their families and friends to make meaning of the illness and improve their communication with one another. The active participation of the therapist differentiates this activity from others associated with memorial quilts, particularly the AIDS Memorial Quilt; however, it integrates with, and intends to complement, related community activities. Although this activity is best documented in relation to HIV/AIDS, similar activities may also serve much the same function for people with other terminal conditions and their families and friends.

Rationale for Use

Although public focus on, and consciousness of, HIV/AIDS has declined with the advent of life-prolonging medical treatment, the epidemic is far from over. On the contrary, the Centers for Disease Control and Prevention's (CDC) most recent estimate is that 1,039,000 to 1,185,000 people are infected with the virus in the United States alone. The CDC further estimates that about 18,000 people in the United States die of AIDS each year (CDC, 2005). Although medical technologies may improve both longevity and quality of life, HIV is still an incurable and deadly virus.

Meaning-making activities may be an important part of both the anticipatory grief process and the mourning process for people with HIV/AIDS and their families and friends (Kerewsky, 1997a,b). This process may be complicated in HIV/AIDS due to cultural stigma associated with the means of HIV transmission, conflicts for gay and bisexual clients between family of origin and family of choice, lack of culturally salient rituals, and bereavement overload in communities hard-hit by HIV/AIDS (Rando, 1993). In addition, many people with HIV/AIDS in the United States are members of disenfranchised or underserved populations. Contributing to the AIDS Memorial Quilt, or quilting with family and friends, may provide an important avenue of expression and connection with others.

For some people, making meaning from grief may take the form of making artwork or other durable creative products (e.g., Jackson, 1991). Activities of this sort are often recommended in the literature on anticipatory and other forms of mourning (e.g., Klein, 2000). As our medical interventions become more sophisticated, people with HIV/AIDS are living longer. While this is a very desirable outcome, it has resulted in a de-emphasis of the terminal nature of AIDS, as well as decreased cultural attention to the avenues for memorializing those who have died or are dying. Thus families and friends, or people with HIV/AIDS themselves, may be less aware of or familiar with useful community resources such as the NAMES Project, which oversees the creation and display of the AIDS Memorial Quilt.

The United States has a rich tradition of social conscience quilts (Atkins, 1994), which raise public consciousness of an issue, and mourning quilts, typically made by a bereaved family, and memory quilts, often contributed to by the person who is dying (Trechsel, 1994). The AIDS Memorial Quilt is a memorial commemorating people who have died of HIV/AIDS. It is composed of 3-by-6 foot panels, each commemorating one or more people who have died of HIV/AIDS, and typically presents their names as well as pictures or symbolic materials. From an initial display of forty panels in 1987 (Ruskin, 1988), it has grown to over 45,000 panels as of June, 2005, presenting over 82,838 names as of October, 2004 (The AIDS Memorial Quilt, 2005). This number represents a fraction of the 524,060 estimated cumulative AIDS deaths through 2003 in the United States alone (Centers for Disease Control, 2005). Chapters of the NAMES Project assist interested people in making panels for the Quilt.

Although the Quilt is "the largest community art project in the world" (The AIDS Memorial Quilt, 2005), the phenomenon of making and contributing panels has not been well studied. Despite many scientific and psychological writers proclaiming the benefits of meaning-making processes, and even using images of the Quilt (e.g., the cover of Kalichman, 1998), few have addressed the Quilt, or quilting in general, as a potentially useful personal and therapeutic activity. Two small-scale qualitative inquiries (Kerewsky, 1997a,b) suggested that HIV-positive gay men found both contributing a panel to the Quilt, and quilting in general, to be important and helpful activities for acknowledging, processing, and communicating with family and friends about their diagnosis. Contributing to the Quilt also appeared to decrease shame and stigma, and was experienced by participants as a positive experience (as, Wadeson, 1980). Anecdotal reports by panel makers and theorists (e.g., Brown, 1992; Ellenhorn, 1997; Gott, 1994; Imber-Black & Roberts, 1993) suggest that family members' and friends' experiences are similar. Working on a memorial quilt provides an opportunity for clients to choose symbols and pictures that represent their experience of the person with HIV/AIDS and to discuss those with the other family and friends making or contributing to the quilt. This is helpful for expressing emotion and discussing the anticipated or actual death.

It is appropriate for therapists and other caregivers to assist clients with HIV/AIDS in locating and engaging in memorializing practices that are emotionally meaningful (Grothe & McKusick, 1993). This may mean providing people with HIV/AIDS and their families and friends with information about the Quilt, asking whether simply making a quilt together might be useful or helpful, or even working with clients and families to create a panel or quilt together. The latter may be especially helpful in communities that do not have a local chapter of the NAMES Project.

Expressive arts interventions may help clients experience and express emotions that are otherwise too difficult or hidden from them. The spectrum of events associated with the production of expressive art includes activity (making the quilt panel), symbolic expression (its meaning for the client and family), and language (the discussion of this meaning and its implications). The panel may serve as a metaphor, or may physically represent metaphors and images that express and cognitively contain the client's affective experience (as, Santostefano, 1985). Discussion of this process, both retrospectively and in the moment (if the client brings the panel to the therapist or works on it in the session), provides access, expression of affect, and a cognitive frame for managing and working with emotions. This latter component, which is important to the therapeutic process, may be missing if the client is socially isolated. For these reasons, quilting in session (or bringing the quilt to session) may serve functions similar to drawing, collage-making, or other expressive activities conducted during a session. As one quilt maker poignantly described a quilt he made shortly after his AIDS diagnosis, "This is a quilt about sadness" (Kerewsky, 1997a). That sadness (or other meanings that the client associates with making a quilt, panel, or other memorial art object) may be more available to the client and in the therapeutic conversation when the quilting occurs during the course of therapy or in the session itself.

The therapist's active participation also may be helpful in decreasing the client's or family's isolation and shame. All who participate in making the quilt or panel affirm symbolically that the relationship with the client is meaningful and endures beyond his or her death (see also Yalom, 1980).

Instructions

Therapists who have not seen the Quilt and are not familiar with it may read about it at The NAMES Project's AIDS Memorial Quilt Web site (www.aidsquilt.org). The Web site includes instructions for making a panel. The film *Common Threads* (Baum et al., 1989) is also extremely useful.

When working with family members or friends who have lost a loved one to HIV/AIDS, or with people with HIV/AIDS who are exploring existential concerns or engaged in anticipatory grief processes, ask whether they are familiar with the Quilt and whether they would like to know more about it. You may wish to look at a book of photographs of panels (e.g., Ruskin, 1988) with your interested client(s) or photos from the NAMES Project's searchable archive (http://www.aidsquilt.org/searchquilt.htm) and discuss their responses. Some clients are not interested in making a panel for the Quilt but may be interested in making a personal quilt, either alone or with family and friends.

If clients express interest in making a panel for the Quilt, first determine the extent to which you are comfortable offering therapist participation based on your preferences, values, theoretical orientation, and the client or family's clinical and interpersonal needs, issues, and welfare. Then within the possibilities that are congruent for you, learn the client's preferences. Since the client or family forgoes their anonymity in making a panel, be sure to explore issues related to the client's privacy and confidentiality. Obtain explicit informed consent for your participation.

Topics of discussion might include where the creation of the panel will take place, sources of help and supplies, and the criteria for panel size and materials. Local AIDS service organizations (ASOs) or chapters of the NAMES Project may be sources of information, support, and assistance. In addition, the NAMES Project's Web site is easy to navigate and includes information on finding a chapter (http://www.aidsquilt.org/chaptermap.htm) and specific instructions for creating a panel (http://www.aidsquilt.org/makeapanel.htm).

If the client completes the panel, it may be helpful to discuss whether the client, friends, or family members will keep the panel for some time, send it to be added to the AIDS Memorial Quilt, or engage in other activities.

Brief Vignette

Horace was a forty-five-year-old biracial gay man who had been HIV-positive for at least twenty years. Many of his close friends had died at the beginning of the AIDS epidemic in the 1980s. His current friends and co-workers had only known him as a person with HIV. Horace had been scrupulous about following health care directives and had been in relatively good health for a number of years. However, in the past two years he had had an increasing number of both opportunistic infections and medication-related cardiac problems and was now on full disability.

Horace came to therapy for help with depression and anxiety related to his health. In the course of his treatment, it became clear that anticipatory grief was an important factor, as was his sense of disconnection from others. He reported that he had tried to talk with his mother and brother about his health problems and belief that he would die soon, but found that his mother changed the subject, while his brother rebuked him for "negative thoughts." After several sessions, Horace reported that he had updated his legal documents and finances but was searching for "a way to say, 'Hey! I was here.'"

Horace had heard of the AIDS Memorial Quilt and had helped make panels for several friends in the late 1980s. After discussion with the therapist, he decided that he did not want to make a panel for himself, but did want a panel made for him, and did want to participate in some way. Because he had friends and family who he hoped would participate, he chose to conduct the activity outside the therapy. He initially asked a trusted former colleague to contact his previous co-workers and current friends to ask them to contribute material or small sections to his panel. After more thought, he asked his mother and brother to contribute as well. Although they initially refused, Horace's co-worker prevailed on them to "visit with us and tell us stories about Horace when he was a kid." Horace's mother agreed to bring her photo album and, after some initial discomfort, soon joined the quilting party when it became clear that despite their good intentions, none of Horace's friends knew how to sew. Horace, who was having respiratory trouble, kept the quilters company, though he was not able to speak above a whisper. His mother told stories of Horace's childhood and adolescence and heard from his co-workers and friends about his life as an adult. Through this mutual conversation, she became more aware of how much Horace's health had declined. In addition to offering to contribute photo transfers of several childhood pictures of Horace to be used on his panel, she shared her new understanding about Horace's declining health with his brother, Ethan. While Ethan was still too uncomfortable to participate in the quilting, he made several trips to visit Horace and offered to write a letter about Horace to accompany his panel to the NAMES Project after he died.

Horace was joined in therapy for several sessions by his mother. They brought his panel with them, both to show the therapist their progress and "to keep us on topic." Horace was able to tell his mother how meaningful it was to have his family acknowledge the extent of his health problems and the likelihood that he would soon die. They discussed his wish to have his full name displayed on his panel and how this might affect his mother, who lived in the same community and had many friends who did not know that Horace had AIDS. His mother expressed her pride in Horace and stated her intention to clarify the nature of his illness to her friends.

Before the panel was completed, Horace suffered a medication-related stroke and died suddenly at home. At his mother's request, the therapist also contributed to the panel by decorating one of the letters in Horace's name. This activity occurred in the therapist's office with Horace's mother and Ethan, who brought Horace's panel and an assortment of permanent markers. During this meeting, the therapist and Horace's family talked about how making the quilt together had increased their intimacy and family communication. About a year after Horace's death, the therapist received a photo of his panel, now a part of the AIDS Memorial Quilt, with a thank-you letter from the mother and Ethan. The mother reported that she had interested some of her church friends in the Quilt and they now met regularly at a local AIDS Service Organization to offer their sewing expertise to other families.

Suggestions for Follow-Up

In addition to creating the panel, clients and their families and friends may wish to keep a scrapbook, journal, or photo album in conjunction with this activity. They also may wish to engage in other meaning-making activities (such as collages) and activities related to dying well (e.g., writing a will, communicating with others, etc.). Clients who have completed a panel for the AIDS Memorial Quilt or a personal quilt may wish to assist others in their community through NAMES Project chapters or by their own initiative.

Clients who are not interested in making a panel may still benefit from exploring these ideas and articulating meaning-making activities that are more developmentally and personally congruent for them. In addition, clients with other terminal illnesses and their families and friends may also wish to make a quilt or other symbolic product together.

Because grief and loss are affectively evocative for the therapist as well as the client, and because symbols and metaphors may stimulate unexpected and less cognitively mediated emotional responses, the therapist should engage in ongoing supervision or consultation throughout this intervention.

If the client dies, family members and friends may require either follow-up sessions or referrals for further services.

Contraindications for Use

Therapists who are not prepared for the emotions that may be aroused by AIDS or grief and loss issues or this specific activity should seek alternative therapeutic strategies or make appropriate referrals. Further, therapists who are not familiar with HIV/AIDS, or with populations to which the client belongs, should educate themselves and utilize consultation.

As noted, therapists should exercise clinical judgment regarding confidentiality. If interpersonal boundary issues are a part of the client's or family's presentation, this activity may be clinically contraindicated, particularly with regard to the therapist's active participation.

This activity should not be used with clients with HIV/AIDS who are not interested in exploring personal responses to dying, or who are unready to approach these issues. Clients and their families who experience "prememorial" activities as tempting fate may find this activity aversive.

For clients with multiple psychological needs, activities from Whitman and Boyd's (1993) *The Therapist's Notebook for Lesbian, Gay, and Bisexual Clients: Homework, Handouts, and Activities for Use in Psychotherapy* (also in this series) initially may be more appropriate interventions.

References

The AIDS Memorial Quilt. (2005). www.aidsquilt.org. Accessed August 31, 2005.

Atkins, J. M. (1994). *Shared threads: Quilting together—past and present.* New York: Viking Studio Books.

Baum, C. (Executive Producer), Couyurie, B. (Producer), Epstein, R. (Producer & Director), Freidman, J. (Producer & Director), Gallin, S. (Executive Producer), Rosenman, H. (Executive Producer), & Sandollar (Executive Producer). (1989). *Common threads: Stories from the Quilt.* [Videotape]. (Available from HBO Video, 1100 Avenue of the Americas, New York, NY 10036).

Brown, J. (Ed.). (1992). *A promise to remember: The NAMES Project book of letters.* New York: Avon.

Centers for Disease Control and Prevention. (2005). A Glance at the HIV/AIDS Epidemic http://www.cdc.gov/hiv/PUBS/Facts/At-A-Glance.htm. Accessed October 24, 2005.

Ellenhorn, R. D. (1997). The AIDS Memorial Quilt and the modernist sacred: Resurrection in a secular world (Doctoral dissertation, Brandeis University, 1997). *Dissertation Abstracts International, 58*(4), A1465.

Gott, T. (1994). *Don't leave me this way: Art in the age of AIDS.* Canaberra, Australia: National Gallery of Australia.

Grothe, T., & McKusick, L. (1993). Coping with multiple loss. In J. W. Dilley, C. Pies, & M. Helquist (Eds.), *Face to face: A guide to AIDS counseling* (updated edition) (pp. 376-379). San Francisco: AIDS Health Project.

Imber-Black, E., & Roberts, J. (1993). *Rituals for our times: Celebrating, healing, and changing our lives and our relationships.* New York: HarperPerennial.

Jackson, S. (1991). The HIV/AIDS Project. *Dulwich Centre Newsletter, 2,* 19-23.

Kalichman, S. C. (1998). *Understanding AIDS: A guide for mental health professionals* (2nd ed.). Washington, DC: American Psychological Association.

Kerewsky, S. D. (1997a). The AIDS Memorial Quilt: Personal and therapeutic uses. *The Arts in Psychotherapy, 24*(7), 431-438.

Kerewsky, S. D. (1997b). HIV+ gay men's processes of making their own AIDS Memorial Quilt panels (Doctoral Dissertation, Antioch University/New England Graduate School, 1997). *Dissertation Abstracts International, 58*(09B), 5192.

Klein, S. J. (2000). Anticipatory mourning in HIV/AIDS. In T. A. Rando (Ed.), *Clinical dimensions of anticipatory mourning: Theory and practice in working with the dying, their loved ones, and their caregivers* (pp. 455-476). Champaign, IL: Research Press.

Rando, T. (1993). *Treatment of complicated mourning.* Champaign, IL: Research Press.

Ruskin, C. (1988). *The Quilt: Stories from the NAMES Project.* New York: Pocket.

Santostefano, S. (1985). Metaphor: Integrating action, fantasy and language in development. *Imagination, Cognition and Personality, 4,* 127-145.

Trechsel, G. A. (1994). Mourning quilts: That distress, by industry, may be removed. *Piecework: All This by Hand, 2,* 52-57.

Wadeson, H. (1980). *Art psychotherapy.* New York: Wiley.

Whitman, J. S., & Boyd, C. J. (Eds.). (1993). *The therapist's notebook for lesbian, gay, and bisexual clients: Homework, handouts, and activities for use in psychotherapy.* Binghamton, NY: The Haworth Press.

Readings and Resources for the Professional

Rando, T. (1993). *Treatment of complicated mourning.* Champaign, IL: Research Press.

Rando, T. A. (Ed.) (2000). *Clinical dimensions of anticipatory mourning: Theory and practice in working with the dying, their loved ones, and their caregivers.* Champaign, IL: Research Press.

Wadeson, H. (1980). *Art psychotherapy.* New York: Wiley.

Bibliotherapy Sources for the Client

The AIDS Memorial Quilt. (2005). www.aidsquilt.org. Accessed August 31, 2005.

Brown, J. (Ed.). (1992). *A promise to remember: The NAMES Project book of letters.* New York: Avon.

Ruskin, C. (1988). *The Quilt: Stories from the NAMES Project.* New York: Pocket.

Chapter 18

Family-Oriented Diabetes Management: Good Nutrition and Portion Control

Carol Pflaffly

Type of Contribution: Psychoeducational Therapeutic Intervention, Handout

Objective

This activity is designed to support and encourage diabetic patients and their families to communicate more openly about the impact diabetes has on each family member by focusing on one aspect of meal-time decision making, specifically the importance of portion control. In addition, it allows the diabetic family member to share expertise and educate others about the dietary challenges faced on a daily basis. It is intended for families with a diabetic member, but can be modified for a multifamily therapy group; it can also be used with families experiencing other chronic illnesses with specific dietary considerations, such as hypertension, heart disease, or obesity.

Rationale for Use

Chronic illnesses, such as diabetes, significantly impact individuals and their families. Conversely, the quality of family life and the level of functioning within the family greatly influence the ability of the individual to cope with chronic illness (McDaniel, Campbell, Hepworth, & Lorenz, 2005). Research on diabetic patients and their families shows that adequate control of diabetes is strongly linked to healthy family functioning (Doherty & Campbell, 1988). A family-centered approach to diabetes care that encourages positive family functioning and leads to lower levels of family-related stress is suggested as a useful way to promote optimal health outcomes (Hanson, De Guire, Schinkel, & Kolterman, 1995).

One of the biggest challenges for diabetic patients is following dietary recommendations in the face of potentially competing eating habits and desires of other family members. Individuals with diabetes often feel isolated or singled out because of their nutritional requirements; while others in the family may feel frustrated if they perceive that their own diets may also be restricted. In our fast-paced society we have been conditioned to think that more is better, especially when it comes to food. The goals of this intervention are to highlight the importance of family involvement in the management of diabetes and to allow the diabetic individual to show his or her expertise in making food selections and controlling portion sizes. After completing this exercise, family members will be more able to accurately judge serving sizes and will begin to learn that a "diabetic diet" is really just a well-rounded, low-fat, healthy meal plan that benefits everyone in the family. Participation by family members increases the chances that the diabetic individual will make healthier self-care choices (Wang & Fenske, 1996).

By organizing the family around a very specific set of decision-making tasks, the therapist can draw on individual strengths within the family while encouraging more open communication about a potentially conflictual topic in a controlled way. Simply clarifying each family member's perspective about a set of concrete tasks, such as how to select appropriate foods and control portion sizes, can prove helpful as family members are often able to relax previously entrenched positions when they feel heard in the therapy setting. Once all family members are able to express themselves, it is often easier to identify what needs to be changed without laying blame on an individual. Then, the role of the therapist is to guide the family in establishing some measurable goals for addressing the challenges and encourage them to make the necessary changes.

Instructions

Preparation for the activity includes having an information sheet of weights and portion sizes (see Table 18.1) available for the family to use as a reference. In addition, the therapist will want to purchase two or three types of juice that are acceptable to the family. Other supplies needed are measuring cups for liquids and solid foods, a food scale, a deck of cards, several containers of play dough, and a number of different sizes and shapes of plates and cups.

The diabetic family member is asked to take a few minutes to review the handout on portion sizes while the family sets up the supplies with guidance from the therapist. The handout allows the diabetic person to share expertise and lead the others through the exercises. The diabetic family member has the information readily available so that he or she can demonstrate knowledge on the subject. The role of the therapist is to coach the diabetic individual as the family moves through a series of meal-planning tasks. The therapist will also encourage ongoing dialogue about sensitive issues relating to the challenges of the family's adjustment to the illness. Suggested introductory remarks by the therapist to the diabetic individual include:

> "Meal planning is challenging enough for families without the added dilemma of accommodating to the needs of a family member with diabetes. If it were just you living alone, you could eat what and when you wanted on your own schedule. But when you live within a household, you have to work the rest of the family's needs into your overall diabetes management plan. You want their support, but don't forget they will want some help from you too. Often, a diagnosis of diabetes prompts a person to make a commitment to eat a little differently. This may mean changes for the entire family. Today's exercise is a way for you to get your family members' ideas about your management plan and to practice your skill at judging portion sizes. Most Americans eat large portions, and will often underestimate the quantity they have eaten unless they practice managing portion sizes. Here's a chance for you to help your family increase their awareness regarding how much they eat."

Each small experiment is followed by a discussion question so the family can begin addressing the areas of tension that have developed in regards to food. During the exercise, participants are coached by the therapist to talk about their feelings as openly as possible and to be good listeners when other family members are speaking.

In preparation for the first task, family members arrange four to six cups and drinking glasses of varying sizes on a table. The leader (diabetic individual) instructs the others to fill each container with "one serving" of juice and then to check their accuracy using a measuring cup. The leader has information on the handout that indicates a standard serving of juice is four ounces, but there are some "trick" questions since some juices are more concentrated and serving sizes are smaller. The family is asked by the therapist to come up with suggestions on how they can accurately estimate a serving size of a beverage if a measuring cup is not available.

Before the next task, each family member is asked to describe a "bad food experience" from the past. This might include receiving poor restaurant service, ordering food that the person did not like, or having an embarrassing situation occur. The therapist's role in the discussion is to highlight the strengths of family members in overcoming the bad experiences.

Next, family members are each given a container of play dough and a paper/plastic plate by the diabetic member. Each family member is given a different size plate and is asked to mould the dough into the shape of a serving of cooked meat/poultry. After weighing the portions created and comparing them to the standard three ounce serving of cooked meat, the leader shows family members how to estimate portion sizes of cooked meat using a deck of cards or the palm of their hand. The therapist leads the family members in describing their "comfort foods" and how these foods can fit within a healthy meal plan.

Depending on time, the same format can be used to estimate portion sizes for other foods. Cooked or uncooked pasta and rice are useful for a discussion on portion sizes. Other discussion questions that can be used include: If you were ordering the perfect meal for your spouse or other family member, what would it be? What's the hardest change you have had to make in meal planning? What's one new family ritual you can initiate regarding meal planning?

Brief Vignette

Rick, a forty-four-year-old male recently diagnosed with diabetes, was referred for couple's counseling by his primary care doctor after Rick reported that he and his wife, Lori, were having difficulty adjusting to his changing health care needs. Although Rick reported taking the recommended doses of his medications regularly, his blood sugar levels were poorly controlled at home. When Rick was hospitalized recently and his diet was controlled, his blood sugar levels stabilized without any medication adjustments. Rick completed the requested dietary education meetings with the hospital dietician prior to leaving the hospital. Rick reported to his doctor that his wife was putting a lot of pressure on him to take care of himself, but at the same time, she seemed distant and angry with his attempts to make lifestyle changes. Rick and Lori came for three sessions of couple's counseling and reported some improvement in their ability to communicate in general, but the topic of Rick's diet remained an area of conflict. Lori admitted that she was angry because Rick's illness now dictated mealtimes and influenced where they could dine out. Rick accused Lori of sabotaging his efforts to make the necessary changes for his health. Rick's doctor stated she was still concerned because Rick was gaining weight and his eating habits were inconsistent. The counselor suggested the couple try an experiment in the next counseling session to address tension around meal planning issues.

In preparation for the next session, the counselor made a copy of the portion control handout and assembled the supplies necessary for the activity. When the couple arrived, Rick was asked to review the handout while Lori was instructed to set out all the materials. Both admitted to being a little nervous about "performing" but were reassured by the counselor that this was intended to be a playful activity not a competition or a way to draw attention to deficits in knowledge. With guidance from the counselor, Rick asked Lori to pour out what she considered to be a serving of juice into two different size cups. Lori was asked to repeat the exercise with another variety of juice. The couple was coached by the counselor to measure the amounts in each cup together. This seemingly simple step took a significant amount of negotiation between the two partners since Rick and Lori each had different ideas on how best to accomplish the task. The counselor chose not to intervene since Rick and Lori seemed to be enjoying the debate over how best to measure the juice levels. After they finished, Rick was prompted by the counselor to share what he learned about portion sizes for beverages. They both admitted that this was not something they ever considered when reviewing food choices, but they agreed on the importance of accurately calculating portion sizes for meal planning and weight management.

Rick and Lori were encouraged to brainstorm ways that they could estimate a portion size if they were unable to actually measure the juice. This led to a discussion of what to do when eating out at their favorite restaurants and how they each could be more conscientious about portion sizes. Since the discussion was productive and the couple were effectively working together to find solutions, the counselor chose not to interrupt the discussion to continue the activity before the session ended. The couple expressed disappointment that they did not have a chance to complete the activity so it was carried over to the next appointment.

During the second meeting, the couple reassembled the supplies for the activity, this time focusing on estimating weights and size of food. The counselor's involvement was minimal since Rick and Lori were more confident with the tasks this time and quickly moved through the process of estimating a serving of meat and checking their accuracy with a scale. The counselor posed the question, "What is the hardest change that you have had to make in meal planning?" Lori spoke first about Rick's illness as an inconvenience to both of them but soon moved in to describing what it really meant to her when Rick was diagnosed with diabetes. She spoke openly for the first time about her fear of losing him, especially when she sees him not taking care of himself properly. Rick admitted his own frustrations, and occasional periods of denial regarding his illness that lead him to make poor food choices. The discussion appeared to be a turning point for the two of them and when the session finished, they agreed to have a discussion on their own about establishing some new rituals for meal planning.

The couple attended several more counseling sessions covering other topics over the course of the next month. The tension around meal preparation diminished significantly as reported by both Lori and Rick. At their last session, the couple announced that they were beginning a weight management program together. It was hoped that Lori's enthusiasm for this endeavor would provide Rick with the motivation and support he needed to be more consistent with his health care management.

Suggestions for Follow-Up

Additional family-centered tasks can be suggested by the counselor to target specific areas of concern such as snacking, dining out, holiday meals, and grocery shopping. If family support is not available, the same exercises can be modified to include friends. With the patient's permission, staying in close contact with the primary care doctor is also suggested.

Contraindications for Use

Some family members are unable or unwilling to provide the positive energy needed to support someone with a chronic illness such as diabetes. If there are indications that a family member is going to be resistant or that the person's presence will discourage the diabetic from making healthy self-care decisions, the exercise may not be useful. Children should be included in the suggested activity only if they are old enough to understand the rationale for the exercise, otherwise their presence may be too distracting. Diabetic individuals who refuse to take personal responsibility for their own health care are not likely to benefit from family interventions such as this.

References

Doherty, W., & Campbell, T. (1988). *Families and health.* Beverly Hills, CA: Sage Publishing.

Hanson, C., De Guire, M., Schinkel, A., & Kolterman, O. (1995). Empirical validation for a family-centered model of care. *Diabetic Care, 18,* 1347-1356.

McDaniel, S., Campbell, T., Hepworth, J., & Lorenz, A. (2005). *Family Oriented Primary Care* (2nd ed.). New York: Springer.

Wang, C., & Fenske, M. (1996). Self-care of adults with non-insulin-dependent diabetes mellitus: Influence of family and friends. *Diabetes Education, 22,* 465-470.

Readings and Resources for Professionals

American Diabetes Association, Inc. (1999). *American Diabetes Association complete guide to diabetes* (2nd ed.). Alexandria, Virginia: Author.

Garner, S., & Stuht, J. (2005). CORE tools and patient information: Easy portion-control tips for reducing calories. *Obesity Management, 1,* 113-115.

Seaburn, D., Lorenz, A., Gunn, W., Gawinski, B., & Mauksch, L. (1996). *Models of collaboration: A guide for mental health professionals working with health care practitioners.* New York: Basic Books.

Resources for the Client

American Diabetes Association, Inc. (1997). *Caring for the diabetic soul: Restoring emotional balance for yourself and your family.* Alexandria, Virginia: Author.

American Diabetes Association, Inc. (1999). *American Diabetes Association complete guide to diabetes* (2nd ed.). Alexandria, Virginia: Author.

American Diabetes Association, Inc. (2005). *Nutrition and Recipes.* Retrieved on October 7, 2005, from http://www.diabetes.org/nutrition-and-recipes/nutrition/overview.jsp.

Anderson, J. (Ed.). (2000). *American Diabetes Association diabetes cookbook: Delicious food for people with diabetes.* New York: Doling Kindersley Publishing.

Betschart, J., & Thom, S. (1995). *In control: A guide for teens with diabetes.* New York: John Wiley & Sons.

Leontos, C. (2000). *What to eat when you get diabetes.* New York: John Wiley & Sons.

HANDOUT 18.1.
What You Need To Know About Portion Sizes

Portion size is just as important as basic food choices for your health and for good glucose control.

What is considered a serving of juice or milk?

- A serving of milk is 8-ounces or 1 cup
- A serving of apple, grapefruit, or orange juice is 4 ounces or ½ cup
- A serving of grape or prune juice, however, is only 1/3 cup.

Look at the sizes and shapes of the drinking cups available. How easy is it to guess the appropriate amount without measuring? If you look at glassware in a store or catalogue today, you will see a wide variety of "standard" sizes. If you purchase a take-out drink, pay attention to what is considered a "small" or "regular" size drink, then take the cup home and measure how much liquid it actually holds.

Hints: 1) At home, measure a serving of juice into a measuring cup and then pour it into the size and style of glass you typically use to get a visual idea of a serving size.
2) Practice using your hand wrapped around a drinking glass and use your fingers to measure how much milk or juice to pour to estimate a serving.

How can you tell how many servings are on your plate?

Dinner plates and bowls can be purchased in a variety of sizes. The bigger the plate or bowl, the more likely you are to overfill it. A cooked serving of meat or poultry is generally considered to be about 3 to 4 ounces. Since meat shrinks during cooking, 4 to 5 ounces of raw meat is considered a standard serving. When dining out, a typical hamburger may contain a half pound of ground meat, while some restaurants serve 12 to 16 ounce servings of steak (three to four times the recommended serving size!).

Hints: Common household items that can help you estimate servings:

- The size of a deck of cards is a good estimate for a 3-ounce serving of cooked meat.
- A medium-size piece of fresh fruit is the same size a tennis ball.
- A 2-ounce serving of chips or pretzels is about 2 handfuls.
- One ounce of cheese equals the size of 4 dice or a computer disk

What about foods that swell during cooking?

Foods like rice, pasta, and some cereals expand during cooking. Rice will triple in volume. One cup of raw rice produces 3 cups or 6 servings of cooked rice.

Hints: Use a measuring cup with foods that expand, and only cook as much as you need for the number of servings you are preparing. One-half cup cooked pasta, rice, cereal, or a small bagel equals the size of one hockey puck.

Pflaffly, C. (2007). Family-oriented diabetes management: Good nutrition and portion control. In D. Linville, K.M. Hertlein, and Associates, *The therapist's notebook for family health care: Homework, handouts, and activities for individuals, couples, and families coping with illness, loss, and disability* (pp. 125-130). Binghamton, NY: The Haworth Press.

Chapter 19

Steps to an Ecology of Treatment: A Handout for Clients with Diabetes

Shoshana D. Kerewsky

Type of Contribution: Activity, Homework Assignment, Handout

Objective

Type II diabetes is rampant in developed countries. Although Type II diabetes is on the rise in children, for most people it is a health concern acquired in adulthood. Self-care for diabetes requires attention to diet and exercise and, in some cases, significant changes in these behaviors. Because food and weight have personal, relational, and cultural meanings, clients with diabetes may have difficulty making and maintaining new health-promoting habits. These handouts and related discussion use aspects of Bronfenbrenner's ecological model (1989) to increase clients' and families' awareness of internal and external factors that contribute to or detract from the client's engagement in more salutary practices. A more inclusive handout allows the therapist to explore these issues in more depth for purposes of treatment planning and further inquiry.

Rationale for Use

The Centers for Disease Control and Prevention (2003) estimates that adult diabetes rates in the United States will double by 2050. It is likely that therapists engaged in direct service provision will work with clients for whom diabetes is a concern or whose family members have diabetes. The vast majority of current and projected diabetes cases are of Type II. Most of the information on Type II diabetes currently available to both clients and therapists ignores the larger systemic contexts in which individuals participate and by which they are influenced.

Most recommendations for therapeutic intervention with people with diabetes are directed toward individual changes intended to decrease the risk of the individual's diabetic complications. These materials tend to provide a blend of educational and behavioral recommendations or describe motivational strategies aimed at increasing or decreasing target behaviors. Although many authors address at least in passing the role of family or other microsystems in the client's response to diabetes, fewer address any contexts or systemic influences beyond the individual and his or her immediate microsystems. This dearth of attention to larger systems issues holds true for a wide range of materials intended to facilitate client's self-help efforts as well (see Kerewsky, 2004).

In addition, information on broader contextual factors, such as the availability of services or effects of cultural beliefs, is largely absent from the psychological, medical, and client-directed literature on prevention and intervention. This narrow focus severely circumscribes both clients' and psychologists' potential roles in addressing the projected U.S. epidemic of Type II diabetes. It further fails to account for the worldviews and assumptions that reflect cultural differences, a glaring omission given that members of many U.S. ethnic groups have much higher rates of diabetes than do Caucasian Euro-Americans (CDC, 2003); that the number of non-Caucasian people of non-European origins continues to increase in the United States; and that food and eating have cultural meanings (Purnell & Paulanka, 1998) and are not affectively neutral. Although some authors have presented models that attend to systemic and contextual factors, these attempts are not well integrated in the professional or self-help diabetes literature and tend to lack specific mechanisms for assessing the larger systemic risk and resilience factors that influence the client.

Unfortunately, the therapist's failure to interview adequately about the client's beliefs is often interpreted as a client deficit or as an indication of psychopathology. Ubiquitous yet largely unexamined differences of cultural context and meaning may provide a better explanation for what is described in the literature as treatment "noncompliance" (e.g., Sarafino, 2001, p. 412) or resistance, typically attributed to the client's individual behavioral problems or familial support system deficits. For example, clients from cultures with a fatalistic or nondeath-fearing worldview may have a very different perspective on prevention and ongoing intervention.

Thus, an ecological approach provides an explicit focus on larger systemic contexts in which clients participate and by which they are influenced. Bronfenbrenner's ecological model (Bronfenbrenner, 1989; Chronister, McWhirter, & Kerewsky, 2004) provides a useful means of exploring systemic influences and contexts that affect clients but of which clients may be unaware. In addition, since each individual is situated differently in his or her personal ecology, this model can be used to encourage more explicit conversation about different experiences and their meanings for family members and others supporting the client.

Instructions

It is important that you be able to describe the ecological model to the client. First, read the handout "Basic Ecological Concepts." This provides both technical terminology and more conversational language, as well as descriptions of each aspect of the personal ecology. Next, use the handout "Ecological Risk and Resilience" to explore your own strengths and vulnerabilities related to food, dietary restrictions, and exercise. This will help you identify some of your own beliefs and influences, as well as anticipate which parts of the worksheet may be easier or more difficult for a particular client.

Introduce the activity as a way to explore some of the ways that the client may be influenced by people, the media, and cultural beliefs. Explain that while the client is aware of some of these influences, the worksheet may help identify others. Using one of the two handouts, describe each level of the personal ecology and help the client identify some risk (vulnerability) and resilience (strength) factors that are true for the client at this time. Have the client write these on the handout. For many clients, the handout "Personal Ecology Worksheet" will be most useful. It focuses on beliefs, attitudes, and ideas. For clients who enjoy more indepth and technical exploration, use the handout "Ecological Risk and Resilience" instead. Responses to this handout may include behaviors and relational quality as well as beliefs.

Brief Vignette

Selene was a forty-year-old Euro-American lesbian newly diagnosed with Type II diabetes. In addition to her existential concerns and depression related to this diagnosis, she reported difficulty following the diet and exercise regimens recommended by her doctor. Selene had read a grim magazine article on diabetes and expressed great fear that she would lose her eyesight, have to have her toes amputated, and die young of cardiac failure. However, these fears did not seem to inspire her to change her health behaviors, but made her feel more desperate and fearful.

Exploration of Selene's situation indicated that she was able to identify some relational factors that influenced her behaviors. For example, she noted that her partner Eva supported Selene exercising but because of her work schedule was unable to exercise with her. Selene found that instead of exercising alone, she watched television while waiting for Eva to come home at about 8:00 pm. During this time she snacked, then ate dinner with Eva at 8:30. Her doctor had asked her to keep a food log, but Selene consistently forgot to do so.

The therapist was curious to learn more about Selene's beliefs about diet and exercise. Further, she wondered what advertising Selene might be watching and what its influence on her might be. She decided to use the Personal Ecology Handout to help Selene explore these influences. First, she helped Selene choose a manageable goal, which was to exercise for thirty minutes a day for one week. Selene's responses included the following:

Ecological level	Positives/strengths/ resilience factors	Negatives/vulnerabilities/ risk factors
My health	My feet are okay. I am able to walk for thirty minutes. I don't smoke.	I am overweight. I bruise easily. I'm hungry all the time.
Ideas that come from my relationships	I accomplish what I set out to do (Eva). I look great in a tank top (Eva).	Food = love (mom). We can't afford a gym membership (Eva?). Exercising takes time away from the relationship.
Ideas that come from television, movies, and magazines	You can get in shape (infomercials). Diabetes is manageable (news).	You're depriving yourself if you don't eat everything you want. There are "good foods" and "bad foods." Everyone who exercises on TV is already thin!
Beliefs, sayings, "everybody knows that..."	"Just Do It." Exercise is good for you.	Fat people have no willpower. "You can't beat the system."

Selene was surprised by some of her responses, particularly the vulnerabilities. She agreed to continue adding to the handout as homework. She asked for two additional copies, one for herself so that she could set a diet goal, and one for Eva. The therapist and Selene agreed that Selene would try to exercise for half an hour a day, and that she would notice which of the beliefs that she had identified were influencing her decisions about this.

At the next session, Selene said that she had exercised five of the previous seven days. She reported noticing that she was especially vulnerable to negative thoughts and self-criticism while watching television and absorbing a great deal of cultural information about food, diets, physical activity, and attractiveness. She had discussed this with Eva, as well as sharing her worksheets with her. Eva had filled out the worksheet herself and they had discussed their responses. Eva clarified that the couple could afford a gym membership if they economized. They decided to drop their cable television and try a gym for three months. Since they both endorsed the belief that food = love, they decided to express their love and support for each other by preparing and eating foods that would help each of them be healthier. Selene requested another copy of the handout to discuss with her mother. She reported feeling "less stuck and more hopeful" about her ability to make small, cumulative changes over time.

Suggestions for Follow-Up

After discussing the identified risk and resilience factors, use narrative, solution-focused, or other techniques to develop goals that will help the client to increase strengths and decrease vulnerabilities. Have the client continue to identify these factors as homework and monitor changes over time.

If family members or other supports are involved in the client's therapy, you may wish to describe the ecological model and ask them to fill out the handout in session as well, focusing on their own risk and resilience factors related to food, dietary restrictions, and exercise. Then facilitate a conversation about similarities and differences between responses, asking how these similarities and differences may contribute to problems and solutions for the client and the family or other intimate systems.

You may wish to ask clients to superimpose the beliefs that are at play in their microsystems (family, friends, and significant others) on a genogram or sociogram in order to understand the relational payoffs and consequences of conforming to or resisting these beliefs.

Finally, clients may use this model to evaluate self-help materials to determine their utility and limits.

Contraindications for Use

If the client is feeling overwhelmed with diets, worksheets, cognitive-behavioral tasks, glucose monitoring, etc., you may wish to use this model in conversation rather than adding another task to the client's responsibilities.

While clients with immediate medical needs, strict regimens, and eating disorders may benefit from an examination of their personal ecologies, you may wish to modify the handouts or activities in consultation with their medical providers.

References

Bronfenbrenner, U. (1989). Ecological systems theory. *Annals of Child Development, 6,* 187-249.

Centers for Disease Control and Prevention. (2003). *Diabetes: Disabling, deadly, and on the rise: At a glance 2003.* Retrieved November 11, 2003 from http://www.cdc.gov/nccdphp/aag/aag_ddt.htm.

Chronister, K. M., McWhirter, B. T., & Kerewsky, S. D. (2004). Prevention from an ecological framework. In R. K. Conyne & E. P. Cook (Eds.), *Ecological counseling: An innovative approach to conceptualizing person-environment interaction* (pp. 315-338). Alexandria, VA: American Counseling Association Press.

Kerewsky, S. D. (2004). Materials for teaching Type II diabetes from an ecological perspective. Poster presented at 112th American Psychological Association Annual Convention, Honolulu, HI.

Purnell, L. D., & Paulanka, B. J. (1998). Purnell's model for cultural competence. In L. D. Purnell & B. J. Paulanka (Eds.), *Transcultural health care: A culturally competent approach* (pp. 7-51). Philadelphia: F. A. Davis Co.

Sarafino, E. P. (2001). *Health psychology: Biopsychosocial interactions* (4th ed.). New York: Wiley.

Readings and Resources for the Professional

Anderson, B. J., & Rubin, R. R. (Eds.). (2002). *Practical psychology for diabetes clinicians* (2nd ed.). Alexandria, VA: American Diabetes Assn.
Beaser, R. S. & the Staff of Joslin Diabetes Center (Eds.). (2001). *Joslin's diabetes deskbook: A guide for primary care providers.* Boston, MA: Joslin Diabetes Center.
Husseini, A. (2005). Strategies for prevention of Type 2 diabetes. Retrieved August 31, 2005 from http://www.pitt.edu/~super1/lecture/lec5361/index.htm.
Snoek, F. J. & Skinner, T. C. (Eds.). (2000). *Psychology in diabetes care.* Chichester, West Sussex, England: Wiley.

Bibliotherapy Sources for the Client

American Association of Diabetes Educators (Producer). (2000). *Diabetes home video guide: Skills for self-care* [Motion picture]. (Available Joslin Diabetes Center, 1 Joslin Pl., Boston MA 02215.)
Doherty, B. (2003). *Outsmart diabetes* Emmaus, PA: Rodale.
Touchette, N. (2002). *American Diabetes Association complete guide to diabetes (3rd ed.).* Alexandria, VA: American Diabetes Assn.
Whitaker, J. (2001). *Reversing diabetes* (rev. ed.). New York: Warner.

HANDOUT 19.1.
Basic Ecological Concepts

Individual

- The person himself or herself without social context (genetics, temperament, etc.)

Microsystem

- The people and communities with whom an individual comes into direct contact

Mesosystem

- Interconnections between the different microsystems
- The theory assumes that an individual's development is enhanced if the mesosystem is positive

Exosystem—How can you use this information to meet your goal?

- Settings that do not directly involve the person (e.g., the media, public policy, access to services) but which exert influence on the person

Macrosystem

- The social blueprint: Cultural values, belief systems, societal structure, gender-role socialization, race relations, and national and international resources

Chronosystem

- The development of interconnections among individuals and their environments over time

Further information and practice activities may be found in:

Chronister, K. M., McWhirter, B. T., & Kerewsky, S. D. (2004). Counseling and ecological prevention practice. In R. K. Coyne & E. P. Cook (Eds.). *Ecological counseling: An innovative approach to conceptualizing person-environment interaction* (pp. 315-338). Alexandria, VA: ACA Press.

Kerewsky, S.D. (2007). Steps to an ecology of treatment: A handout for clients with diabetes. In D. Linville, K.M. Hertlein, and Associates, *The therapist's notebook for family health care: Homework, handouts, and activities for individuals, couples, and families coping with illness, loss, and disability* (pp. 131-139). Binghamton, NY: The Haworth Press.

HANDOUT 19.2.
Ecological Risk and Resilience

Identify risk and resilience factors related to the index person's presenting issues or problems at each ecological level.

Kerewsky, S.D. (2007). Steps to an ecology of treatment: A handout for clients with diabetes. In D. Linville, K.M. Hertlein, and Associates, *The therapist's notebook for family health care: Homework, handouts, and activities for individuals, couples, and families coping with illness, loss, and disability* (pp. 131-139). Binghamton, NY: The Haworth Press.

HANDOUT 19.2 *(continued)*

	Risk factors	Resilience factors
Chronosystem; the system's changes over time	1. 2.	1. 2.
Macrosystem; culture, beliefs, grand narratives, social unconscious	1. 2.	1. 2.
Exosystem; media, service delivery structures, public policy	1. 2.	1. 2.
Mesosystem; connections and communication between micro- and exosystems	1. 2.	1. 2.
Microsystem; people and communities in direct contact with person	1. 2.	1. 2.
Individual; genetics, temperament, biology, innate characteristics	1. 2.	1. 2.

Kerewsky, S.D. (2007). Steps to an ecology of treatment: A handout for clients with diabetes. In D. Linville, K.M. Hertlein, and Associates, *The therapist's notebook for family health care: Homework, handouts, and activities for individuals, couples, and families coping with illness, loss, and disability* (pp.131-139). Binghamton, NY: The Haworth Press.

HANDOUT 19.3.
Personal Ecology Worksheet

Each circle represents a different set of influences on your own thoughts and feelings. Fill in each circle with specific quotes and ideas. On the left, list the *beliefs, attitudes,* and *ideas* that help you meet your goal. On the right, list those that make it harder to meet your goal. In the center, list your *physical strengths* and *vulnerabilities* related to your goal.

My goal is:

How can you use this information to meet your goal?:

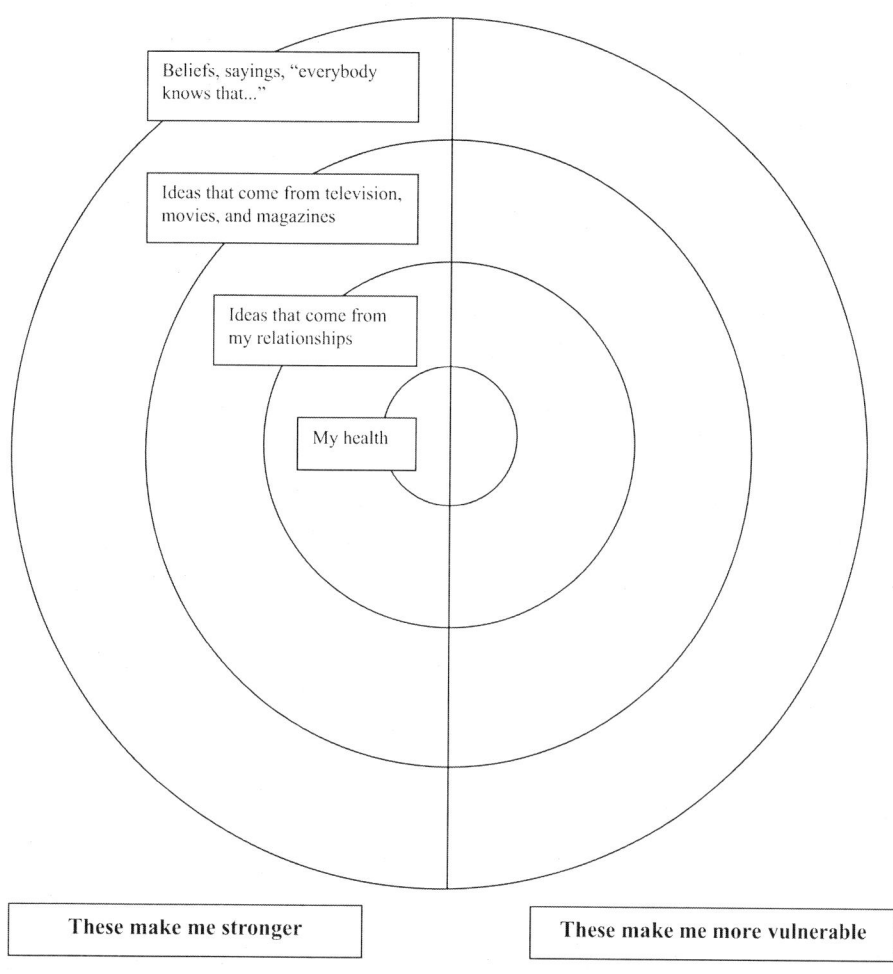

Kerewsky, S.D. (2007). Steps to an ecology of treatment: A handout for clients with diabetes. In D. Linville, K.M. Hertlein, and Associates, *The therapist's notebook for family health care: Homework, handouts, and activities for individuals, couples, and families coping with illness, loss, and disability* (pp. 131-139). Binghamton, NY: The Haworth Press.

Chapter 20

Every Woman's Problem: Self-Assessment for Disordered Eating and Body Image Despair

Margo D. Maine

Type of Contribution: Homework, Self-Assessment, Handout

Objective

This chapter and self-assessment tool increases self-awareness of obsessions regarding weight, eating, exercise, and body image in adult women. It also challenges the myth that these issues only affect teens and college-aged women.

Rationale for Use

Today, despair about eating, weight, and body image are of epidemic proportions, affecting the physical and mental health of more and more women. Eating disorders and body image despair are homogenized throughout all socioeconomic, racial, and ethnic groups, and are now reported in as many as forty countries due to the far-reaching impact of globalization (Gordon, 2001). In other words, this is "every woman's problem."

These issues occur on a continuum from obsessions with appearance, shape, and exercise to chronic and dangerous weight-control practices, including the clinical diagnoses of: Anorexia Nervosa, Bulimia Nervosa, and eating disorders not otherwise specified. When eating disorders or body image conflicts are mentioned, however, the face we imagine is one of youth. It may be a preteen, an adolescent, or a young adult woman, but we rarely visualize an aging face in that picture. Yet more and more older women, approaching or beyond midlife, also struggle with their bodies and their eating habits and need professional help. In fact, in 2003, one-third of inpatient admissions to a specialized treatment center for eating disorders were women over thirty years of age (Davis, 2004). The picture of a young, vibrant teenager who succumbs to an eating disorder is tragic, but eating disorders are just as destructive in the lives of adult women. The sad truth is that *the language of fat* (Friedman, 1997) is spoken by women of all ages, at all stages in their lives.

Although eating disorders are more common than many other serious illnesses, they receive much less attention in the health care system (Powers & Bannon, 2004). It is common to suffer from significant eating and body image problems for years and never be diagnosed. Due to the stereotypic beliefs that these problems only affect young women and teens, health care professionals often fail to recognize these conditions in adults. Furthermore, adult women are not likely to disclose their eating and body image concerns, as they also believe these are problems that they should have outgrown. They tend to have a deep sense of shame and embarrassment, feeling they "should know better" and fearing that health professionals will not take their problems seriously.

Research is sparse on topics related to eating and body image disorders in adults; however, what we do know is compelling. Surveys of adult women's dieting and body image concerns, precursors to clinical eating disorders, reveal that 43 million adult women in the United States are dieting to lose weight at any given time and another 26 million are dieting to maintain their weight (Gaesser, 2002). Other studies find comparable levels of dieting and disordered eating across young and elderly age groups (Hetherington & Burnett, 1994). In fact, when asked what bothered them most about their bodies, a group of women aged sixty-one to ninty-two said weight was their greatest concern (Clarke, 2002).

Although these statistics suggest that body dissatisfaction, severe and dangerous dieting practices, exercise abuse, and related rituals are now normative, few women understand the potential risks of these behaviors when taken to the extreme. In fact, among psychiatric conditions, eating disorders have the highest health risk, with an estimated 10 percent of women dying after being sick for ten years (Sullivan, 2002) and 20 percent dying after twenty years (American Psychiatric Association, 2000). Thus, regardless of what issues bring a woman to treatment, clinicians should incorporate self-assessment tools to raise her consciousness of the serious impact of unhealthy ideas and behaviors related to food, weight, and body image on the quality of her life. This could save her life.

The Context of Adult Eating and Body Image Concerns

In the past quarter century, cultural roles and expectations for women have transformed more rapidly than ever before. Globalization has introduced a powerful and relentless consumer culture, with expectations about appearance and beauty as well as dramatic revisions in women's social role (Gordon, 2001). This consumer culture thrives by making women feel "hungry" for things to purchase and ways to spend money to change themselves and prove their worth to this global economy.

Contemporary western culture consistently values women's bodies and appearance above other attributes (Maine & Kelly, 2005). Sexualized images of female bodies saturate everyday media, constantly creating a standard few can or should attain. Today's women are always on display, endlessly criticized for being too sexy or not sexy enough, and completely dismissed when they no longer look young. Rarely do we see an older face, be it in film, fashion, advertising, print media, or television. Thin, young bodies seem to have more value and credibility, so most women struggle with the natural physical changes associated with aging and fight against nature instead of honoring and accepting it.

In this age of body technology, when cosmetic plastic surgery can be purchased at a mall during a lunch hour, women are sold the myth that they can (and should) be in complete command of their bodies. The female body has never been more exposed while its natural processes, such as the symptoms of menopause, are to be completely masked or corrected. The rhythmic cycles of the female body, many of which are associated with weight gain, such as premenstrual bloating, pregnancy, and the slower menopausal metabolism, are great challenges in this era of body control and unrealistic beauty images. If a woman's power is still defined in terms of beauty and a youthful body, the eight to twelve pounds she naturally gains at menopause (Waterhouse, 1997) can be a source of great distress and anticipated disempowerment.

While social changes always create stress, those associated with globalization may especially impact women, increasing the risk for body image and eating problems (Gordon, 2001). For example, because of greater access to education and increased involvement in the workplace, women are competing with one another and with men in ways previous generations have not experienced. Women's roles outside the home have grown, yet women's bodies must be smaller to meet today's standards. At the same time, today's hectic but sedentary lifestyle and western diet, filled with prepared foods higher in calories and fat, have led to an increase in obesity. In this context, the body reality and the beauty ideal clash head-on, no matter what a woman's age. It becomes easy to believe *The Body Myth* that the "perfect body" will help a woman to succeed in her work, her social environment, in her relationships, and in managing the challenges of everyday life (Maine & Kelly, 2005).

The fast-paced life inherent in current postmodern culture emphasizes adaptation, achievement, and appearance, leaving little time to reflect on these new roles and expectations. Instead of identifying, exploring, or describing their complex emotions, needs, and appetites, contemporary women are taught to translate these into the language of fat. Given little permission for negative feelings, and surrounded by a sociocultural environment that has labeled fat as bad, "feeling fat" is now the cover for all discomfort, anger, disappointment, and other "bad" feelings.

For many women, extreme dieting, obsessive exercise, and other rituals related to food, weight, and appearance, have become automatic and unconscious ways to cope with stress (Maine & Kelly, 2005). Having internalized unreasonable cultural standards of beauty, they may not report these to their medical providers or psychotherapists. For some, the symptoms may feel ego-syntonic while for others, they may cause deep shame; in either case, denial may preclude open admission and exploration of their relationship to food and to their bodies (American Psychiatric Association, 2000). A self-assessment tool integrated into the early phase of therapy will help a woman to become more conscious of these behaviors and may improve her physical health as well as her psychological well-being.

Instructions

Introduce the importance of understanding and addressing a woman's relationship with food and her body since so many women struggle with these issues today. Stress the notion that this is "every woman's problem," but that for some women, these behaviors can become dangerous to their health, both physically and psychologically. Ask the client to utilize the "Self-Assessment for Eating and Body Image Concerns Handout" to raise her consciousness about how these problems may play out in her life and that she share her reactions and responses with you. Explain the importance of reflecting on the feelings she may have when considering these questions, as they may stir up unresolved or unconscious issues. Ask that she write these down and talk about them in session. Also suggest that she explore these insights or concerns with trusted friends.

Together examine the pattern of her responses. If most are in the "Never-Rarely" categories, her concerns are very manageable. It may be useful to discuss some of these in therapy, but they are unlikely to be the focus of treatment. If most fall in the "Sometimes, Often, or Usually" categories, it is likely that her body, food, and weight concerns are interfering with her life. Invest the time to understand what her answers reveal about her relationship to her body. Help her to commit to be more respectful and accepting of its needs and nature.

Before using this tool with clients, all therapists should complete it and examine their own potential concerns in these areas. With such self-awareness, clinicians will be more capable of understanding the unconscious links among eating, body image, and emotions and will be better able to guide clients through this process.

Brief Vignette

Susan was being treated for depression and anxiety. She identified many stressors in her life: marriage to a successful but self-absorbed man who relied on her to do all the parenting and emotional care of her own family and extended family; raising her children in a very competitive community; and a demanding job. She was constantly exhausted and overwhelmed, feeling totally out of control of her life. Her therapist gave her support and validated her experience and Susan agreed to take antidepressants as well. While she valued the time with her therapist, she was still very depressed and anxious; as she wasn't making "progress," she felt undeserving of the therapy and more inadequate.

Over the year of treatment, Susan was never asked about her behaviors related to exercise or eating, but in fact was eating less than 800 calories per day. (Less than 1,500 calories is considered starvation.) She was also exercising one to three hours every day.

Susan's disordered eating and obsessive exercise were not identified until she had lost twenty pounds and she was sick constantly. Incorporating some self-assessment tools regarding obsessions around food, body image, or exercise early in her treatment may have helped Susan to address these issues sooner and avoided the physical problems she developed due to her poor nutritional status. Had she continued her ritual of restricting her food intake while exercising excessively, she might have had a cardiac arrhythmia, a heart attack, lost consciousness, or developed osteoporosis among other serious health issues. Susan's antidepressants probably had no impact on her brain chemistry as she was not consuming enough fat for her body to effectively utilize them. Regardless of medication and the increased insight she derived in psychotherapy, her depression and anxiety could not improve due to the impact of starvation on brain chemistry and mood. She was increasingly feeling like a failure, in her words "hopeless," as she was following treatment recommendations but not getting better.

Susan began addressing her eating and exercise abuse by working with a therapist and a dietitian specializing in eating disorders. She was able to see how these rituals had been attempts to control other problems in her life that she felt she could not control; gradually she was able to address the underlying problems and to let go of her eating and exercise rituals. Her mood improved and her anxiety became manageable.

Health and mental health professionals often ignore the individual's relationship to food, body image, and weight issues. When we do ask a woman if she is dieting, she may say no, despite the fact that she is doing many things to restrict her intake and trying to lose or "manage" her weight. These behaviors have become "normal" to her, when they could be signs of disordered eating, even anorexia or bulimia. Had Susan's therapist included the "Self-Assessment for Eating and Body Image Concerns Handout" in her initial assessment and treatment, she may have suffered far less.

Suggestions for Follow-Up

Ask the client to share her reactions to the self-assessment process. Inquire about which of the topic areas or questions aroused the most discomfort. It can be very difficult for a woman to talk about these issues; be sensitive to this by asking how she feels talking with you about her eating and body image. Review the self-assessment together in a session, providing support and empathy. If her problems are significant (with most responses in the "Sometimes, Often, or Usually" categories) and you have not worked with eating disorders and related issues effectively in the past, consider referring her to a specialist for an evaluation, consultation, or treatment. A consultation with an eating disorder expert will also determine if she needs a higher-level of care or a specialized program that treats body image issues and eating disorders. If you have been working effectively with her in other areas and have skills and experience with eating and body image issues, you may be able to continue your work and add other components such as nutritional counseling with a dietitian and experiential therapies with a body image specialist.

There are many resources available today, including a growing self-help literature. Help your client to access these. Contact the National Eating Disorders Association (www.nationaleatingdisorders.org) for general information about eating disorders and related problems. They also have a referral list for treatment. Visit Gurze Books at www.bulimia.com to find self-help resources and books. My Web sites www.mwsg.org or www.thebodymyth.com also have links to many others.

Contraindications for Use

Anyone with a serious eating disorder (symptoms such as: purging; abuse of diet pills, diuretics, or laxatives; weight loss, inability to concentrate; depression; difficulty sleeping; irritability; chest pain or tightness; dizziness; extreme fatigue; hair loss; irregular periods) should access professional services with a specialist in eating disorders and body image issues right away. Self-help alone will not be enough. A thorough medical evaluation is necessary to rule out any other illness and to treat any acute problems and plan appropriate medical monitoring. Often periods of residential treatment, hospitalization, or day-hospital treatment are necessary.

Readings/Resources for Professionals

American Psychiatric Association (2000 January). Practice Guideline for the Treatment of Patients with Eating Disorders (Revision). *American Journal of Psychiatry, 157*(1), 1-39.

Clarke, L. H. (2002). Older women's perceptions of ideal body weights: The tensions between health and appearance motivations for weight loss. *Ageing and Society, 22,* 751-773.

Davis, W. (2004). Personal communication.

Friedman, S. S. (1997). *When girls feel fat: Helping girls through adolescence.* Vancouver, Canada: Salal Books.

Gaesser, G. (2002). *Big fat lies: The truth about your weight and your health.* Carlsbad, CA: Gurze Books.

Gordon, G. (2001). Eating Disorders East and West: A culture-bound syndrome unbound. In M. Nasser, M. A. Katzman, R. A. Gordon, (Eds), *Eating Disorders and Cultures in Transition* (pp. 1-16). New York: Brunner-Routledge.

Hetherington, M. M., & Burnett, L. (1994). Ageing and the Pursuit of Slimness: Dietary Restraint and Weight Satisfaction in Elderly Women. *British Journal of Clinical Psychology, 33,* 391-400.

Knapp, C. (2003). *Appetites: Why women want.* New York: Counterpoint.

Maine, M., & Kelly, J. (2005). *The body myth: Adult women and the pressure to be perfect.* New York: John Wiley.

Powers, P. S., & Bannon, Y. (2004). The Last Word: Meeting the Challenge of Eating Disorders. *Eating Disorders: The Journal of Treatment and Prevention, 12,* 91-95.

Sullivan, P. (2002). Course and outcome of anorexia nervosa and bulimia nervosa. In Fairburn, C. G., Brownell, K. D. (Eds.) *Eating Disorders and Obesity* (2nd ed.) (pp. 226-232). New York: Guilford Press.

Waterhouse, D. (1997). *Like mother, like daughter: How women are influenced by their mother's relationship with food and how to break the pattern.* New York: Hyperion.

Web Sites

www.aedweb.org—The Academy for Eating Disorders is a professional organization that provides training and education to clinicians and dedicates itself to improving the research, treatment, and prevention of eating disorders.

www.ANAD.org—National Association of Anorexia Nervosa and Related Disorders provides information, referrals, education, and support groups regarding eating disorders.

www.bulimia.com—Sponsored by Gurze Books, this Web site is both a bookstore and a resource for information about eating disorders.

www.edreferral.com—The Eating Disorder Referral and Information Center has free information and referral lists for treatment of eating disorders.

www.iaedp.com—The International Association of Eating Disorders Professionals provides education and training to professionals.

www.nationaleatingdisorders.org—The National Eating Disorders Association is the largest national organization providing educational materials and referral information, sponsoring the annual Eating Disorders Awareness Week, offering educational programs and materials. A great resource for both the public and professionals.

Bibliotherapy Sources for Clients

Costin, C. (1996). *The eating disorder sourcebook: A comprehensive guide to the causes, treatment, and prevention of eating disorders.* Lincolnwood, IL: NTC Publishing.

Freedman, R. (2002). *Body love: Learning to like our looks and ourselves.* Carlsbad, CA: Gurze Books.

Gaesser, G. (2002). *Big fat lies: The truth about your weight and your health.* Carlsbad, CA: Gurze Books.

Hall, L. (1993). *Full lives: Women who have freed themselves from food and weight obsession.* Carlsbad, CA: Gurze Books.

Hall, L., & Cohn, L. (1999). *Bulimia: A guide to recovery.* Carlsbad, CA: Gurze Books.

Hall, L., & Ostroff, M. (1999). *Anorexia Nervosa: A guide to recovery.* Carlsbad, CA: Gurze Books.

Hutchinson, M. G. (1985). *Transforming body image.* Freedom, CA: The Crossing Press.

Johnston, A. (2000). *Eating in the light of the moon.* Carlsbad, CA: Gurze Books.

Maine, M. (2000). *Body wars: Making peace with women's bodies.* Carlsbad, CA: Gurze Books.

Maine, M. (2004). *Father hunger: Fathers, daughters, and the pursuit of thinness.* Carlsbad, CA: Gurze Books.

Maine, M., & Kelly, J. (2005). *The body myth: Adult women and the pressure to be perfect.* New York: John Wiley.

Rabinor, J. R. (2002). *A starving madness: Tales of hunger, hope, and healing in psychotherapy.* Carlsbad, CA: Gurze Books.

Waterhouse, D. (1997). *Like mother, like daughter: How women are influenced by their mother's relationship with food and how to break the pattern.* New York: Hyperion.

HANDOUT 20.1.
Self-Assessment for Eating and Body Image Concerns

Handout

For these self-assessments, honestly pick the most accurate reflection of your thoughts and behavior on these items. Pick:

A for Always; *F* for Frequently; *S* for Sometimes; *R* for Rarely; and *N* for Never.

Part I: Dieting
____ I skip meals or go as long as possible between them.
____ I have strict rules about food.
____ I weigh myself daily or more often.
____ I drink liquids or chew gum to avoid eating.
____ I count calories and fat, carbohydrate, and protein grams.
____ I eat secretly.
____ I am so worried about food that I can't concentrate or get things done.
____ I feel guilty after eating.
____ I take pills such as laxatives, diet pills, metabolism boosters.

Part II: Exercise
____ My self-worth each day is based on my exercise.
____ I exercise even if I am injured or sick.
____ I put exercise ahead of social life or other obligations.
____ I become very upset if I cannot exercise.
____ I always feel I should do more when I exercise.
____ I calculate how much I need to exercise to burn up what I ate.
____ People who care about me think I exercise too much.

Part III: Body Image
____ My self-worth is based on my weight and clothing size.
____ I constantly compare my body with others.
____ I cannot take a compliment.
____ I won't wear a bathing suit or other revealing clothes.
____ I constantly check myself in the mirror.
____ I want to have plastic surgery to improve my appearance.
____ I wear clothes to hide or cover up my body.
____ I am never satisfied with my body.

Part IV: Social Interactions
____ I talk about weight, exercise, and appearance with friends.
____ I am jealous of women who may be thinner or more attractive.
____ I avoid social settings due to my body image concerns.
____ I don't like to be touched, even by my partner.
____ I judge people based on their weight or appearance.
____ I feel judged by others based on my weight and appearance.
____ I cannot relax when I am with others.
____ People's affection for me is related to my appearance.

Maine, M.D. (2007). Every woman's problem: Self-assessment for disordered eating and body image despair. In D. Linville, K.M. Hertlein, and Associates, *The therapist's notebook for family health care: Homework, handouts, and activities for individuals, couples, and families coping with illness, loss, and disability* (pp. 141-147). Binghamton, NY: The Haworth Press.

Chapter 21

Put a Wrench in It

Nicole M. Childs
Stephanie R. Burwell

Type of Contribution: Homework, Handout, Activity, and Intervention

Objective

This contribution provides a unique opportunity for clients to determine where and how they discontinue the cyclical nature of a presenting problem. The example provided in this chapter was used with a woman who presented with bulimia. Given the systemic nature of this intervention, it can be adapted and applied to other common problems such as depression, anxiety, and relational distress. It is also flexible enough to be used as an activity or intervention within the therapy room, or as an assignment to complete outside of the session.

Rationale for Use

Body weight and body image are common concerns, especially among women. According to the American Psychiatric Association (2000), almost 90 percent of those who suffer from eating disorders are women. According the Diagnostic and Statistical Manual of Mental Disorders IV-TR (American Psychiatric Association, 2000), some essential characteristics of bulimia include binge eating and inappropriate means for maintaining weight (e.g., purging, use of laxatives, and excessive exercise). Women with bulimia evaluate their overall self-concept and worth based upon their weight. Another major characteristic of bulimia is a sense of loss of control. This is especially apparent during binges where women report having no ability to control the amount or quality of food they eat.

Because eating disorders are largely considered to be a woman's health issue, theories grounded in the feminist perspective have served as a major framework in the understanding and conceptualization of eating disorders (Faith, Pinhas, Schmelefske, & Bryden, 2003). Although there are various forms of feminism, feminists generally believe that women should have "full economic, political, and social participation" in the social order (Leupnitz, 1988, p. 14). Other core concepts of feminism include the belief that gender is not biologically determined, but rather is socially constructed and that patriarchy limits both men and women. Feminist theory asserts that it is imperative to connect the experiences of women within the broader sociopolitical context by examining the impact of the political and social messages from the patriarchal society (Brown, 1994; Israeli & Santor, 2000). Women are encouraged to "become aware of power dynamics in her life context, develop skills for achieving control over her life, use this control without impinging on the rights of others, and work toward empowerment of others" (Cummings, 2000, p. 48). By becoming more aware of the social injustices that the patriarchal society places upon both men and women, women can make active changes that limit problems associated with the internalization of destructive social roles and realities.

This stance on gender and society has been applied to the clinical conceptualization and treatment of eating disorders. Feminists have examined and made hypotheses about the impact society has on the gendered nature of eating disorders (Katzman & Lee, 1996). According to this perspective, "gender significantly influences how a person experiences her life and defines what is valued in the size, shape, or age of human bodies" (Faith, Pinhas, Schmelefske, & Bryden, 2003, p. 306). Some theorists have asserted that society and culture actually produce and maintain the existence of eating disorders, which can be life threatening (Bordo, 1993; Gatens, 1996). Feminist therapists who treat women with eating disorders often focus on the profound impact that culture has on the conceptualization of body image, and self-worth, and women's health (Faith et al., 2003). Thus, in the work of feminist therapists, the eating disorder is deconstructed within a social and political context. Eating disordered women are urged to explore the impact of patriarchy on their values and beliefs and process how the sociopolitical environment has influenced their cognitions about body image and femininity.

Another important goal in the feminist treatment of eating disorders is to foster client empowerment and control (Brown, 1994; Faith et al., 2003). A feminist-informed approach offers a collaborative treatment for women that emphasizes the importance of negotiating the process of therapy so that the client shares equal power with the therapist. Feminist-informed therapists recognize that each eating disordered woman has expertise that should be used to inform her treatment. By creating a therapeutic relationship that is empowering, the client is able to experience a sense of control, which supports her ability to identify solutions and exceptions to the eating disorder. Because eating disorders are typically about control, clients are encouraged to experience and maintain control in therapy. This provides a new way of experiencing control, as compared to restricting food intake or vomiting. As the treatment progresses, the therapist becomes less of a leader or director of context and more of a catalyst for change (Brown, 1994).

Instructions and Brief Vignette

Before using this intervention as homework, a handout, or activity, the therapist and client must collaboratively map out the cyclical nature of the presenting problem. In the first author's initial session with Jane (named changed to maintain confidentiality), problematic patterns related to bulimia were mapped out. This process can include other family members or significant partners to help provide information about the pattern. This is especially relevant when a family member or partner influences the client's pattern. Jane's pattern involved binging and purging behaviors and their associated triggers including negative cognitive distortions, feeling uncomfortable and fat, feelings out of control, and negative body image. This is visually presented in Handout 21.1. Once this pattern was drawn on a piece of paper or blackboard, Jane identified where she needed to "put a wrench in it." What this means is that the client decides where to do something different to alter the pattern. This provides an opportunity for the client to take control by deciding how and where the changes occur. In doing this, not only does the client obtain a sense of empowerment and control, but she is also able to recognize her own capabilities of change (Brown, 1994; Faith et. al., 2003). For instance, Jane was initially not able to stop the process of binging. However, she was able to "put a wrench" in the pattern before the binging occurs by modifying the repetition of self-deprecation that is maintained through negative thought patterns. The location that the client places the wrench is where the therapist and client focus on changes needed for the wrench to perform its function by stopping that part of the pattern. As shown in Handout 21.1, the wrench is placed between negative internal thoughts and binging. Jane knew that she was not yet able to alter her negative internal thoughts but desired the termination of binging and the repercussions that followed. Rather than relying on binging as a form of coping and sense of control, Jane and the therapist collaboratively created different ways to cope with negative cognitive distortions. In this particular case, Jane named several other strategies that included calling a friend, using positive self-talk, and practicing relaxation techniques to help battle negative cognitive distortions instead of binging. Feedback and support can also be garnered from family members during this process as they provide additional information and strategies to alter the client's problematic behavior.

The goal of therapy is to keep moving the wrench to different places in the cycle to ensure that all parts of the pattern are identified and eventually confronted. The wrench should be moved in a counter clockwise direction so that the client is able to reach all parts of the process in a matter that is not counterproductive to forward change. For example, in Handout 21.1, Jane would not want to put the wrench in the cycle and change binging behavior one week, just to move it forward in the cycle to allow for binging the next week. The next step in Jane's treatment would be to place the wrench in between negative internal thoughts and binging with the goal of identifying the negative cognitive distortions and where they originated. In Jane's case, the feminist perspective on the impact of society and gender on self-worth and esteem was especially relevant (Faith et al., 2003). She was urged to explore the impact of patriarchy on values and beliefs, discussing how the sociopolitical environment has influenced her cognitions about body image and femininity. This discussion would also be helpful in the context of family therapy to understand behaviors (e.g., comments made about client's food intake) that may be contributing to the client's problem. In collaboration with her therapist, Jane then determined what she would do differently that would minimize feeling worse about herself, thus allowing the pattern to be altered.

A diagram of a "wrench" is included as Handout 21.2. This can be used during the session as an intervention, or can be given to the client to take home and complete. Thus, the client would bring home a picture of the mapped out cyclical nature of the problem, along with the wrench handout. The wrench diagram provides a space for the client to complete what it is going to take to put a wrench in the pattern (e.g., distraction from usual behavior). When formulating the components of their wrench (i.e., what it is going to take to alter the pattern), clients are able to organize their thoughts about how they see themselves making appropriate changes. Consistent with the empowerment approach, it is important for the client to "hold the wrench," as this facilitates control over change. Again, this is very powerful for women with bulimia because they not only are able to control their medium of change but also attain a sense of empowerment. As they begin to feel empowered, an increase in self-esteem and self-worth can foster endurance needed to continue successful change in defeating bulimia.

Suggestions for Follow-Up

If bulimic symptoms reappear, it is appropriate to revisit the problematic cycle and triggers that led to the resurfacing of the symptoms. In that way, developing an entirely novel systemic pattern of behavior might be especially appropriate for clients who relapse. Two reasons for revisiting this process include: (1) The system may have changed from the initial stages of therapy so that the mapped out cyclical nature of the problem is no longer accurate or acceptable, and (2) The original map may have been an incorrect representation of the cyclical nature of the problem. At this time it would also be beneficial for both the therapist and client to identify the components of change that seemed to work previously and compare them to those that did not. By focusing on the dynamics of these contrasts, unique facets may emerge that were not recognized.

One issue therapists may want to attend to is second order systemic change (Bateson, 1979). As the bulimic client gains more control over her symptoms and health care homeostasis is altered. This may facilitate relational changes such as role shifts. For example, as her power and self-esteem increase, her partner or family member may experience a loss of power. In this example the therapist can help the couple and family adapt to these shifts.

In addition, it is beneficial for therapists to collaborate with the client's primary physician and other available health professionals. This way the client is provided access to many forms of guidance and support. In addition, the therapist can serve as advocate in helping the client navigate her own health care by becoming more assertive and empowered (McDaniel, Hepworth, & Doherty, 1992). Through this process, the client develops and strengthens her voice in her relationships with medical providers. This can foster a more open patient-doctor communication and treatment compliance.

This intervention can be used to help clients with a variety of concerns such as major depression, diabetes management, and medication adherence. If women are able to successfully use this intervention for bulimia, they can then apply the same process to other problematic areas in their lives. In this way, they can create their cyclical pattern of the problem, make a copy of the wrench, and place it in their desired areas. Being able to use this tool independently will continue to increase the competence and worth of the client in that she will have the confidence in knowing that she can appropriately handle future problems.

Contraindications for Use

This intervention focuses upon client competence and control and assumes the client wants to make an effort to change her behavior. Therapists should be sensitive to clients' motivation for change and level of understanding of having a potentially life-threatening disorder. If the client thinks that her illness is not impacting her life in any way and has no desire to change, other forms of treatment that are more comprehensive or empirically supported should be applied.

References and Resources for the Professional

American Psychological Association (2000). *Diagnostic and Statistical Manual of Mental Health Disorders, Fourth Edition,* Text Revision. Washington, DC: APA.

Bateson, G. (1979). *Mind and nature: A necessary unity.* New York: Dutton.

Bordo, S. (1993). *Unbearable weight: Feminist, Western culture, and the body.* Berkeley, CA: University of California Press.

Brown, L. S. (1994). *Subversive dialogues: Theory in feminist therapy.* New York: Basic Books.

Cummings, A. L. (2000). Teaching feminist counselor responses to novice female counselors. *Counselor Education & Supervision, 40,* 47-58.

Faith, K., Pinhas, L., Schmelefske, J., & Bryden, P. (2003). Developing a feminist-informed model for decision making in the treatment of adolescent eating disorders. *Eating Disorders, 11,* 305-315.

Gatens, M. (1996). *Imaginary bodies: Ethics, power, and corporeality.* London: Routledge.

Goldner, V. (1985). Feminism and family therapy. *Family Process, 24,* 31-47.

Goodrich, T. J., Rampage, C., Ellman, B., & Halstead, K. (1988). *Feminist family therapy: A casebook.* New York: W.W. Norton.

Hare-Mustin, R. C. (1978). A feminist approach to family therapy. *Family Process, 17,* 181-193.

Israeli, A., & Santor, D. (2000). Reviewing effective components of feminist therapy. *Counseling Psychology Quarterly, 13,* 233-247.

Katzman, M., & Lee, S. (1996). Beyond body image: The integration of feminist and transcultural theories in the understanding of self starvation. *Journal of Eating Disorders, 22,* 385-394.

Luepnitz, D. A. (1988). *The family interpreted: Psychoanalysis, feminism, and family therapy.* New York: Basic Books.

Martz, D., Handley, K., & Eisler, R. (1995). The relationship between feminine gender role stress, body image, and eating disorders. *Psychology of Women Quarterly, 19,* 493-508.

McDaniel, S. H., Hepworth, J., & Doherty, W. (1992). *Medical family therapy: A biopsychosocial approach to families with health problems.* New York: Basic Books.

Walters, M., Carter, B., Papp, P., & Silverstein, O. (1988). *The invisible web: Gender patterns in family relationships.* New York: Guilford Press.

Bibliotherapy Sources for the Client

Fallon, P., Katzman, M., & Wooley, S. (1994). *Feminist perspectives on eating disorders.* New York: The Guilford Press.

McCabe, R., McFarlane, T., & Olmstead, M. (2004). *Overcoming bulimia: Your comprehensive, step-by-step guide to recovery.* Oakland, CA: New Harbinger Publications.

Rhodes, C. (2003). *Life inside the thin cage: A personal look in the hidden world of the chronic dieter.* Colorado Springs, CO: WaterBrook Press.

Schaefer, J. (2003) *Life without ED: How one woman declared independence from her eating disorder and how you can too.* New York: McGraw-Hill Books.

Weiner, J. (2003). *A very hungry girl.* Carlsbad, CA: The Hay House, Inc.

HANDOUT 21.1

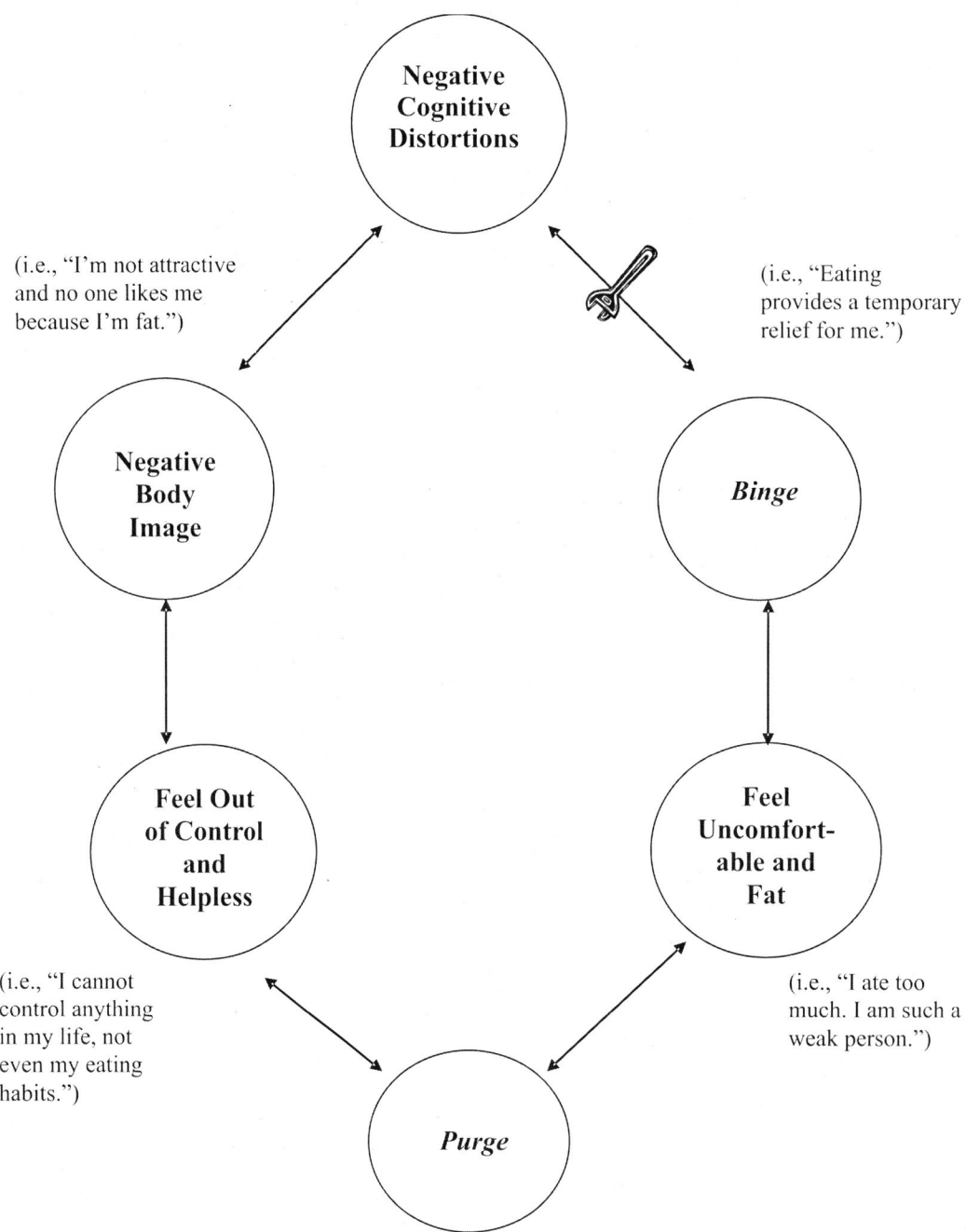

Childs, N.M., & Burwell, S.R. (2007). Put a wrench in it. In D. Linville, K.M. Hertlein, and Associates, *The therapist's notebook for family health care: Homework, handouts, and activities for individuals, couples, and families coping with illness, loss, and disability* (pp. 149-155). Binghamton, NY: The Haworth Press.

HANDOUT 21.2.
Components of the Wrench

(i.e., "This is my option. I can purge all of the negative
thoughts and feelings about myself when I vomit.")

1. _____
2. _____
3. _____
4. _____
5. _____
6. _____
7. _____
8. _____
9. _____
10. _____

Childs, N.M., & Burwell, S.R. (2007). Put a wrench in it. In D. Linville, K.M. Hertlein, and Associates, *The therapist's notebook for family health care: Homework, handouts, and activities for individuals, couples, and families coping with illness, loss, and disability* (pp. 149-155). Binghamton, NY: The Haworth Press.

Chapter 22

Women Caring for Partners with Dementia: A Contextual Model

Christine A. Fruhauf
Jennifer T. Aberle

Type of Contribution: Assessment as Intervention, Handout

Objective

The objective of this assessment model is to provide a basis for intervention to support women caregivers. Specifically, this model emphasizes the variables pertinent to women caring for partners with dementia or a form of dementia (i.e., Alzheimer's disease and related disorders). This contextual model provides therapists with a broad understanding of the important issues that may directly influence clients' well-being and presenting therapeutic issues. Underlying this model is the belief that good therapy and support include comprehensive, sensitive, and contextual assessment of the client's worldview and meaning-making practices. By assessing well-being throughout the therapeutic process, therapists offer a client-centered intervention that respects differences and takes into account a wide range of approaches in easing clients' stress, depression, mental strain, and other presenting problems of women caregivers.

Rationale for Use

As scholars in family gerontology and marriage and family therapy, we recognize the need to assist women who are providing care to their partners. Female caregivers often have multiple roles (i.e., partner, sister, mother, employee, volunteer, etc.) while caregiving that can be overwhelming. In addition, the nature of dementia-type illness can result in unacknowledged losses and grief to a family system, resulting in unresolved grief for caregivers. In this chapter, we present a supportive intervention for family therapist to use when helping women careproviders identify and learn to cope with their caregiving and losses due to their spouses' illnesses. Specifically, we introduce a model for assessing a women's context of caregiving and in this way offer intervention by addressing issues of role conflict, loss and grief, and attuning to resources that are helpful and meaningful to clients.

Caregiving for Individuals with Alzheimer's Disease

The caregiving literature does not hesitate to suggest that caregivers' level of stress is highly related to physical, emotional, and lack of social support status (Biegel & Schulz, 1999; Cahill & Shapiro, 1998; Gallant & Connell, 1998; Kosloski, Young, & Montgomery, 1999). Caregiver stress is often due to lack of sleep, loss of social support, inadequate coping skills, decrease in personal health, and the lack of resources for nutritious foods (Gallant & Connell, 1998). Moreover, when women caring for spouses with dementia experience a decline in their own physical health, there often is a decline in their emotional health and vice versa.

As family therapists, we may not have clients presenting role strain or caregiving as the main reason for therapy. More likely, female caregivers will seek support for symptoms of depression that often stem from the outcomes of multiple roles within a family and/or guilt and multiple losses (e.g., financial loss, loss of "the future," loss of who the partner was, etc.) associated with caregiving. The client's chance of experiencing depression increases by the social pressures to provide care to a partner. Potential complicating factors can be the initial shock of the dementia diagnosis, lack of direction for the future as a couple, and the possible neglect of self. Therapists help clients by recognizing and normalizing these losses and the role conflicts.

By taking a constructivist and contextual perspective about women's caregiving situations, therapists honor their clients' worldviews, expectations for their family, and goals for relieving stress and grief associated with providing long-term care. In this way, assessing women careproviders' unique contexts is essential to appropriate and enduring treatment options.

Assessing Women's Worldview and Life Experience

There is a lack of understanding in the literature about the contextual nature of caregiving and specifically, the issues women face in this role. Understanding the unique concerns, needs, and resources of female clients is important in helping them cope with their situation and make appropriate changes. Like all clients we work with, it is necessary to unfold the layers of influence that bring them hope as well as discouragement in their lives and with the presenting problems. It is important to take into consideration a woman's worldview in order to evade assumptions based on overgeneralized female stereotypes, research findings, our own personal experiences, or commonalities with other clients. If we do not ask the question, "How has your life as a caregiver been for you as a women?," we are ignoring the unique lived experience of that woman. While we believe this question is essential in work with all people of minority statuses (i.e., race, class, sexual orientation, levels of education, etc.), for our purposes we are emphasizing the experience of being a woman. As a therapist using this contextual model to support female caregivers, please include race and all identity experiences when appropriate.

Instructions

Assumptions of Our Assessment Contextual Model As an Intervention

Our contextual model of assessing women's caregiving situations has three primary goals: (1) to consider women's meaning making of current, past, and future variables influencing them, (2) to recognize and augment resources, and (3) to allow for self-reflection to aid in discovery and the creation of energy for change. When we developed this model for assessment we considered the intimate experiences of women's caregiving roles to their partners' as the common interest of all who might use this model. However, we recognize the diversity of women's lives and how they assume their roles as caregivers; hence, this model structures therapy and the view of clients' experiences as emergent and constructed. The distinct nature of one woman's life becomes the foundation for therapy—her situation, what that situation means to her, and her resources for change.

The first goal of this model is to provide the therapist and clients with a broad picture of many (probably not all) of the contextual issues that may be influencing the client's current situation. At times, we may believe that one client is like many others when the presenting problem and surface issues seem similar. The assessment/intervention model presents a more detailed picture of clients' lives, from elements of what influences clients' meaning making to how they cope and internalize socialization of roles and gender expectations. Family and couple therapists often come from training and experience their practice from a systemic orientation. From this perspective a contextual model for understanding women caregivers is a necessity.

The second goal of the assessment model is for the client's own self-reflection and discovery. Many people seek therapy for urgent needs or presenting problems with the hope of establishing a quick resolution. Not all conflict and trouble clients experience are entirely recognizable by them or by therapists in the first few sessions (Gottman & Silver, 1999). Clients require an efficient way to explore their current experiences that takes into account a wide-range of influences. Facilitating clients' self-exploration helps them gain a sense of where their story has been shaped and where they want to go now that they are taking time to reflect.

In the context of caregiving, offering women a way to reflect on their situation is critical to supporting them in therapy. Women in caregiving roles often seek therapy with the purpose to resolve role conflict or disenfranchisement of their experience. They seek therapy for depression or as a result of a physician's referral after being treated for a somatic symptom. By giving women the opportunity to look at the map of their lives through the use of a contextual model, they can explore the salient factors causing the friction or stress in their lives.

The final goal of the model is to help clients recognize and build upon their resources. The model empowers women to make choices that benefit their coping and meaning-making strategies. When women caregivers are given space and time to take into account the many divergent influences in their lives, they may gain a new awareness of helpful patterns and areas in their lives that provide them strength. We call these areas resources. When one is bombarded with tensions and the stresses that caregiving for a loved one produces, it can be difficult and almost impossible to recognize and call upon these resources. Assessing resources is a critical part of the interventional support of this assessment model.

Using the Contextual Model of Women Caregivers for Assessment and Intervention

The Contextual Model of Women Caregivers (CMWC) was developed from a constructivist perspective. The model recognizes the assemblage, manipulation, and creation of meaning based on lived experience (Hoffman, 1988; Watzlawick, 1984). In the context of caregiving for a partner with dementia, women require the respect that a model of these types offers in support of their presenting problem. With this in mind, the assessment and gathering of information enhances therapeutic practices based in almost any theoretical framework. Therapists using brief therapy may find it helpful in denoting the exceptions to depression or any presenting problem. Narrative therapists will note how the assessment of the clients' context unfolds the unhelpful or restrictive story while emphasizing tenets of the preferred story. Cognitive therapists will recognize thought patterns and events that stimulate unhelpful meaning-making processes. Therapists with a strategic orientation will easily be able to map behavioral, event, and thought patterns that produce unhelpful outcomes for clients. Therapists from all orientations can devise intervention that fit their style and understanding of the client's situations.

In this section, we outline the basic elements of the model (see Handout 22.1) and give suggestions for their use. There are five main areas of influence in the model. The first is the woman caregiver as herself. Second are the variables that describe and influence the woman's partner with dementia. Third are the factors that influence and detail the nature of the couple's relationship. Next, we take into account the social influences that affect the client. Finally, we account for the resources of the woman caregiver, both internal and external. The model denotes interconnectedness of all aspects of the female caregiver with circular arrows. As you consider the variables in model, ask yourself these questions:

- What questions and issues would I add?
- What questions and issues are not relevant to my client?
- How does one area of influence affect or change another area?
- What are primary forces in this woman's life?
- What is the interconnectedness of the variables?

Female client as caregiver. This is the primary category of the model as it includes the identifying features and characteristics of the woman herself. With a circle, we hope to represent women caregivers as endlessly constructing meaning, integrating this meaning and transforming as she builds upon her experiences. Clients may not see themselves this way, and we find it empowering to offer them this view through the exploration of the category.

We ask them about the following aspects of their lives:

1. Roles. What roles are you filling right now? What do you do in these roles? How do these roles relate in your life? Or not relate? What roles would you like to keep? Give up?
2. Culture. What is your culture? What is your ethnicity? Who is part of your culture? How is your culture helpful and unhelpful to you?
3. Age/Development. When were you born? How does your age and the historical context in which you have lived influence you today? What meaning have you made of life based on these contexts? How do your developmental needs influence your sense of self and caregiving right now?
4. Self-Care. What is self-care? How do you take care of your self? What supports your self-care?
5. Response to Partner's Illness. How do you feel about your partner's illness? What has this illness been like for you? If the illness was in the room right now, what would it say to you? What would you say to it?
6. Burdens/Losses. What burdens or losses are you currently experiencing? What has this been like for you?
7. Internal Resources. What are your belief systems that give you hope? What brings you courage? What of your experience is a resource to you right now? What do you like most of yourself?
8. Coping Strategies. What is coping? How do you cope? What are coping strategies? What are your most helpful ways of coping? What do you wish of your coping?
9. Additional. Please tell me all that you find important about yourself that we have not covered. What can I know more about in order to understand your life right now?

Partner with dementia. Understanding the partner with dementia will help you better understand what your client is going through as a caregiver. In particular, it is important to understand what symptoms of the illness the care recipient is experiencing as well as the stage of the illness. This section can be used as a way to reassure the client that she is meeting her partner's needs. It may also shed light on how to meet the needs of the client within the context of her partner.

1. Identity of Partner. All about partner—age, developmental needs, culture, resources, coping strategies, enjoyments, dreams, previous experience, etc. These questions are focused on unfolding the client's current view of who her partner is, was, and will become.
2. Nature of Diagnosis. What is your partner's diagnosis? When was your partner diagnosed? Tell me about this time? What was that like for you? Has anyone in your family experienced this before?
3. Trajectory of Illness. What has this illness been like for your partner? For you? How is the illness progressing?

4. Symptoms. What symptoms does your partner display? How do you feel about these? How does your partner feel about these symptoms? (This may be layered in a timeline context.)
5. Medical Care. What is the nature of medical care your partner requires? Who is involved? How do you relate to this medical care?
6. Coping with Losses. How is your partner interpreting losses? How is your partner coping with loss and illness?
7. Additional. Please tell me all that you find important about your partner that we have not covered. What can I know more about in order to understand your partner right now?

Couple's Relationship. Understanding how your clients conceive the meaning of their partnership is essential to your assessment. Some clients may find the grief of their losses in the relationship the most difficult aspect of caregiving. Other clients may describe their relationship as unsatisfactory and the aspect of caring for their partner brings up a lot of confusion about their commitment. The questions in this area of influence unfold clients' understanding of their relationship and how they see themselves in it. Ultimately this section offers tremendous information about how your client relates to her partner—for good and for bad, and all in between.

1. Nature of Relationship—length, ways of relating before and after diagnosis, satisfactions, difficulties, etc. How long have you been in a relationship with your partner? What has this been like for you? What are the best moments of your relationship? What have been some of your struggles? How has your relationship been influenced after the diagnosis of the illness? (These questions may offer an opportunity to witness some of the losses your client is grieving—work to be comfortable with the grief work needed here.)
2. Client in Context of Relationship. How have you seen yourself in relationship with your partner? What do you like about yourself in this relationship? What do you want to be different about yourself in this relationship or about the relationship itself?
3. Major Life Events. Describe the timeline of your relationship–what has happened in your time together? What are the major events, struggles, celebrations in your life together?
4. Future Plans. What future plans did you and your partner have before the illness? What are your plans now if they have changed?
5. Family System. Tell me about your immediate family? Who is important to you and who is important to your partner? How about your extended family? Who are key people for your? Your partner? Who else is your family?
6. Additional. Please tell me all that you find important about your relationship with your partner that we have not covered. What can I know more about in order to understand your relationship right now?

Historical and societal influence. The historical and social contexts in which our clients find themselves can be pivotal information in discerning major influences of their thinking and being. Woman who grew up in the 1950s and 1960s may experience themselves differently than women who were young in the 1970s. The differences are not what is important. Rather, understanding how meaning is made according to powerful historical and social influences can offer clients agency and community.

1. Historical Contexts. On top of the major timeline of your relationship with your partner, what historical events have been significant in your lifetime? How have these shaped you? What is/has been important to you?
2. Social Constructions and Stereotypes. What ideas from society do you value? What notions of women are important to you and how do these affect your identity as a woman?

What stereotypes of women are unhelpful to you? In what ways have these influenced you? What about society is influential to you?
3. Beliefs about seeking help. What do you believe about asking for support? Who do you ask for support? How do you feel about this?
4. Intergenerational Policy. How have governmental, medical, and social policy and law influenced you? What is helpful and what is unhelpful?
5. Media. In what ways do TV shows, movies, books, magazines, and other media influence you? What media do you most interact with? What about it do you like?
6. Additional. Please tell me all that you find important about how society influences you that we have not covered. What can I know more about in order to understand your sense of the world right now?

Resources. Resources come in many shapes and sizes. We want to emphasize here that what might be a resource to one of your clients may be a hindrance to others. It is important that you first ask your client how she defines resource and what she would name as her most significant resources. From here, you can continue with the variables in this section to gain a deeper understanding of her meaning and interpretations of resources. This area of influence can be a shifting point to start a dialogue of intervention. For both information and formal support, be sure to assess the nature of resources from these aspects of the woman's life: family, social, emotional, behavioral, physical, cognition, etc.

1. Informal Support. Who supports your roles? Who supports your culture? Who supports your partner? How? Where do you go for support?
2. Formal Support. What organizations or groups support you (and in what roles)? What do they offer? What do you want more of from these groups? What organizations or groups support your partner? How is this helpful or unhelpful to you? What do you want more of from these groups?
3. Financial. How does your financial situation influence your experience of caregiving?
4. Medical. Describe the medical support that you and your partner receive? Who is on your medical team that is a resource to you and your partner? What medical needs do you have? How are they being met?
5. Spiritual. What gives you courage? What brings you hope? What offers you strength? What gets you through your tough days?
6. Additional. Please tell me all that you find important about resources that we have not covered. What can I know more about in order to understand your resources right now?

Brief Vignette

A client, who understands herself as a partner and a primary careprovider to her spouse struggling with dementia, may have conflicting thoughts and be unresolved about how to behave as a partner in a relationship that has become less fulfilling and unsatisfactory and perhaps is much more demanding than ever before. Understanding her perceptions of familial and nonfamilial roles, culture, self-care, etc., will allow for the client to believe the therapist is taking her seriously as well as provide a solid foundation for the client to begin making meaning with her caregiving experiences. Examining the person with dementia and his or her experiences with the illness as well as prior to, will also allow the therapist to better meet the needs of the client. For example, if the partner with dementia is at an advanced stage of dementia and has struggled with the illness prior to therapeutic intervention, this may present itself with more challenges than if the partner with dementia is in the early stages of the disease or did not struggle earlier.

Exploring with the female caregiver the many variables that have emerged to shape her new relationship with her husband in the context of the dementia illness will allow the client to be able to also reshape her needs, capacities, and willingness to take on a new role in the relationship. If the couple seeks therapy together and their primary goal is to maintain and/or increase marital satisfaction in the midst of the dementia illness, the therapist will need to consider both partners' experiences of these relationship factors. In this case, the therapist will want to expand all factors for both clients in effectively assessing the influence of context and meaning making on the couple's lives. Finally, historical and social context may impact the female caregiver and her partner if both were socialized to not ask for help and do things on their own. It may mean that the therapist will have to reassure that seeking therapy is a good decision as opposed to those clients who were not influenced by that social phenomenon.

In this way, the contextual intervention helps the couple understand each other's sense of who they are (individually and as a couple), what the illness is, and the myriad of factors and resources at play that have and will influence their future. The contextual intervention allows the couple to explain and discover their situation from each individual's point of view, and recognize differences and similarities among their meaning making and put into play coping strategies for achieving their martial satisfaction goal in the context of one partner's dementia illness.

Contraindications for Use

Female caregivers may also be experiencing conflict with children and/or other family members that may impact their success while in therapy. It might be necessary for the therapist to use this model when meeting with the client one-on-one. It is recommended that the therapist follow up with the activity listed in Chapter 29 to support the entire caregiving system especially when the partner with dementia is nearing his or her end of life.

References

Biegel, D. E., & Schulz, R. (1999). Caregiving and caregiver interventions in aging and mental illness. *Family Relations, 48,* 345-354.

Cahill, S. M., & Shapiro, M. M. (1998). "The only one you neglect is yourself": Health outcomes for carers of spouses or parents with dementia. Do wives and daughters carers differ? *Journal of Family Studies, 4,* 87-101.

Gallant, M. P., & Connell, C. M. (1998). The stress process among dementia spouse caregivers. Are caregivers at risk for negative health behavior change? *Research on Aging, 20,* 267-297.

Gottman, J., & Silver, N. (1999). *The seven principles for making marriage work: A practical guide from the country's foremost relationship expert.* New York: Three Rivers Press.

Hoffman, L. (1988). Constructing realities: An art of lenses. *Family Processes, 29,* 1-12.

Kosloski, K., Young, R. F., & Montgomery, R. J. V. (1999). A new direction for intervention with depressed caregivers to Alzheimer's patients. *Family Relations, 48,* 373-379.

Watzlawick, P. (Ed.). (1984). *The invented reality.* New York: Norton.

Readings and Resources for the Professional

Martin-Cook, K., Trimmer, C., Svetlik, D., & Weiner, M. F. (2000). Caregiver burden in Alzheimer's disease: Case studies. *American Journal of Alzheimer's Disease, 15*(1), 47-52.

Roberto, K. A., Richter, J. M., Bottenberg, D. J., & Campbell, S. (1998). Communication patterns between caregivers and their spouses with Alzheimer's disease: A case study. *Archives of Psychiatric Nursing, 12,* 202-208.

Wright, L. K. (1993). *Alzheimer's disease and marriage.* Newbury Park, CA: Sage.

Bibliotherapy Sources for the Client

Mace, N. L. & Rabins, P. V. (1999). *The 36 hour day: A family guide for caring for persons with Alzheimer's disease, relating illnesses, and memory loss in later life.* New York: Warner Books.

Mittleman, M. S., & Epstein, C. (2003). *The Alzheimer's health care handbook: How to get the best medical care for your relative with Alzheimer's disease, in and out of the hospital.* New York: Marlowe & Company.

Smith, D. C. (1997). *Caregiving: Hospice-proven techniques for healing body and soul.* New York: Macmillian.

HANDOUT 22.1.
Contextual Model of Women's Caregiving Experience

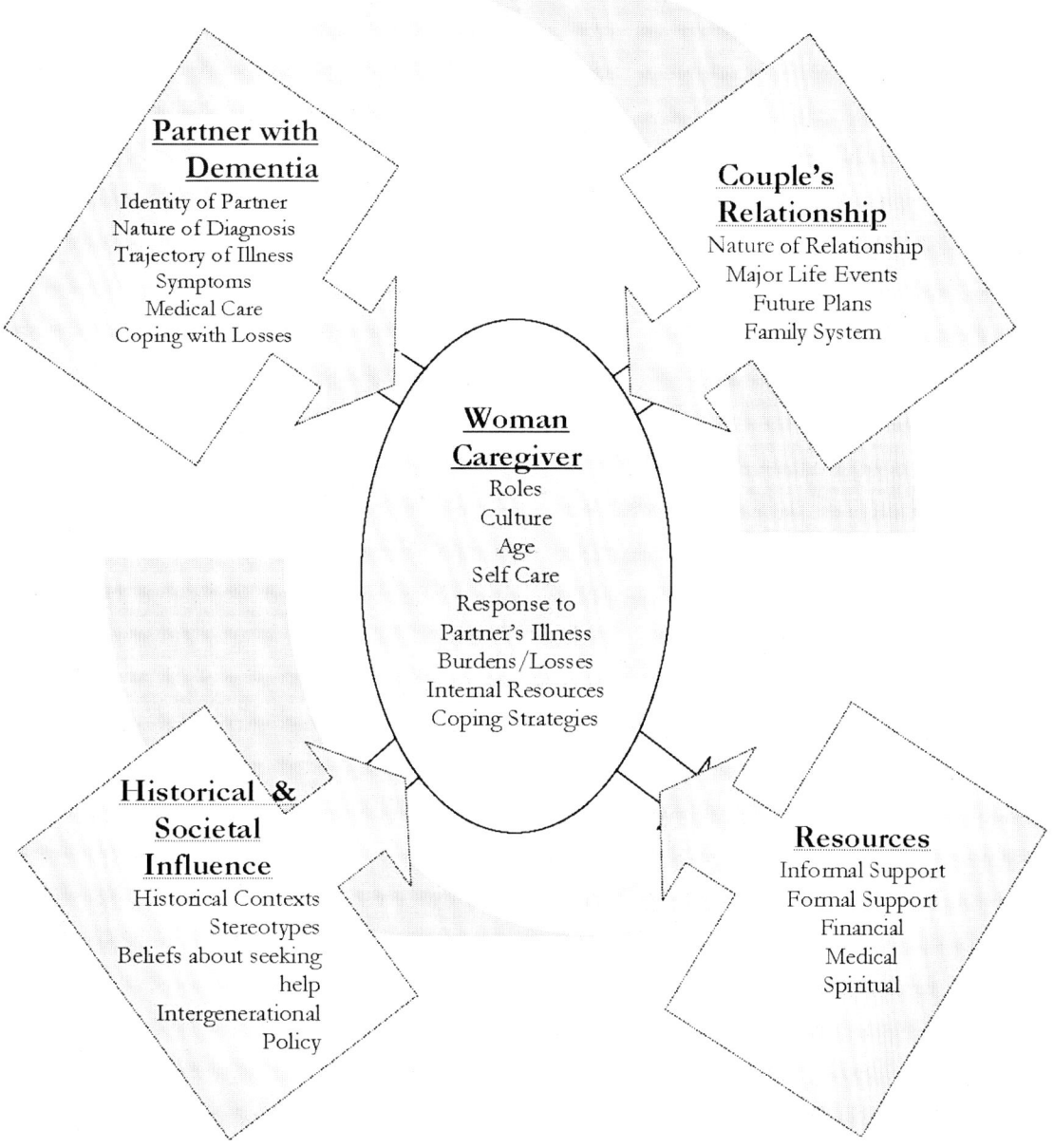

Fruhauf, C.A., & Aberle, J.T. (2007). Women caring for partners with dementia: A contextual model. In D. Linville, K.M. Hertlein, and Associates, *The therapist's notebook for family health care: Homework, handouts, and activities for individuals, couples, and families coping with illness, loss, and disability* (pp.157-165). Binghamton, NY: The Haworth Press.

Chapter 23

Inviting Resiliency to Join the Family's Journey with Cancer

Anne Prouty Lyness

The faces of the people in my office were pale. Not just the typical New England white of their stalwart, French-Anglo culture, but withdrawn and drained. I sensed a tension, the protective type, as my typical joining questions were met with short, quiet answers from the two, tall, athletic, teenage boys. After several minutes, the forty-year-old mother with the new diagnosis of breast cancer broke the silence by saying, somewhat loudly, "I'm still here and you boys are just going to have to get used to the idea of growing up." New England pragmatism had joined us and would open the door to this family's journey with cancer.

Type of Contribution: Intervention

Objective

The purpose of this chapter is to introduce family therapists to one use of a feminist-informed construction of resiliency as an organizing principle for therapy with families as they find themselves beginning an unpredictable medical treatment regime, one that is often unpredictable in its course and in its effects on the patient and the family.

Rationale of Use

Talking about cancer develops differently in families. The word *cancer,* the diagnosis, and the wide variety of meanings and treatments can pose an endless morass for families. Some become frozen, rigid in a familiar or new and unfamiliar structure. Some become chaotic in structure, flexible in leadership, flexible in goals, finding or never finding a balance. Some use staunch or paper-thin denial; others rally to a battle cry. Most families with whom I've worked have had a variety of responses. It is important to help families to get a mindful start to the journey of living alongside a chronic illness and its treatment: so as not to overwhelm their system by organizing solely around the illness for too long. Slowing the process, or even giving people permission to acclimate a bit slower than light speed (too prevalent a mandate in American popular culture) and then helping them to take a brief meta-look at their old patterns, and choices for new patterns has worked well to help families to construct a personal understanding of their style of resiliency.

The construct of resiliency is not new within family intervention and family research literature. McCubbin and McCubbin (1988) proposed a "Resiliency Model of Family Stress, Adjustment, and Adaptation" that included family schemata as a central construct in coping with stress. Family schema involves the meaning a family assigns to stressful events such as illness and the patterns of functioning they develop around that meaning (McCubbin, McCubbin, & Thompson, 1993). Others have talked about a family's world view (Patterson & Garwick, 1994), belief system (Antonovsky, 1979, 1987), and family paradigms (Reiss, 1981; Reiss & Oliveri, 1980). Researchers increasingly consider resilience to be a family-level construct because of the importance of family interactional processes and shared beliefs in the health of family members. Family researchers have pointed to several family level variables that appear to distinguish well-functioning from dysfunctional family patterns, such as: cohesion, flexibility, open communication, and problem-solving abilities (Beavers & Hampson, 1990, 1993; Epstein, Bishop, Ryan, Miller, & Keitnor, 1993; Moos, 1986; Olson, 1993; Olson, Russell, & Sprenkle, 1989). Building upon this, Hilton (1993, 1994, 1996) developed basic qualitative inquiry into how families talk about breast cancer. I found Hilton's research intriguing because she proposed that denial was potentially an aspect of resiliency for some families.

It is also important that resiliency not be confused with invulnerability or rugged individualism (Walsh, 1998), concepts too often revered in white American culture. I prefer more interpersonal and flexible constructions of resiliency such as, "relational hardiness" (Walsh, p. 4), "struggling well" (Walsh, p. 5), interdependence, shared efforts at shifting and reshifting interpersonal boundaries and responsibilities, and sharing of emotional work. These more interpersonal constructs of resiliency have often been valued in African-American families and in cultures around the world (Boyd-Franklin, 2003; McGoldrick, Giordano, & Pearce, 1996). Many of my clients, facing different issues, have reported that they resonate with the concept of "struggling well." Walsh's phrase seems to validate, normalize, and honor people's experiences, giving them permission do be doing well while still being in pain and being in the middle of their lives' stressors. These interpersonal constructions of resiliency allow for the *integration* of the crisis (Walsh, 1996) into the emotional unit of the family, so that resiliency becomes a process along the journey, not an endpoint. I have found these constructions to fit well with looking at families' propensities to shift in amounts of cohesion, flexibility/adaptability, and methods of problem solving and communication—because all of these interpersonal processes shift over normal development as well as during times of crisis.

Instructions

1. Pre-First Session Assessments: FACES-III, FCOPES, and Emotion Work Scale

Often, as a part of my joining and getting to know the family's interpersonal style, I ask families to complete three short assessment tools that I believe give me information from which to help them get back in touch with or to craft their style of relational hardiness: FACES-III (Olson, Portner, & Lavee, 1985); Family Crisis-Oriented Personal Evaluation Scale (F-COPES) (McCubbin, Larsen, & Olson, 1985); and the Emotion Work Scale (Wharton & Erickson, 1995). I ask all adult and teen members to bring the completed assessments to the first session. By doing this, I set the stage for therapy to be a group effort that will include everyone's perspectives. I also start clients thinking about their perspectives regarding coping with stress, closeness, distance, adapting to change, and emotional work strategies and preferences within their family. I believe it helps people begin to take a metaperspective.

2. First Session: Explore everyone's perspectives of who they were, as a family, prior to the cancer diagnosis and how they envision the cancer treatment potentially changing their family's routines and relationships

During the first session, I focus on hearing where the family has been: what they have enjoyed and with what they have already struggled. We discuss how each of their experiences is influenced by people and systems (schools, medical, work, etc.). We begin to talk about the cancer diagnosis and how each of them understands and feels about it. I have found that I can help families begin to get in touch with their style of resiliency by discussing, mapping, or sculpting how they have addressed major challenges in the past and how this might inform how they will live with cancer and its treatment. I feel this provides a compass for their journey into the unknown—only they know their family and their social system.

3. Draw a genogram and ecogram to locate and emphasize resiliency

In the second and/or third sessions, the family draws an intergenerational family genogram (McGoldrick, Gerson, & Shellenberger, 1999) within an ecomap (e.g., Hartman, 1995): A family tree of relational patterns situated within the community systems they define as the most influential community systems. When the definition of family is extended to important people and animals, most of the people with whom I've worked have readily included kinship networks, close friends, and pets or horses. Then, they have discussions about which larger systems are the most influential and how. Usually, schools, churches, work, and the new medical contacts are chosen as primary. This process of mapping, talking, and focused noticing (punctuation) often helps families develop skills at metacommunication to connect with one another about their relationships and priorities. We begin a gentle investigation (via curiosity and gentle questions, direct and circular) about the family's historical style of resiliency—usually pervasive within their history, but not always part of their previous dominant story (see narrative therapy, e.g., Freedman and Combs, 1996). I may or may not, depending on how overwhelmed they report feeling, send a copy of the in-process genogram project home with them to add to between sessions. If they wish to do so, I may assign small projects. For example, I may ask a family to notice and make a list of the things they each do, and what they notice others doing, to live alongside cancer this week (see, for example, Lipchick, 2002).

Brief Vignette

This case description provides an example of a family developing their story of resiliency. To facilitate finding this story, I used three assessment instruments, a genogram, and an ecogram. The family was able to join together to *begin* their journey with cancer. This stage is sometimes referred to as the crisis stage of cancer (Rolland, 1994), and this family was able to begin by *establishing an experience* of their family's legacy of resiliency: being able to have faith in their family to live with the emotional and physical challenges that cancer treatment might bring them.

Intake. Sharon, a fifty-year-old, working-class, French Catholic woman and her two sons, John, twelve, and Michael, fourteen, called for family therapy at the suggestion of Sharon's primary care nurse practitioner. The father had died in surgery when John was two and Sharon was scheduled for surgery, for what she hoped would be a lumpectomy, in two weeks. During the phone conversation to set the first appointment, Sharon reported that they were in shock about her diagnosis, and she thought the boys needed to talk about what they were feeling not only about her diagnosis, but also to do some grieving about their father—something the family had not discussed much. She wanted to have at least two sessions before her surgery. We set up two family therapy sessions, and I sent her the packet of family assessments by mail.

Looking at the Assessments and Formulating Questions. Remarkably (I very rarely see this in families with teens), the boys and Sharon had very similar FACES-III scores. They all agreed they lived in the flexibly (borderline chaotic) enmeshed range prior to the diagnosis, with the boy's ideal families being slightly less connected, and Sharon's ideal family remaining the same as their current one. The FCOPES revealed that Sharon's major forms of coping were spiritual/church, family, friends, and faith in her family to deal with problems. Both of the boys checked friends, sports, watching television, and faith in their family to deal with problems.

Only Sharon had completed the Emotional Work Scale, as she thought the boys would give her too big a hassle over it. She rated herself as providing significantly more emotional work for the boys than they did for her, but that they did a bit more for each other by being good friends and encouraging each other around sports. Perhaps because this was a single-parent family, Sharon indicated that there was no one within the family unit with whom she could share her innermost thoughts and feelings, provide her with compliments, do her favors without being asked, express concern for her well-being, or discuss their relationship future.

First Session. I introduced myself and the therapy process and ethics, briefly looked over the assessments, and then proceeded to tell the boys that I knew about the cancer but that it would be helpful to tell me about their family first. The boys each said a few words about the sports they liked, and Sharon talked about her work, her book club, and her church activities. Then there were several minutes of silence. After their initial quiet and Sharon's suggestion that the boys needed to address growing up as a means to deal with her illness and its treatment, I suggested that it might be helpful if they thought back to other experiences they'd had with big changes, transitions, and illness. The boys talked about changing schools and moving to the next town when they were in middle school. They talked about joining teams and changing sports throughout the seasons. Sharon talked about changing jobs. It was during this discussion that I interwove the clarification questions about what Sharon had identified as their family preferences on the FCOPES and Emotional Work Scale. They were able to talk about their facility making new friends, Sharon's sister's family, and their holiday rituals, and Sharon's involvement with her parish and her spiritual life. The boys said they believed in God, but they didn't go to mass nor did they have a family patron saint.

Almost at the end of the first session, Mike brought up his dad's death and absence. This initiated a family talk about their fear of losing Sharon, and how angry the boys felt that they might now lose their mom after already losing their dad. We briefly talked about our culture's lack of models for grieving and fear, and how dad's death and legacy within each of his sons has probably meant a little something different to both of them over the years. I wondered aloud how this initial thought, this initial connection with their father's life, death, and legacy might affect their family. Might their husband/father help them to connect to resources (inside and outside their family) they had not habitually noticed until now? Might their father and his death lend some inspiration to discovering how they wanted to navigate, together, through this cancer surgery and their future? Might they have some kind of family ritual to honor his absence, invite his presence, and mark their embarkment into their future?

Second Session. When they returned three days later, the boy's baseball caps were off and I could see their eyes. They talked about Sharon having made a birthday cake for their dad and the boys putting on candles that relit despite being blown out. They talked about eating most of the cake in one sitting. We discussed how each of them felt while preparing for and doing this ritual and what each of them had begun to think about since. Because they were mostly talking about connections to other people, I began a family tree within a diagram of their community support systems (a genogram within an ecogram) so I could reflect back to them their connections and barriers to their dad and the other important people and resources in their lives. I integrated questions from the information I had gathered from the assessments about their preferred methods of coping and how they might use them to emotionally and practically prepare for Sharon's surgery.

In the course of a longer discussion during which they took turns adding to the diagram on the wall, Sharon told the boys that she had called her lawyer and was updating her will. She verified with them that they wanted her sister and brother-in-law to be their guardians in case she died. She also told them that her brother-in-law had volunteered to stay with them while she was in the hospital. The boys decided to each tell one friend and their favorite coach what was happening in their lives. Mom talked with the parish priest who said he would be sure to visit her prior to and after surgery. I started to reframe all the connections they were forming and the steps they were outlining as evidence of their resiliency emerging in regard to living their lives alongside cancer, and whatever it might bring with it.

This family was able to define resiliency as: recognizing ways they had dealt with past challenges; accessing resources to continue their life as a family; and having faith that they might struggle, but much like playing an unknown number of innings (they were into baseball), they would win a few and sometimes feel pretty winded and bruised, but unlike a sporting event, only they got to decide what winning meant. They wondered if the game might at times take on a Jumanji-like (Van Allsburg, 1981) twist, but they'd decide what those twists would mean for them as they appeared. I remember John wondering aloud what they would be like this time next year; he had a sense that they'd be similar but different. At the end of session, somewhat out of the blue, Michael suggested they clean up more and start doing their chores to help mom out more—more pragmatism. I integrated that into my end of session summary and wonderings.

I summarized the resiliency themes for the session and then suggested: (1) Sharon: I wonder if each of the boys were to have his own, special, support person, who were options she trusted? Was there something of their father's she might give to each boy? Was there something of hers? (2) Boys: What might you want your mom to know? How will you let your friend, coach, family know when you need support? What kinds of support might you need? What tasks can you learn to do around the house to begin to share the workload?

Suggestions for Follow-Up

I have found that facilitating the experience of resiliency as an interpersonal process, a journey of living alongside cancer and its treatment, is easily extended throughout family therapy during the various stages of treatments for serious illnesses and chronic illnesses. Resiliency is not an all-or-nothing concept; it permeates a person and a family's being in the world. They can have bad days, weeks, and months and still be able to see themselves as struggling well. I have also found that families have been able to see themselves as resilient, even when the loved one dies, because resiliency remains in their experience of their entire journey.

Contraindications for Use

I have found that assessments, genograms, and ecograms help facilitate people's ability to equilibrate to a constructive therapeutic tempo. Whatever the family system needs—to go slower, faster, to be more focused, or more flexible—they take what they need from the process and use it to get them where they need to go. Like all visual interventions, if clients have difficulty processing visual information, these tools might need to be adjusted or they may be contraindicated. If clients cannot read, or if the assessments are not in their primary language, the therapist could cover the same information during a more structured first session, or you may need the instruments translated into the dialects of the languages spoken in your area. If the children are of preschool age, these methods might be contraindicated and more age-appropriate therapy that includes play as the mode of communication and reality construction might be better. I have used similar interventions (assessments, genograms, and ecograms to find resiliency patterns) with families struggling with understanding how to live alongside major mental illnesses in a hospital setting, so I do not believe that severe mental health struggles pose a contraindication to this therapy focus or these methods, although the assessments may need to be adjusted or delayed.

References

Antonovsky, A. (1979). *Health, stress, and coping: New perspectives on mental and physical well-being.* San Francisco: Jossey-Bass.

Antonovsky, A. (1987). *Unraveling the mystery of health: How people manage stress and stay well.* San Francisco: Jossey-Bass.

Beavers, W. R., & Hampson, R. B. (1990). *Successful families: Assessment and intervention.* New York: W.W. Norton.

Beavers, W. R., & Hampson, R. B. (1993). Measuring family competence: The Beavers Systems Model (pp. 73-103). In F. Walsh (ed.), *Normal family processes* (2nd ed.). New York: Guilford.

Boyd-Franklin, N. (2003). *Black families in therapy.* New York: Guilford.

Epstein, N. B., Bishop, D. S., Ryan, C., Miller, I., & Keitnor, G. (1993). The McMaster model: View of healthy family functioning (pp. 138-160). In F. Walsh (Ed.), *Normal family processes* (2nd ed.). New York: Guilford Press.

Freedman, J., & Combs, G. (1996). *Narrative therapy.* New York: W. W. Norton.

Hartman, A. (1995). Diagrammatic assessment of family relationships. *Families in Society, 76,* 111-112.

Hilton, B. A. (1993). Issues, problems, and challenges for families coping with breast cancer. *Seminars in Oncology Nursing, 9*(2), 88-100.

Hilton, B. A. (1994). Family communication patterns in coping with early breast cancer. *Western Journal of Nursing Research, 16,* 366-391.

Hilton, B. A. (1996). Getting back to normal: The family experience during early stage breast cancer. *Oncology Nursing Forum, 23*(4), 605-614.

Lipchik, E. (2002). *Beyond technique in solution-focused therapy.* New York: Guilford.

McCubbin, H. I., Larsen, A., & Olson, D. H. (1985). F-COPES: Family crisis oriented personal evaluation scales. In D. Olson, H. McCubbin, H. Barnes, A. Larsen, M. Muxen & M. Wilson (Eds.), *Family inventories* (revised edition). St. Paul, MN: Family Social Science, University of Minnesota.

McCubbin, H. I., & McCubbin, M. A. (1988). Typologies of resilient families: Emerging roles of social class and ethnicity. *Family Relations, 37,* 247-254.

McCubbin, H. I., McCubbin, M. A., & Thompson, A. I. (1993). Resiliency in families: The role of family schema and appraisal in family adaptation to crises (pp. 153-177). In T. H. Brubaker (Ed.), *Family relations: Challenges for the future.* Newbury Park, CA: Sage.

McGoldrick, M., Gerson, R., & Shellenberger, S. (1999). *Genograms: Assessment and intervention.* New York: W. W. Norton.

McGoldrick, M., Giordano, J., & Pearce, J. K. (1996). *Ethnicity and family therapy.* New York: Guilford.

Moos, R. H. (Ed.) (1986). *Coping with life crises: An integrated approach.* New York: Plenum Press.

Olson, D. H. (1993). Circumplex Model of marital and family systems: Assessing family functioning (pp. 104-137). In F. Walsh (ed.), *Normal family processes* (2nd ed.). New York: Guilford.

Olson, D. H., Portner, J., & Lavee, Y. (1985). *FACES III*. St. Paul: Family Social Science, University of Minnesota.

Olson, D. H., Russell, C. S., & Sprenkle, D. H. (Eds.). (1989). *Circumplex Model: Systemic assessment and treatment of families*. Binghamton, NY: The Haworth Press.

Patterson, J. M., & Garwick, A. W. (1994). Theoretical linkages: Family meanings and sense of coherence (pp. 71-89). In H. I. McCubbin, E. A. Thompson, A. I. Thompson, & J. E. Fromer (Eds.), *Sense of coherence and resiliency: Stress, coping, and health*. Madison WI: University of Wisconsin Press.

Reiss, D. (1981). *The family's construction of reality*. Cambridge: Harvard University Press.

Reiss, D., & Oliveri, M. E. (1980). Family paradigm and family coping: A proposal for linking the family's intrinsic adaptation capacities to its responses to stress. *Family Relations, 29*, 431-445.

Roland, J. (1994). *Families, illness, and disability: An integrative treatment model*. New York: Basic Books.

Van Allsburg, C. (1981). *Jumanji*. Boston: Houghton Mifflin.

Walsh, F. (1996). The concept of family resilience: Crisis and challenge. *Family Process, 35*(3), 261-281.

Walsh, F. (1998). *Strengthening family resilience*. New York: Guilford.

Wharton, A. S., & Erickson, R. J. (1995). The consequences of caring: Exploring the links between women's job and family emotion work. *Sociological Quarterly, 36*(2), 273-296.

Chapter 24

Exploring Mood Differences: Sports Car and K-Car Metaphor

Nancy Taylor Kemp

Type of Contribution: Activity, Homework, Handout

Objective

This activity was created for families in which one or more members have bipolar disorder (manic-depressive illness). The goal of this activity is to increase understanding between family members diagnosed with bipolar disorder and family members who may not struggle with mood instability. This activity can be especially useful for shifting family member's focus from criticism and blame to viewing contrast with curiosity, ultimately leading to acknowledgements of each family member's strengths and contributions to the whole.

Rationale for Use

Bipolar disorder is a chronic, cyclic mood disorder effecting approximately .4 to 1.6 percent of the population (American Psychiatric Association, 2000). Although individuals are often first diagnosed with bipolar disorder (BPD) in their early twenties, an increasing number of children and adolescents are being diagnosed with the disorder, in what appears to be the same incidence rate as adults (Evans, Beardslee, Biederman, Brent, Charney, Coyle, et al., 2005). The onset of BPD typically occurs during the normal developmental phase in which adolescents are individuating from their nuclear family. Bipolar disorder is a cycling mood disorder that has periods of depression (a deeply depressed or irritable mood with compromised function) and at least one of period of mania (a highly euphoric or irritable mood with compromised function). Early in the illness many individuals experience an intermingling of these symptoms in what is labeled a "mixed" episode. Two-thirds of individuals with BPD experience months, if not years, of normal mood and functioning between the mood episodes. In fact, many people with BPD are quite bright, creative, and high achieving. During episodes of the illness, family members often report frustration, confusion, and helplessness related to the changes in the functioning level (and interpersonal interactions) of the person with BPD.

There appears to be a genetic component in bipolar disorder and many families have both a parent and a child with the illness (American Psychiatric Association, 2000). In fact, families with a child with BPD (onset before age fifteen) are twice as likely as to have an additional relative with bipolar disorder than families in which BPD has an adult onset (Leboyer, Henry, Paillere-Martinot, & Bellivier, 2005). Understanding of the illness, coping strategies, and positive communication skills are essential for all families with a BPD member, as research has shown that maintaining noncritical family relationships leads to fewer symptoms of the disorder over time (Johnson & Meyer, 2004).

Children with bipolar disorder often struggle with extreme mood fluctuations, which for some can include rages leading to threats or acts of violence against siblings or parents. They also may have periods of hypersexuality, report vivid nightmares of a macabre quality, and when feeling blue report thoughts of death or suicide. Children with BPD vacillate between periods of high functioning when they may accomplish a great deal of goal-directed activity and excel in their schoolwork, and other periods when parents note that they appear unwilling or incapable of focusing on their homework, and avoid prosocial play activities. At these times, their social interactions may have a quality of hyperactivity, sullenness, or aggression. For many children with BPD, social and academic performance is ever fluctuating, leading parents to infer that problems are related to poor motivation or deliberate misconduct.

Recognizing BPD in adolescents can be a challenge, as even normal teen years are commonly fraught with mood swings, limit testing, and behavior changes as a result of peer group influences. As well, adolescent alcohol and drug use can mimic the symptoms of BPD. Adolescents with BPD mania may experience high surges of energy that last for days if not months at a time. They often report little to no need for sleep (which is uncommon in non-BPD adolescents) and exhibit rapid and pressured speech with difficulty maintaining silence and involvement in numerous projects without adequate follow-through to completion. An adolescent with bipolar depression may withdraw from social activities, miss classes, sleep too much, appear preoccupied with death, and struggle with intense irritability that may erupt into rage. Both children and adolescents may experience hallucinations or develop distorted perceptions of reality (delusions) when their manic or depressive episodes become severe.

One of the greatest challenges for BPD families is developing coping strategies and crisis plans without losing the healthy identity of the BPD individual by overidentifying the individual with the illness. Parents become frightened on their child's behalf and may become hypervigilant to any signs of mood changes that could indicate instability, which creates tension between the parent(s) and the individual with BPD. The risks to BPD families are very real: strong suicidal feelings are common during depressive episodes, and up to 15 percent of BPD individuals ultimately complete suicide. Prevention efforts are appropriate, as suicide is the third leading cause of death for adolescents in the United States (Evans, Beardslee, Biederman, Brent, Charney, Coyle, et al., 2005).

Balancing symptoms of mood episodes with affirmation of and respect for the individual's strengths and contributions helps to strengthen a child or adolescent's self-image and sense of value in the family unit. Often in therapy, family members report anger and frustration related to the BPD individual's behaviors, and this can lead to pathologizing of the BPD member, which can easily move to defensive stances and a breakdown in family communication. Criticism and negating responses can quickly and negatively escalate, and emotional responses can lead to moving into defensive postures. As the family members polarize, communication breaks down and no gains occur around the creation of coping strategies for the illness, nor understanding of each member's experiences and perspectives. In their research on family interaction patterns and symptom management of bipolar illness, Miklowitz and Goldstein (1997) found that criticism, hostility, emotional overinvolvement, and conflictual interactional patterns were correlated to higher rates of relapse in BPD.

This intervention was created to enhance communication between family members in family focused treatment for bipolar disorder. The goals of family focused treatment (FFT) are to assist family members (including the patient) in six areas: Integrating experiences associated with episodes, accepting a vulnerability to future episodes, accepting the need for psychotropic medication, recognizing and coping with stressful events that can trigger episodes, distinguishing between the person and the disorder, and re-establishing functional family relationships (Miklowitz & Goldstein, 1997).

The specific target of FFT is to reduce tension in the family relationships, improve internal communication to increase understanding, and to assist in developing problem-solving strategies. In their research of family interaction patterns, Miklowitz and Goldstein (1997) found that "parents of bipolar patients are more likely to exhibit a specific form of communication deviance, that is, 'contorted, peculiar language'.... Their messages are understandable but jumbled, with many unnecessary words or words used out of order. We suspect that these kinds of speech errors occur when family members or patients are anxious, hurried or perhaps ambivalent about the message they are conveying" (p. 51). FFT's "communication enhancement training" uses exercises to express positive feelings, increase active listening, and change the structure and function of family relationship interaction patterns. By helping family members to increase their curiosity about the other's views and meaning, and by making specific, positive requests for change, family members have a better outcome for success (Miklowitz & Goldstein, 1997).

The following activity encourages the family to clarify its communication and move away from engaging in generalized (of personality rather than to specific behaviors) critical comments that result in defensive responses and negative escalation. It allows all family members to acknowledge both strengths and weaknesses which normalize that everyone has struggles and/or symptoms (the *spreading the affliction* intervention) which in turn helps to destigmatize the individual(s) with BPD. This activity helps to balance potential distorted simplifications of the illness (overidentification leading to hypervigilance around symptoms, or under-identification denying the illness and finding personal fault) with accurate information related to strengths and to symptoms. It also provides an arena to discuss role disputes between family members in a narrative context (via metaphor) that allows the nondefensive investigation of realistic options (Frank & Swartz, 2004). The ultimate goal is decreasing stress within the familial environment, as research supports that a posthospital patient returning to a stressful family environment is more likely to experience reoccurrence of an episode (Miklowitz & Goldstein, 1997).

Instructions

Before introducing this exercise, the therapist should assess the general affective tone (criticism, sorrow, compassion) between the family members to determine if enough goodwill exists to allow members to participate fully in the exercise. The therapist may wish to identify specific goals for the family's struggles ("a lot of mind reading is occurring, and this exercise will help give a more accurate picture of what the other people are thinking"), or specific instructions in precise terms if communication difficulties are resulting from overly vague language. If the family is having difficulty defining problems clearly and then resolving the problem, it is better to conduct the exercise in session with facilitation by the therapist.

Introduce this activity in midsession when family members begin to become polarized around how an event or situation "should have" been handled. This activity is most effective when "stable" family members are expressing frustration or disbelief about a BPD individual's inconsistent functioning and symptom set. Begin by stating that at times it is easier to explore differences between people by thinking about how we easily accept differences between things, such as the vehicles we use. Continue: "For example, at times we need a car that can carry many people, and at other times we may need a truck for hauling. Most types of cars have benefits and drawbacks at different times. If you think about engines and performance, it is sometimes helpful to think of an individual with BPD as being like a sports car. When they are in tune, they are high-performance vehicles that can outperform most other vehicles in speed, ability, and flare. The downside of many sports cars is that they need regular maintenance and tinkering, and they need repairs more often. Non-BPD individuals may relate more to being a K-car, an everyday sedan that will run each morning and meet basic needs, but isn't a flashy performer."

Ask each family member to identify the type of vehicle that he or she most relates to or identifies with and why. Have members identify the strengths of each vehicle, and facilitate a discussion of how the different vehicle types interplay as a family fleet. As a homework assignment, ask the family members to complete the "What type of vehicle are you and why?" handout individually, then share each of their vehicle types and strengths with one another. After the strength-building exercise, ask the family to discuss how they can work together as a fleet of vehicles to meet all of the family's needs. Ask the family to create specific strategies to use the fleet most effectively, with the least wear and tear on all vehicles. With late adolescents with BPD, this exercise can be extended to explore what options or strategies need to be in place when the family fleet is no longer as available because the individual is living alone or otherwise individuated.

Brief Vignette

Janna, a twenty-two-year-old Euro-American female, had been in individual therapy for four weeks because of severe depressive symptoms, including sleeping much of the time, social withdrawal, missing her college classes, and heavy binge drinking. She had been attending college for three-and-a-half years, with only two years of college credit to show for her efforts. Janna had been diagnosed with Bipolar I Disorder three years earlier. Several of her college terms had been interrupted by extreme mood symptoms that contributed to failing grades and late course withdrawals that resulted in tuition money spent without earning any credits. Although her parents were supportive of her the first term this occurred, the family relationships had become strained around the cost of Janna's education, her (perceived) destructive behaviors, and everyone's dashed hopes. Janna had become increasingly ashamed about her performance and withdrew from communicating with her parents. She reported that the idea of suicide was a more attractive option than "hearing another speech about how I'm not disciplined, have bad judgment, and don't try hard enough."

Janna requested that her mother join her for a family therapy session focused on her bipolar illness and the struggles she was having in school. At the family session, Janna's mother shared openly her frustration with her daughter's "inability to stay focused on her studies when she was the brightest student in her high school," and then stated that the family could not afford to pay college tuition "forever." Janna responded defensively with "But I can't study when I'm depressed," and her mother replied that she herself had worked full time and put herself through school, so she knew that it could be done by someone as bright as Janna with a little consistency and effort. Janna slumped back in her chair, folded her arms, and responded "You just don't get it, and you never will." Janna's mother turned to the therapist and said, "I don't know why I even try to get through to her."

Recognizing that both family members had taken on defensive postures and were no longer responding to the concerns of the other, the therapist suggested that the problem might be more easily explored in looking at the differences between the two women rather than deciding what "should have" occurred. The therapist shared that sometimes it is easiest to think of a metaphor that exemplifies basic differences between individuals. The therapist surmised that living with bipolar disorder can be a bit like being a sports car: When one is running well, it can outpace any other car at premium performance, but alas, it gets out of tune easily, and needs a lot of tinkering. The therapist then shared with the mother that "most people are a bit more like K-cars, the more pragmatic midrange sedans without the extra bells and whistles." She continued, "K-cars start up every morning and get the basic job done. They are reliable, but generally aren't very flashy."

The therapist asked the two to compare how each is similar to and different from a sports car and a K-car. Janna laughed and said, "I'm a sports car alright, but I've totally broken down."

Janna's mother nodded and stated that "Janna is an amazing girl." The mother then shared that in college she could always keep going, no matter how tired she was, but that she was never the stellar student Janna could be. As the two drew the metaphor out further, each was able to name the strengths that their own style brought both to the world and to their family. Laughing again, Janna turned to the therapist and said, "I think my dad is a tank." Coming to his defense, her mother stated that much of the time he is just worn out from working so hard. The therapist reminded them that all models have their strengths, and the two women agreed that dad actually was more of a pickup truck that could transform into a powerful tank during family crises.

The mother and daughter were sent home to flesh out the metaphor further by identifying different strengths of each vehicle type and determining how their family could utilize their fleet most efficiently. They were also asked to develop a plan based on reasonable expectations for each type of vehicle (clarifying that the pragmatic vehicles cannot be overutilized or they will not last). The therapist reminded Janna that it is an extra challenge to have a sports car as one's only vehicle. The ride can be incredible, but there must be a back-up plan for when the car isn't running very well.

The following week Janna returned to therapy with her mother. They reported that they had come to a compromise about funding and that Janna would get a small part-time job to subsidize her educational costs. Janna reported that during the strength-building portion of the homework exercise she realized that she actually broke down less whenever she had a job. She remarked that this was probably because it forced her to go out and be social, and gave her something positive to do when she couldn't concentrate as well on her studies. Janna further said that she felt proud to be a sports car, and that she and her mother had spent time talking about career choices that might fit a sports car the best. Janna acknowledged that she strongly relies on her mother's stability. She stated that she didn't know what she would do without her mother's K-car nature. Janna made a commitment to manage her medications and sleep more responsibly, to help to keep her car in running condition. Janna's mother agreed to read *Touched with Fire* (Jamison, 1993), a book about all the talented individuals with bipolar disorder, as a way to remember that although her daughter struggled at times, she remained capable of great things. Janna and her mother identified that Janna didn't need advice about what she should be doing, because she already knew. Janna did ask that her mother continue to provide emotional support for the pain and frustration she experienced. At the end of the meeting, Janna's mother reported that she had also decided to purchase bicycle for Janna, both because Janna loves bicycling, and because she knows that exercise might also help to avoid future breakdowns. She joked, "Shouldn't everyone have a bike in their trunk in case of a breakdown?"

Suggestions for Follow-Up

The therapist can follow-up by asking the family the following: (1) What strategies or back-up arrangements might assist the client or her family when she is not in top condition? For example, can she arrange to work at home on these days, have a mechanic (psychiatrist) on call, or a can of carburetor cleaner (additional medication) available? (2) Ask the family to work together to identify the major contributors to the sports car beginning to run roughly, and ask if any routines or expectations could change to reduce wear and tear on the sports car. (3) Are there certain journeys that are especially hard on the car? Are there journeys that the other vehicles are making that the sports car is better suited to make?

The therapist may also ask the family to work on a protocol for responding to a sudden and complete breakdown of the sports car. What are the diagnostics that can guide whether to wait and see, add some carburetor cleaner (additional medicine), or to take the car in for a complete servicing (hospitalization)? Whose job is it to get a mechanic involved and when?

Another follow-up activity is to have the family examine if their fleet is not meeting certain necessities (for example, if the fleet is comprised of specialty vehicles) and have them create a plan for getting these needs met. Are they going to rent additional vehicles (hire someone to do the task), live without the necessities, or take turns using their vehicles for unintended purposes and deal with the wear and tear? The therapist may need to work with the family around creating clear problem statements, coming to compromises, and developing concrete action plans.

Families may also develop their own metaphors. If they are useful for clarifying the situation, help them to extend their own metaphor.

Contraindications for Use

This exercise is appropriate for use with any family where alterabled individual's strengths and ways of coping need to be further understood and honored. This exercise is likely to be ineffective for young family members who cannot understand the concept of vehicle differences embedded in the metaphor. As alluded to in Janna's comment about her father, this exercise is not recommended for families displaying a great deal of contempt between members, as the metaphor will likely be used for further criticism of the individual with BPD.

This activity is most suited to families where members have highly distinct differences in levels of mood stability. For families in which some members have health conditions that consistently and severely limit activities of daily living without periods of partial to full remission, creating a vision of one "family car" in which members provide different components (the entertainment system, the drive train, etc.) may be more effective than separate vehicle identities.

References

American Psychiatric Association (2000). *Diagnostic and statistical manual of mental disorders (DSM-IV-TR)* (4th ed., text rev.). Washington, DC: Author.
Evans, D. L., Beardslee, W., Biederman, J., Brent, D., Charney, D., Coyle, J., et al. (2005). Defining depression and bipolar disorder. In D. L. Evans, E. B. Foa, R. E. Gur, H. Hendin, C. P. O'Brien, M. E. P. Seligman, & B. T. Walsh (Eds.), *Treating and preventing adolescent mental health disorders: What we know and what we don't know* (pp. 3-27). New York: Oxford.
Frank, E., & Swartz, H. A. (2004). Interpersonal and social rhythm therapy. In S. L. Johnson & R. L. Leahy (Eds.), *Psychological treatment of bipolar disorder* (pp. 162-183). New York: Guilford Press.
Jamison, K. R. (1993). *Touched with fire: Manic-depressive illness and the artistic temperament.* New York: Free Press.
Johnson, S. L., & Meyer, B. (2004). Psychosocial predictors of symptoms. In S. L. Johnson & R. L. Leahy (Eds.), *Psychological treatment of bipolar disorder* (pp. 83-105). New York: Guilford Press.
Leboyer, M., Henry, C., Paillere-Martinot, M., & Bellivier, F. (2005). Age at onset in bipolar affective disorders: A review. *Bipolar Disorders* 7(2), 111-118.
Miklowitz, D. J., & Goldstein, M. J. (1997). *Bipolar disorder: A family-focused treatment approach.* New York: Guilford Press.

Readings and Resources for Professionals

American Psychiatric Association (2002). Practice guideline for the treatment of patients with bipolar disorder (revision). Available: www.psych.org/psych_pract/treatg/quick_ref_guide/Bipolar_org.pdf.

Frank, E. (2005). *Treating bipolar disorder: A clinician's guide to interpersonal and social rhythm therapy.* New York: Guilford Press.

Johnson, S. L., & Leahy, R. L. (2004). *Psychological treatment of bipolar disorder.* New York: Guilford Press.

Miklowitz, D. J., & Goldstein, M. J. (1997). *Bipolar disorder: A family-focused treatment approach.* New York: Guilford Press.

Bibliotherapy for Clients

Copeland, M. E. (2003). *Living without depression & manic depression: A workbook for maintaining mood stability.* Oakland: New Harbinger Publications.

Fast, J. A., & Preston, J. D. (2004). *Loving someone with bipolar disorder.* Oakland: New Harbinger Publications.

Fawcett, J., Golden, B., & Rosenfeld, N. (2000). *New hope for people with bipolar disorder.* New York: Prima Publications.

Jamison, K. R. (1993). *Touched with fire: Manic-depressive illness and the artistic temperament.* New York: Free Press.

Jamison, K. R. (1995). *An unquiet mind.* New York: Knopf Press.

Miklowitz, D. J. (2002). *The bipolar disorder survival guide: What you and your family need to know.* New York: Guilford Press.

Papolos, D. M., & Papolos, J. (2002). *The bipolar child: The definitive and reassuring guide to childhood's most misunderstood disorder (rev. ed.).* New York: Broadway Publishing.

Web Sites for the Family

Child & Adolescent Bipolar Foundation www.bpkids.org
Depressive and Bipolar Support Alliance www.dbsalliance.org
National Alliance for the Mentally Ill www.nami.org

HANDOUT 24.1.
What Kind of Vehicle Are You and Why?

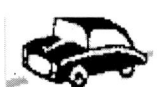   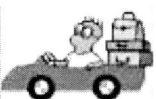   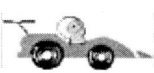

Standard K-car   Hatchback   Sports car

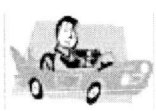   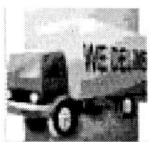   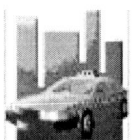

Convertible   Truck   Taxi

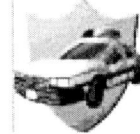   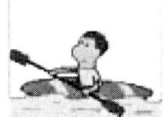   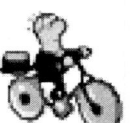

Emergency Vehicle   Kayak   Bicycle

What are your strengths and benefits?

What are your drawbacks or weaknesses?

Do you have additional alternative vehicles as well? When are they used?

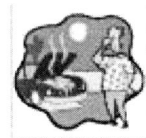   What is your plan for when you break down?

Kemp, N.T. (2007). Exploring mood differences: Sports car and K-car metaphor. In D. Linville, K.M. Hertlein, and Associates, *The therapist's notebook for family health care: Homework, handouts, and activities for individuals, couples, and families coping with illness, loss, and disability* (pp. 175-183). Binghamton, NY: The Haworth Press.

HANDOUT 24.2.
The Family Fleet

I. What is your fleet of vehicles? What assets does each bring?

II. List the basic needs of the family. Which vehicles meet which needs?
   (Money, fun, socializing, love, future stability, pride, problem solving, knowledge, creativity, etc.)

   <u>Needs</u>   <u>Vehicle(s)</u>

III. Are there needs that your fleet doesn't meet? Are some vehicles being used more than others? List specific areas or needs that your fleet must find a way to cover. How will you cover these needs?
   (Hire someone outside the fleet to do them? Learn a skill to meet them? Share the burden across the fleet?)

Kemp, N.T. (2007). Exploring mood differences: Sports car and K-car metaphor. In D. Linville, K.M. Hertlein, and Associates, *The therapist's notebook for family health care: Homework, handouts, and activities for individuals, couples, and families coping with illness, loss, and disability* (pp. 175-183). Binghamton, NY: The Haworth Press.

SECTION IV:
INTERVENTIONS FOR WORKING WITH GRIEF AND LOSS

Chapter 25

Story Squares: Creating a Dialogue with Grieving Children

Tiffany B. Brown

Type of Contribution: Activity, Handout

Objective

The purpose of this activity is to provide a child with the means to communicate his or her experience of a death in a safe manner. By giving children the tools to share their experiences, the dialogue regarding their grief can begin to unfold. This is also an intervention that may be used in therapy with siblings and family sets.

Rationale for Use

The purpose of this activity is to present the child and the clinician with an opportunity to create a dialogue about grief. The death of a loved one impacts our lives in various ways, whether the death is anticipated or unexpected. We live in a "death denial" culture as it is not characteristic to discuss our experiences of a death with one another (McGoldrick, 1991). While most clinicians agree that a large percentage of their clients have experienced the phenomena of grief and loss, there is still a scarcity of resources for clinicians on how to handle grief in session. Professionals may be mirroring the experience within a family; death can be difficult to discuss and many are not sure where to begin. McDaniel, Hepworth, and Doherty (1992) discuss how many clients may want to talk about death, although the discussion may be uncomfortable. As a society we have a hard time approaching the topic of grief and loss and the therapy room is often not an exception.

Children are not exempt from struggling with grief and loss and they may experience grief as intensely as adults. Children often lack the emotional vocabulary to express their grief with others (Nida & Pierce, 2000). When a death occurs in a child's life the feelings and emotions attached to the loss can be difficult to communicate. It is common for the needs of children and adolescents not to be properly acknowledged or understood by adults (Corr, 1999). Moreover, important adults in children's lives are often grieving alongside the children so it can be hard for them to accurately see how the grief is impacting the child. As McGoldrick and Walsh (2005) point out, children will often cover up their own grief in order to protect their bereaved parents

---

This activity is adapted from Courageous Kids, a grief support program for children and adolescents in Eugene, Oregon.

from more anxiety. Adults may turn to clinicians to assist in helping their child and family cope with the overwhelming experience of a loved one's death.

In this activity, the child is given a means for expressing his or her grief in a developmentally appropriate way. The expression of feelings through an art project can be a useful way to share what can otherwise be challenging to do verbally. The therapist is given the opportunity to see what the child knows regarding the death and how he or she experiences the loss.

There is a therapeutic value in using realms of play therapy with children. As Gil (1994) points out, the main approach with children in therapy is play because it is an innate mode of self-expression. Art has long been used as a way to express oneself; more specifically, it serves as an excellent means of expression for children. In therapy, it provides a useful tool in understanding the world of the child and gives the child an opportunity to express emotions. It also allows children to share their truths and their experiences—their stories.

Therapists have long attempted to access the story the individual or family has created. The Mutual Storytelling Technique (MSTT) is aimed at hearing an original story from the child (Gardner, 1993). In addition, narrative therapy reflects a similar focus, seeking to understand the stories clients have created in order to reconstruct new and more productive stories (Nichols and Schwartz, 2002).

Instructions

This activity is designed to be an in-session task and is relatively simple to organize. It could be used as an assessment tool and/or as an intervention at a designated point in the therapy process. Therapists first need to gather materials and create a workspace for the child prior to the session. A large piece of art paper is desired, approximately 11" × 14" works best. Also needed is an array of art supplies such as crayons, markers, pens, pencils, colored pencils, oil pastels, etc. It is important to have choices available so that children are able to find their own means of expression.

The paper is to be folded in half, and then half again, creating four equal squares. Each square will serve a different purpose in this project. The upper-left quadrant will represent the question "Where were you when it happened," the upper-right quadrant will represent "What happened," the bottom-left quadrant will represent "What was it like," and finally, the bottom-right quadrant will represent "How are you now." See Handout 25.1 for a diagram.

The option of drawing or writing is offered to the child in order to give him or her the freedom of expression in the form that is most comfortable. The therapist then allows the child the space to complete the project independently. It is important for the child to have the opportunity to work without suggestions or ideas from the therapist. Often in the process of grief there is an expectation that one should be "doing it the right way." To counter this expectation during projects related to the process of grief, a child should be given the control back to direct his or her own experience. As the therapist, it is helpful to remind yourself that there is no right or wrong way to express grief and that you should be respectful of the personal process that is associated with this project.

It is likely that a child will not be able to complete one of the squares. For example, the child may not remember where he or she was when it happened (upper-left quadrant), or have the information yet of how the death occurred (upper-right quadrant). Noticing whether the child completes all four squares may be helpful to see what the child knows and does not know. At this point in the therapy, it may be useful to include other family members who can share additional information with the child, if that is what the child wants. It may also be a useful time to include other family members in order to create in-session dialogue about shared grief associated with the death. This dialogue is likely to leave the therapy room and continue at home.

Dependent on the child's comfort level, it might be appropriate for the therapist to also participate in this project. Although it would require some self-disclosure on the part of the therapist, it would be an opportunity to share experiences of grief. For a child to see an adult who has had a similar experience is a powerful gift. Such revelation may begin a process of normalizing the experience of grief and may begin to challenge the tendencies to deny death. The therapist may work on his or her own story squares at the same time as the child. It is important for therapists to be aware of their own personal process so as not to supersede the child's experience. For example, the therapist's process may overtake the session if he or she is unable to stay connected to the child's work due to the intense focus on their own. In addition, it would be detrimental if the emotions of the therapist overwhelmed the session and the child was put in the position of caretaker.

Upon completion of the project, a discussion regarding the content and the process is appropriate. Some questions could be:

- Tell me about your project.
- What words come to mind when you are looking at your squares?
- How would you describe what it was like when it happened?
- How would this look different if your mom (or dad, sibling, grandparent, friend, etc.) did this project?
- Is there anything you would like to add now that you have taken a break from working on it?
- What was it like to work on this project?
- What kinds of feelings did you have as you worked on this project?

It is important that the therapist not attempt to make interpretations as to what the child must mean with different drawings. If the therapist is curious about particular parts of the story square, he or she should ask the child if it is okay to ask a few questions about the picture. The interpretations therapists are likely to make are based on their own assumptions and may not be an accurate depiction of the child's process. The therapist should also allow time for the child to ask questions regarding the therapist's story square if he or she participated in the project. Giving the child the freedom to ask questions of the therapist can be a very significant addition to the joining process. This dialogue may open up other therapeutic topics regarding the child's grief.

Based on the therapist's understanding of the child's comfort level, a conversation about the project is encouraged. Therapists are also encouraged to engage other family members in this discussion if it makes sense for the particular case. It may also be appropriate to do this project with the entire family, with each member doing his or her own story square and sharing it with the family in therapy. The therapist should consider the involvement of the family as a means to share the grief experience of the child. Including the family should be considered as a means to discus how each member experiences the grief process. It may benefit the family to understand each person's perspective and how this experience relates to the entire family process. This will also give the therapist the opportunity to learn more about the experience of grief in the family and how that may impact the child. Regardless of the constellation that presents in therapy, this project may serve as an appropriate means to open the dialogue about each person's grief process.

It is okay if the child does not want to talk about the drawing. He or she will do his or her own processing while engaging in the project. It is important to respect the unique way each child engages or does not engage with the project. Once the child feels safer in the therapy room, it may make sense in subsequent sessions to revisit the story square.

Brief Vignette

Thomas phoned requesting services for his daughter, Jennifer, age eight, following the death of her paternal grandmother from cancer. Thomas was separated from his partner and was the primary caregiver to Jennifer. He mentioned in the initial phone call how the death of his mother has been particularly hard for him and he felt he had not been able to be as supportive of Jennifer as he would have liked. Thomas reported that Jennifer was having difficulty in school and had withdrawn from her friends and other adults. He requested that she come to therapy to talk about her grandmother to someone who would not "break down crying." The first appointment was scheduled as a family session and most of the session was spent introducing therapy to the clients and building a therapeutic relationship. Jennifer was relatively withdrawn in session and did not share much about her grandmother. Thomas did most of the talking as he discussed how hard the death had been and the difficulties he had functioning at work. He also expressed his concern for Jennifer and her "not dealing with the death." He stated he was unsure how she was doing and did not know how it was affecting her. Jennifer did not have much to say about the death, as it seemed she had difficulty explaining her feelings. At the end of the session, Thomas requested that Jennifer attend alone next session. Jennifer agreed and was scheduled for an individual session.

Recalling the experience of the first session, the therapist planned to use the story square activity to give Jennifer an alternative way to express her grief. When Jennifer arrived for the session, a few pieces of art paper were out and an array of art supplies was displayed. The beginning of the session was spent talking about school and how the week went in order to continue the joining process. The therapist asked Jennifer if she would like to do an art project and she excitedly agreed as she noticed the variety of art supplies available.

The therapist explained to Jennifer how to fold the paper, folding once and then folding in half again to create story squares. The therapist told Jennifer what each square represented, "The first square is to draw or write about where you were when your grandma died. The second square is for you to draw or write what happened to your grandma. The third square is for what it was like for you and the fourth square is for how you are doing now." The therapist answered the questions Jennifer had about which art supplies she could use by telling her they were all available. The therapist told Jennifer she could write or draw in each square and to request if she needed a bigger piece of paper or different art supplies. The therapist then started to build her own story square and worked simultaneously with the child.

Upon completion of the project, the therapist asked Jennifer to tell her about her picture. Jennifer shared how she was at school when she found out that her grandma died and how her dad picked her up after lunch. She talked about how her dad was crying a lot when they drove home and she remembers having pizza that night for dinner. Jennifer explained that was why she drew a picture of her school and pizza. Jennifer continued sharing and said she did not know much about how it happened, other than that she was at the hospital for "a really long time." The therapist asked if she ever went to visit her and Jennifer talked about the times she was able to visit the hospital and play games with her grandma. A conversation unfolded about the visits at the hospital and what they were like for Jennifer.

The therapist asked Jennifer to talk about how she is doing now. Jennifer had drawn many pictures of sad faces in her square and one happy face. Jennifer explained that her happy face is because she knows her grandma does not have to be sick anymore, but it still makes her really sad that she died. She continued to explain that it makes her sad to see her dad cry so she works really hard to stay happy.

Toward the end of the session the therapist asked Jennifer if she had any questions for her about her story square. Jennifer asked a few questions about how the therapist felt when her friend died. The therapist shared how she felt really sad and confused and missed her friend a whole lot. Jennifer said that is how she feels and did not know others felt that way, too.

The session concluded with an agreement to continue talking about these ideas. The therapist also asked Jennifer if she would like to work on this project in the future to which she agreed. Subsequent sessions included deeper discussions about how much she loved her grandmother and what she is going to miss the most. Toward the end of the therapy process Thomas was brought in and participated in family sessions. The two of them were able to begin talking about how they are going to honor Jennifer's grandmother and keep her memories a part of their life. Jennifer was also able to start sharing how she was feeling with her dad without feeling guilty about making him sadder.

This activity was a good experience for this client as evidenced by her engagement in a dialogue about her grief experience. The activity gave Jennifer a means to express herself and allowed her the opportunity to talk about the impact of her grandmother's death. It also gave some relief to her father as he was having a difficult time with his own grief. Giving Jennifer the opportunity to tell her story normalized her feelings and emotions regarding the death.

Suggestions for Follow-Up

There are a few suggestions for follow-up for this activity. It may be used as an assessment tool to give the therapist some information about what the child knows regarding the death. Prior to termination, this activity may be again used to gauge what has changed over the course of therapy. It may be a useful way to show the child his or her own growth and progress with the grief. The child may have learned new things about the death, or may feel differently about how he or she is doing now.

The therapist may include the entire family in the story square activity; a child may be more willing to participate if the family also does a story square. When the activity is used in a family session, it is best if the entire family participates to avoid singling out one member.

It may also be valuable to have the child take his or her drawing home to share with the family. However, it would be necessary to follow-up with the child in a subsequent session about how it went and how he or she experienced sharing with the family. This may not be appropriate for all clients, as it would depend on the presence of a safe environment at home.

If using this activity in a family session, homework assignments could be given to the family to discuss in more detail the elements of the story square. Certain topics may emerge in the therapy room, such as what each family member needs or how they are experiencing their grief. Again, any way to extend the conversation from the therapy room to home will assist in normalizing the discussion of the person who's died and the process of grief.

Contraindications for Use

This activity may not be useful for a client who was not engaged in a relationship with the individual when they died. For example, it may not be helpful for a child with a death of a parent whom they never met. In such cases, there may be other activities that better address the client's circumstances. Like all activities in therapy, the safety of the client is most important. The therapist should assess the environment and make a decision about how this activity will impact them emotionally.

Even if a child does not know much about the death, if the child had a relationship with the person who died, the activity may be useful. The lack of information about the death may end up being a place to start in processing the grief experience.

In working with children with disabilities, it is best to consider the adaptive methods the child has already employed to compensate for his or her disability. If the child has a vision disability it may be appropriate to verbally go through each square asking what the child would draw and what that would look like. The visual imagery may be a new way for the child to discuss his or her grief. In addition, if the child lacks motor capabilities he or she may have the use of a mouth pen that may be used for this project. In the case of any disability, it is best to consult with the parent(s) and discuss the adaptive methods the child has and discuss how to best modify activities in session.

References

Corr, C. A. (1999). Children, adolescents, and death: Myths, realities, and challenges. *Death Studies, 23,* 443-463.

Gardner, R. (1993). Mutual storytelling. In C. E. Schaefer & D. M. Cangelosi (Eds.), *Play therapy techniques* (pp. 199-211). New Jersey: Jason Aronson.

Gil, E. (1994). *Play in family therapy.* New York: Guilford Publications.

McDaniel, S. H., Hepworth, J., & Doherty, W. J. (1992). *Medical family therapy: A biopsychosocial approach to families with health problems.* New York: Basic Books.

McGoldrick, M. (1991). Echoes from the past: Helping families mourn their losses. In F. Walsh & M. McGoldrick (Eds.), *Living beyond loss: Death in the family* (pp. 50-78). New York: W. W. Norton & Company.

McGoldrick, M., & Walsh, F. (2005). Death and the family life cycle. In B. Carter & M. McGoldrick (Eds.), *The expanding family life cycle: individual, family, and social perspectives* (pp. 185-201). New York: Allyn & Bacon Classics.

Nichols, M., & Schwartz, R. (2002). *The essentials of family therapy.* Boston: Allyn & Bacon.

Nida, R., & Pierce, S. (2000). Children's social and emotional development: Applications for family therapy. In C. Everett Bailey (Ed.), *Children in therapy: Using the family as a resource* (pp. 428-474). New York: W.W. Norton and Company.

Walsh, F., & McGoldrick, M. (1991). Loss and the family: A systemic perspective. In F. Walsh & M. McGoldrick (Eds.), *Living beyond loss: Death in the family* (pp. 1-29). New York: W. W. Norton & Company.

Resources for the Professional

Dougy Center for Grieving Children. (1999). *35 ways to help a grieving child.* Portland, OR: The Dougy Center for Grieving Children.

Fogarty, J. A. (2000). *The magical thoughts of grieving children.* New York: Baywood Publishing Company.

Lamberti, J. W., & Detmer, C. M. (1993). Model of family grief assessment and treatment. *Death Studies, 17,* 55-67.

Rycroft, P., & Perlesz, A. (2001). Speaking the unspeakable: Reclaiming grief and loss in family life. *Australian and New Zealand Journal of Family Therapy, 22,* 57-65.

Webb, N. B. (2002). *Helping bereaved children.* New York: The Guilford Press.

Bibliotherapy for the Client

Buscaglia, L. (1982). *The fall of Freddie the leaf: A story of life for all ages.* New Jersey: SLACK Incorporated.

Heegaard, M. (1988). *When someone very special dies: Children can learn to cope with grief.* Minneapolis, MN: Woodland Press.

Krasney Brown, L., & Brown, M. (1996). *When dinosaurs die: A guide to understanding death.* NY: Little, Brown Young Readers.

Mundy, M. (1998). *Sad isn't bad: A good-grief guide book for kids dealing with loss.* St. Meinrad, IN: Abbey Press.

Simon, N. (1986). *The saddest time.* Morton Grove, IL: Albert Whitman & Company.

HANDOUT 25.1

Where were you?	What happened?
What was it like?	How are you now?

Brown, T.B. (2007). Story squares: Creating a dialogue with grieving children. In D. Linville, K.M. Hertlein, and Associates, *The therapist's notebook for family health care: Homework, handouts, and activities for individuals, couples, and families coping with illness, loss, and disability* (pp. 187-194). Binghamton, NY: The Haworth Press.

Chapter 26

Open Up a Window

Miriam Claire Godwin

Type of Contribution: Activity

Objective

The purpose of this activity is to encourage couples who have recently experienced a loss or the diagnosis of an illness or a disability to explore how the loss or diagnosis has or will influence their couple relationship through a Biopsychosocial-spiritual lens. This activity is based on the saying, "When God closes a door, He opens a window." This activity may take several sessions to complete.

Rationale for Use

The saying, "When God closes a door, He opens a window" has been used in times of despair, sadness, and many other difficult emotions that result from news of illness or a disability of a loved one or oneself. The phrase is used to comfort people that feel as if God has "closed a door" or if there has been a loss of something, whether it be the loss of a loved one through death, the loss of an idea, or the loss of a dream for a child's life that is changed with the diagnosis of an illness or disability. The phrase "opens a window," intends to offer comfort by telling individuals that another opportunity or "window" will come into their life.

This activity is intended to encourage the couple to explore what the "door" is being closed on, as well as what is outside their "window," or rather their future. By exploring what is outside a "window," clients may begin to see the possibilities that await them and support them in strengthening a sense of hopefulness about the illness or loss they have experienced. This use of reframing in discussing an illness or loss can assist the couple in viewing the challenge in a "different light" and help them see the positives in their situation more clearly. Reframing is an important part of many family therapy theories, but it is most often used in narrative therapy. Narrative theorists use reframing to help clients change their "negative stories" into their "preferred" stories, which often include positive elements (Freedman & Combs, 1996).

Instructions

The activity can be conducted simply by conversation, or it can be facilitated through the use of art. The couple can be encouraged to paint, draw, or sculpt what they "see outside of the window" during the activity. If art is chosen, the clinician will need the typical supplies for the art technique choosen. Paper, paints, and brushes are needed if the couple chooses to paint. If the couple chooses to draw, needed supplies are pens, pencils, colored pencils, and paper. Finally, if a couple chooses to sculpt, then clay or play dough is needed.

In this activity, the "door" is a metaphor for anything the couple is facing that poses a challenge to them in some way (such as a loss or medical diagnosis). The "closing of the door" can also mean the ending of some sort of hope or dream for the couple (example, a couple recently lost their young son in a car accident, so the "door closing" for them might represent the loss of their hopes and dreams for their son's life).

In this activity, the "window" represents a new possibility for the clients (such as their future together). To "look out the window" can mean to look into the future and see the possibilities that await the couple in their life after the diagnosis or loss has occurred (example, a couple recently found out that their oldest daughter has been diagnosed with multiple sclerosis, so to "look out the window" for them might represent looking into the future of their family and thinking of ways in which the illness will influence their family functioning). The purpose of using the "window" metaphor is to help clients view their world through a biopsychosocial-spiritual lens so that they may fully appreciate the impact the illness or loss will have on their lives.

The clinician should begin the activity by discussing with the couple the saying "When God closes a door, He opens a window." The couple's feelings and thoughts about the saying should be explored and how they feel it applies to their current situation.

After discussing the phrase, the clinician processes with the couple what the "closing of their door" was in their lives (the diagnosis of illness or a loss) and their thoughts and feelings about the experience. The clinician explores with the couple if they have noticed any changes in their couple relationship since the diagnosis of illness or loss.

The clinician should then explore with the couple what is "outside their window." Clients are given the opportunity to openly express their thoughts about the concept and what they "see" outside the "window" after the "door" has been "shut." The clinician works with the couple in using their words or an art technique (mentioned previously) to explore and describe what is outside their "window." If the couple chooses to use art, they should create the work together to promote a sense of connection and teamwork in relation to the diagnosis or loss.

The clinician asks the couple to identify a room in their house that symbolizes their friends and family in some way (i.e., "What room comes to mind when you think of gathering with friends or family?"). The couple should then be asked to "look out" the window in that room. The clinician might ask them questions such as, "How does the 'door shutting' influence your family and how you as a couple are a part of the family? What do you see out of the window of this room? What is your future as a family going to be like after learning of the diagnosis or loss?"

The couple is then asked to identify a room in their house that symbolizes their marital relationship (i.e., the bedroom, the living room) and then they should "look out" the window of that room. The clinician might ask them questions that encourage them to focus on how the diagnosis/loss has or will influence their marital relationship. The "windows" in the rooms that symbolize their friends, family, and couple relationships should focus the couple on how the diagnosis or loss will influence them socially.

The clinician should then focus the couple on the biological influence the diagnosis/loss will have on their relationship. The couple should identify a room in their house that symbolizes their health in some way (i.e., the bathroom) and "look out" the window in that room. The clinician should process with the clients how the diagnosis/loss has or will influence their physical health by asking questions such as: "Have you noticed any physical changes in yourself or your partner since learning about the diagnosis or loss? What physical changes might you expect to encounter as you begin coping with the illness or loss? How have or how will these physical changes influence your relationship with each other?"

Next, the clinician engages the couple in a dialogue about the psychological influence the diagnosis/loss will have on their relationship. The couple can identify a room in their house that is a place they can seek privacy or be alone with their thoughts. The clinician asks the couple to "look out" the window in that room and share how the illness or loss has or will influence their psychological well-being. The clinician could ask, "Have you noticed any emotional changes since learning about the illness or loss? Have you noticed any emotional changes in your partner? How might the illness/loss change your thought processes? How will these changes influence your relationship as a couple?" The clinician should assess for safety if a client states he or she is thinking of harming themselves or others and ensure the client does not have a plan to commit a harmful act.

Lastly, the clinician should focus the couple on processing how the diagnosis/loss will influence their spirituality. The clinician should ask the clients to pick a room in their house through which they could imagine viewing their place of worship. The couple should then "look out" that window and the clinician should ask them how the illness/loss will influence their spirituality/religiosity as a couple. The clinician could ask questions such as: "How has your spirituality influenced your ability to cope with the illness or loss? Has your involvement with your place of worship increased since your diagnosis or do you anticipate it will? Have you noticed any spiritual changes in your partner? How will the illness/loss influence the spiritual component of your couple relationship?"

Brief Vignette

Brack and Bev G. came to therapy because they recently lost their son, Jack, in a hunting accident. Their therapist, Judi, discussed with them the phrase, "When God closes a door, He opens a window." Judi encouraged the couple to process how the phrase related to their recent loss and how they have been coping with the loss. Judi processed with the couple what their "door closing" was (the loss of their son) and what "windows" have opened in their lives (becoming closer as a couple through the loss).

Brack and Bev decided they wanted to work with Judi in completing the "Open Up a Window" activity and they chose to paint together throughout the activity. Judi supported the couple in painting what they "saw out of their windows" as they looked into their future. Judi worked with the couple in anticipating how the loss would affect them in relation to their physical health, their emotional/mental health, their social relationships, and their spirituality.

Judi asked the couple to choose a room in their house that represented their physical health in some way. The couple decided their kitchen represented health and then they were asked to look out the "window" in that room and discuss how the loss of their son has or will impact their physical health. The couple worked together in painting a picture of them appearing very skinny and "weak" and shared that they felt the loss had negatively impacted their physical health and diminished their appetite. The couple anticipated that they would continue to decline in physical health while coping with the loss of their son.

Judi asked the couple to choose a room in their house that represented their emotional or mental health. The couple chose their bedroom because they said it was where they felt privacy and time to be "alone." The couple was asked to "look out the window" in this room and discuss how they felt the loss of their son was going to impact their emotional or mental health. The couple worked together in painting a picture depicting them as being very "sad" and "upset." The couple shared that the loss of their son would continue to negatively impact their emotional health for many years to come.

Judi then asked the couple to choose a room in their house that represented their social relationships. The couple chose their living room because they said it was where they gathered with friends and family during holidays and other special occasions. Judi asked the couple to "look out of the window" in that room and share how they felt the loss would impact their social relationships. The couple painted a picture of them surrounded by friends and family members, sitting on their living room couch. The couple shared that they felt their social relationships would improve in the future because their friends and family had already demonstrated a desire to "be there for us" and maintain close contact after their loss.

Judi asked the couple to choose a "window" in their house through which they could imagine viewing their place of worship. The couple chose their living room window and painted a picture of their church. The couple shared that they felt their spirituality would grow and strengthen in the future as they relied more and more on their "church family" to support them in coping with their loss. The couple shared that they felt they had already grown spiritually together since their loss as they often prayed together.

In subsequent sessions, Judi used the paintings the couple had completed together to process with them their coping skills and how they wanted to strengthen those skills and build new ones.

Suggestions for Follow-Up

If the couple used an art technique to create what they saw out of their "windows," the clinician should process with them their thoughts and feelings about their creations. The clinician could ask, "How do you feel about what you created?," "Are you satisfied with your creation, or would you change anything?," or "Does anything about your creation surprise you?"

If the couple did not use art to express themselves, then they should process what the discussion was like for them and what they gained from the activity. The clinician could ask, "What was helpful about your discussion?," "What was not helpful about your discussion?," "Did anything in the discussion surprise you?," or "What will you take away from this activity?"

The clinician should give the couple an opportunity to share with each other what they need in relation to coping with the diagnosis or loss. The clinician could ask, "Can you share with your partner anything that you need from him/her that will help you cope more effectively with the diagnosis?" or "In what way can your partner best support your coping efforts?"

In future sessions, the clinician could have the couple explore the "windows" that did not have a positive "view" and what they plan to do to change that "view." The clinician could say, "The view outside of your kitchen window seemed gloomy. What do you plan to do together to change that view?" or "What needs to change so that the view is a little sunnier?"

Contraindications for Use

This activity is to only be used with a couple that has expressed a desire to use religious/spiritual concepts in their treatment. The use of such an activity with couples in treatment that are not comfortable using their spiritual beliefs, have different spiritual beliefs, or who are atheist can be offensive.

This activity should only be used with clients that are able to understand metaphors. If the therapist does not feel certain that the clients can understand the metaphor and how it applies to their lives, then the use of this activity is not suggested.

Reference

Freedman, J., & Combs, G. (1996). *Narrative therapy: The social construction of preferred realities.* New York: W.W. Norton & Company.

Readings and Resources for the Professional

Barth, J. C. (1993). *"It runs in my family": Overcoming the legacy of family illness.* New York: Brunner/Mazel.

McDaniel, S., Hepworth, J., and Doherty, W. D. (1992). *Medical family therapy: A biopsychosocial approach to families with health problems.* New York: BasicBooks.

Bibliotherapy Source for the Client

Whitbourne, S. K. (2004). *Adult development and aging: Biopsychosocial perspectives.* New York: John Wiley.

Chapter 27

Threading the Strengths of Families Through Loss and Grief

Miriam Claire Godwin
Angela L. Lamson

Type of Contribution: Activity

Objective

The purpose of this activity is to assist a client and/or family through their mourning process after the loss of a loved one and create a physical reminder of their loved one that they can hold on to when they are experiencing grief.

Rationale for Use

A number of amazing clinicians, academics, and researchers have written or presented on issues of death, dying, grief, and bereavement. Certainly each person and professional has his or her unique way of addressing these issues. However, we believe that the work of Elizabeth Kübler-Ross (1981, 1969) and Terry Hargrave (1997) have been most influential when working with clients who are managing the loss of a loved one.

Kübler-Ross is perhaps best known for her creation of the five stages of grief: denial, anger, bargaining, depression, and acceptance. She believed that individuals and families explored their experiences with loss through these stages. Some would move quickly through the stages, others more slowly, and rarely if ever would a person go through these stages in order. In fact, most encounter these stages several times as they go through a single grief experience. Regardless of the pace or order, the hope is that those who grieve will eventually be able to reorganize their lives in a healthy way given the loss experience.

Hargrave uses four factors (type of relationship, balanced and fulfilled versus unbalanced and unfilled, sudden and unexpected versus gradual and expected, and in time with life cycle versus out of time with life cycle) to explain how loss invades our emotional well-being. He describes how loss of an individual when the death was unexpected and out of time with life cycle sequence may include more conflicted and confusing feelings associated with grief. His factors allow others to consider how the loss of a close family member may be experienced differently than the loss of a co-worker or the loss suffered in a traumatic event in another state or country.

The work of Kübler-Ross and Hargrave supports the rationale for this activity by promoting the need for individuals and families to address their grief experiences as they encounter or have encountered the five stages. With the knowledge that each loss experience is unique, the four factors allow clinicians to consider what attributes are most influential to the loss experience.

Using this knowledge, the clinician can begin to assist families by figuratively weaving in emotional components often associated with loss while the family literally weaves together materials that create a pillow or blanket that reflects their loved one who has passed on.

This activity most closely represents the intertwining of experiential family therapy model and Adlerian psychology. Experiential theorists emphasize the importance of expressing emotions to support healthy family functioning and believe that the purpose of the family is to support the emotional growth of each member (Satir, 1972). Adler promoted the concept of people needing to feel connected to others and to develop social interest as the cornerstone of mental health (Adler, 1992). This activity encourages the participants to express emotions and build connections with others in order to address grief experienced after the loss of a loved one.

The purpose of this activity is to bring families and perhaps friends together to talk about the grief and personal memories associated with a loved one who has passed on while creating a symbolic or material memento that reminds them of that person. The authors specifically selected blankets and pillows as two items that could be created by families through the therapy process. A blanket symbolizes warmth and comfort to an otherwise unsheltered experience, while pillows provide a familiar place for our heads and minds to relax or when hugged may represent an embrace that might have been given to the loved one who has passed on. Families have stated that a pillow is easier to transport from one place to another; this option may be especially important for a child who seeks relief from an object that represents something familiar.

Instructions

The family should first decide which activity they would like to create, a blanket or pillow. This choice may be based on where the pillow or blanket will be kept (some may store the item for legacy purposes, while others will want the item always physically close), their intended use of the memento (to sleep on/with or for emotional comfort), ages of children, or ability to transport the memento in times of need. The family is asked to reflect on which item they want to create, while the clinician explores what they plan to do with the blanket or pillow and how it can be helpful when they are experiencing feelings of sadness or loneliness. Questions from the clinician could include: "How can this blanket or pillow be useful to you when you feel sad or lonely?" "Can you describe a time when this memento would have been helpful in the past?" or "When can you see yourself using this blanket or pillow?"

After a decision has been made on which item to complete, the clinician should ask the client/ family to bring fabrics to the next session that best represent the lost loved one (e.g., a favorite color, texture, shape) and are acceptable to use for this project. Some clients have used clothes that belonged to their loved one. Others have pinned memorabilia to the blanket or pillow so that they could easily be removed if necessary.

At the start of the session designated for the activity, the clinician should instruct the clients to cut the selected fabric into large square pieces that when sewn together will make a 4' × 5' blanket with a 2" seam allowance on each side (if making a blanket). When making a pillow, the fabric should be of equal width and length (and will differ based on clients' need) with a 2" seam allowance on each side. The participants can appoint a "cutter," or can work as a team. The decision-making process during this stage can allow the clinician to begin observing group or family dynamics that may be present.

The clinician should then instruct the clients to work together in placing the pieces of fabric in a pattern that can be sewn together to create the blanket or pillow. This, as well, can be a key observational opportunity for the clinician. The design of the pillow or blanket should be determined by the family/group and not by one person. If the family feels that certain pieces of fabric have special meanings, they should be encouraged to share those meanings and use them to determine the placement of the piece of fabric in the design. If there is a disagreement during this stage about the pattern, the clinician should encourage the family to use problem-solving skills to work out the situation. The clinician should also process with the family what the arguments represent and mean to them.

The clinician should assist the family in sewing the edges of the pieces of fabric together when making the blanket (only the front side should be formed at this time) or pillow (all but one side of the pillow should be sewn). As the family members are sewing the fabric together, the clinician should encourage them to openly share memories and feelings about their lost loved one. Everyone should participate in the sewing process. Small children, elderly, or disabled clients may need assistance from another family member/client throughout the design, cutting, and sewing process.

When finishing the blanket, the participants should be instructed to cut the fabric that will be used to back the blanket and begin sewing it to the front side of their memento. The family should further personalize the blanket by adding plastic sleeves for photos or by sewing on special tokens.

For families who chose to create a pillow, a pillow form should be inserted into the shell (the three sides of the pillow that have been sewn together) followed by sewing up the final side of the pillow. Again, the family should decide if any additional personal items should be sewn onto the pillow.

The clinician should process with the family what it felt like to create something that reminded them of their loved one. Some questions might be, "What was the best part about creating the blanket or pillow?" "What was the worst part about creating the blanket or pillow?" "Do you feel this was a positive experience and why?" "How was the creation of this item helpful or not helpful with your grief process?"

Lastly, the clinician should make a point to discuss with the family the hypothetical perspective of the lost loved one, as it relates to the creation of the blanket or pillow. This could be done by asking "What do each of you think your loved one would say about this pillow/blanket?" "What would your loved one say about how you talked as a family while making this memento?" "What would your loved one say about your grief experience?" This can be an opportunity for the clinician to gain a better sense of where the family members are in their grief. It can also give the family another perspective about the work they have already accomplished. This reflection will allow the therapist to tap into the relevance of Hargrave's four factors of grief as well as explore the intensity of the Kübler-Ross stages.

Supplies

The clinician should support participants in selecting fabrics that best represent the lost loved one (e.g., a favorite color, texture, shape) and are acceptable to cut up and use for the project. Some clients have used clothes that belonged to their loved one instead of throwing them away or donating them; they used them to help in their healing process.

The clinician should provide needles and thread, embroidery floss and embroidery needles, or yarn and tapestry needles (may work best for small children because it is easier to handle than the typical needle and thread). Craft scissors or fabric scissors should also be used. "No-sew" materials (fabric glue or iron-on stitching replacement) could be used to connect the pieces of fabric together if skill, time, or age (may be easier for younger children) are an issue.

A premade pillow form (if creating the pillow) can be purchased at any major craft store. They are available in various sizes. Plastic sleeves can also be sewn onto the pillow to secure a photo or other special tokens. The plastic sleeves can be purchased at local craft stores to suit different sizes of photos.

Material to back the blanket (if creating the blanket) should be fleece or another durable and soft fabric. It should be cut 4' × 5' for a typical throw-type blanket, with a 2" seam allowance on each side. Premade quilts can also be used and decorated with symbols that best represent the lost family member or friend. Photographs can be transposed onto the quilt by using a computer scanner, a printer, or an iron-on transfer paper.

Brief Vignette

Beverly G. came for treatment after the death of her beloved dog. She had already been through the Kübler-Ross grief stages of denial, anger, and bargaining and was now moving into the acceptance stage. During the first session, Beverly had decided to invite her sister, Mary, to join her for the next session in which she would create a pillow that reminded her of her lost pet, Roscoe.

The clinician asked Beverly to bring some of the old sweaters, T-shirts, and bandanas her dog had worn. Throughout the second session, Beverly and Mary cut the various fabrics into square pieces and began creating a pattern with Roscoe's favorite camouflage T-shirt as the focal point of the design. The clinician encouraged Beverly and Mary to share the meanings attached to the fabrics while creating the final pattern.

As Beverly and Mary stitched the pieces of fabric together, the clinician facilitated a discussion about their fondest memories of Roscoe and what he meant to their lives. Beverly expressed her feelings of joy when thinking about Roscoe barking and running to meet her when she came home from work every day. Mary shared that it makes her smile when she thinks about Roscoe jumping into the ocean over and over again until he could barely stand from exhaustion.

Beverly and Mary finished the pillow they had been working on during their third session and the clinician encouraged them to share what had been helpful about the project and how they saw themselves using the pillow when experiencing feelings of grief. Beverly shared that she had not realized how much Mary loved Roscoe until they worked together on the pillow and shared their feelings about him. Mary said she gained a better sense of what Beverly had been dealing with when she heard about the difficult emotions Beverly had experienced. Beverly shared that she planned to place the pillow against the headboard of her bed, where she often found Roscoe laying in the afternoons. She also discussed how she could imagine herself hugging the pillow as she had hugged Roscoe in the past.

Suggestions for Follow-Up

In subsequent sessions, the clinician should encourage the participants to describe times when the blanket or pillow had been helpful for them. The clinician could ask, "When you felt sad last Thursday night, did you use the pillow to comfort you or did you do something else?" The clients should also be encouraged to share where the blanket or pillow was placed in their home. The clinician may ask, "Was the blanket placed on the wall and used as a wall hanging?" or "Was the pillow used like a regular pillow or just for decorative purposes?" This will allow the clinician to explore the intended use and usefulness of the memento (as explored during the design and creation sessions) versus actual use/usefulness of the memento.

The clinician could also encourage the clients to think of other items they could create, such as a memory box full of pictures and mementos related to the lost loved one. The clinician could ask, "Are there other items you could create that would help comfort you?" or "Are there other things you miss about your loved one that weren't captured in your pillow/blanket-making activity?" and encourage them to make a physical object that will support them when they are missing that particular thing about the lost loved one. For example, they may miss the loved one's humor, so they could be encouraged to create a video of others telling some of the lost loved one's favorite jokes.

The clinician and family may also want to discuss future thoughts about grief and the use of the mementos, including whether the family intended on sharing memories about the loved one with others, expressing feelings about the lost loved one, or describing the usefulness of the blanket/pillow with others. The participants should be encouraged to continue sharing memories and feelings throughout the healing process. The clinician might ask, "In the next month, when or where do you see yourself sharing memories about your loved one or the value of your blanket/pillow?" or "When do you feel your pillow/blanket will be most helpful for you in the future?"

Contraindications for Use

The clinician should assess where the client and/or family is in their grief process. This activity might not beneficial soon after the loss; the timeliness for application of the intervention is at the discretion of the clinician. For example, if the client is in the Kübler-Ross stage of anger, this activity might not be as beneficial as if the client were in another of the stages. The client may be so angry about the loss, that he or she is unable to remember pleasant memories about the lost loved one.

Clinicians must always assess for unhealthy coping patterns, suicidal ideations, or abusive measures to managing grief. By becoming aware of unhealthy coping patterns, the clinician can assist the client in maintaining safety by addressing these issues and taking proper reporting measures. If the client is in danger due to unhealthy coping patterns, this activity should be postponed until safety is consistently maintained and grief work is appropriate.

The activity does require some sewing, but if the clinician is not comfortable with the technique, a "no-sew" method is suggested. Comfort with sewing is based on the past experiences and abilities of the clinician. A clinician who has never sewn may be a perfect candidate for using "no-sew" materials or a premade quilt. If the clinician has had minimal experience with sewing, he or she may wish to practice the technique prior to using it in an intervention. The clinician must feel confident enough to instruct clients who have little or no sewing experience and wish to complete this activity. The activity should be proposed to the clients first and then they should make the final decision about whether to proceed. Some clients have no interest in sewing or crafts. Their needs and preferences are more important than that of the clinician's and should be used to determine whether the project is going to be beneficial in their healing process.

If the clinician is not comfortable with creating a large blanket due to the amount of material available, time allowed, or ability to complete a large project, a small blanket would be suitable. Perhaps working with the client and/or family in creating smaller pieces would be more manageable for some clinicians. This activity can take several sessions and depending on the size of the family, the clinician may suggest that the family take the project home to work on and then process with the family during subsequent sessions what their experience was like outside of the office setting.

References and Resources for the Professional

Adler, A. (1992). *Understanding human nature*. Oxford: Oneworld Publications. (Original work published in 1927.)

Carroll-Parker, C. (2003). *Surviving a hero: A clinician looks at family loss*. CA: Authorhouse.

Hargrave, T. D. (1997). *New directions in family grief and loss*. Workshop presented at the 55th Annual Convention of the American Association of Marriage and Family Therapy, Atlanta, Georgia.

Kübler-Ross, E. (1969). *On death & dying*. Simon & Schuster/Touchstone.

Kübler-Ross, E. (1981). *Living with death & dying.* Simon & Schuster/Touchstone.
Satir, V. M. (1972). *Peoplemaking.* Palo Alto, CA: Science and Behavior Books.
Walsh, F., & McGoldrick, M. (2004). *Living beyond loss: Death in the family* (2nd ed.) New York: W. W. Norton & Company.
Worden, J. W. (2001). *Grief counseling and grief therapy: A handbook for the mental health professional* (3rd ed.). New York: Springer Publishing Company.

Bibliotherapy Sources for Clients

Bernstein, J. R. (1998). *When the bough breaks: Forever after the death of a son or daughter.* Kansas City, MO: Andrew McMeel Publishing.
Umberson, D. (2003). *Death of a parent: Transition to a new adult identity.* Cambridge: Cambridge University Press.
Zonnebelt-Smeenge, S. J. & Devries, R. (1998). *Getting to the other side of grief: Overcoming the loss of a spouse.* Massachusetts: Baker Books.

Chapter 28

A Creative Encounter with Anticipatory Loss

Claudia Grauf-Grounds

Type of Contribution: Homework, Activity

Objective

This exercise empowers terminally ill patients to say good-bye to their young children in meaningful ways, and for a transitional object of love to be left for each child.

Rationale for Use

Terminal illness often strikes at times when younger family members do not have the cognitive or emotional ability to understand what is occurring. Parents who are dying have limited opportunity to share meaningfully with their young child in the present. Sometimes patients make video or audiotapes to be left for their children to watch and listen to after their death. This exercise provides another way to create connections between a dying parent and his or her child that can be used in the future, and processed in the present.

Rituals and transitional objects can facilitate better closure when someone dies and can often be associated with healthy grieving (Imber-Black, Roberts, & Whiting, 1988). Rituals include tangible objects which are filled with meaning. Allowing the patient who is dying to "leave" a specific object for his or her child can be a very important process in the bereavement. Receiving the "gift" from a dying family member can also allow for grief to be processed at developmentally appropriate times as the child grows older. Change and loss can help to transform feelings of powerlessness to those of agency or efficacy, as noticed in resilient families (Walsh, 1998). When illness discussions are filled with meaning and stories, the family shares a preferred experience of loss (Seaburn, Lorenz, Campbell, & Winfield, 1996).

Instructions

The task for the patient is to determine what "things" he or she possesses that might serve as a special gift for each child. This task can be accomplished in many creative ways. Explore with patient which items he or she possesses that are filled with value and meaning, and if anything had ever been "passed down" to him or her with special positive significance. Many families have "collections," or pieces of jewelry, or furniture, or art, or prized dinnerware that would be appropriate. The importance here is not the "value" of the item but the item's connection to the child as understood by the parent. The patient needs to confirm with his or her spouse or partner about the gift selected so that they agree and commit to "saving" the item for that particular child.

Next the patient writes a note for the child to read when he or she is older. In the note, the patient makes some association between the "gift" and the child. For example, "I selected this beautiful porcelain vase that was my grandmother's because you are beautiful and strong just like this vase." Explore with the patient a time "in the future" when the note would be read by the child and for the patient to write the note, imagining the child at that age. I usually suggest ages eleven to thirteen (close to the start of adolescence) as a good time frame for the note to be read/written. The parent can project into the future some words of wisdom and hopes for the child as he or she begins to move toward adulthood. This is also a common time for grief to be revisited by the child. The note is written directly to one child at a particular time, for example, "Katie, you will be reading this note from me when you turn twelve." It is also important that there is not a significantly different monetary value between each gift when given to multiple siblings. Sometimes smaller, less financially valuable items are better than those with lots of objective worth.

The note and the gift note are then wrapped in a special box or package, if possible, or the note is just placed in a moderately sized package. In large print on the outside of the package, write the words: "To be opened by _____ (fill in name) at age ____ (fill in age/date). A larger package size with the note inside the box ensures that the gift and letter will not get lost over the years.

The patient's partner or another family member or friend is then designated to be the "holder" of the package until the appropriate time (written on the outside of the box). At the selected time, the child is given the gift and note.

Brief Vignette

A client came to my therapy office to help her work on behaviors associated with an alternative medicine regime. After being very curious about her agenda for therapy and taking a thorough psychosocial and medical history, I came to the startling realization that she was probably dying of liver cancer. However, my client was unable to directly verbalize this; she could only say that she thought she "might" be very sick and that her husband and children had no idea about her "fears." I requested a release of information from her medical professionals so I might be more informed about how to help her. She concurred that this would be a good idea. The physicians I contacted did confirm the grim diagnosis. I asked the client to bring her husband to the next meeting so we could work on things together.

The following week the client came with her husband. I asked the client to review (outloud) her goals in therapy and to explore thoughts and feelings about her medical condition. During this session, my client disclosed to her husband that she believed she was dying and that she had been too scared to tell him. She told us how she "hid" the news from him when the doctor had asked her to invite him in for a follow-up appointment. A teary session followed with many fears expressed about their four children, all under the age of nine.

Our therapy then shifted to grieving and making preparations (e.g., considering hospice care) as my client's functioning was probably going to deteriorate. Again, a key concern for my client was "leaving" her children at such a young age and not being able to talk with them as they grew older. Since this topic was so central to my client, I suggested that she might want to "leave" something for each of her children for when they got older and to write a brief letter (she did not like to write) about how she particularly selected the "gift" for that child. During our next session the client told me that she had been "inspired" to leave some meaningful and valuable family jewelry to each of her children—items that had been treasured by her family and had been "passed down" to her. As she had placed several items on her bed, she said she felt "drawn" to each item as having a "characteristic" of one of her children. We discussed her joys about the unique qualities of each of her children and how they were associated with the gift.

Within three months of this meeting, my client was in home hospice care and highly medicated, no longer able to think clearly or write. I would do home visits and therapy with the children on occasion and attended the funeral two months later. The husband commented to me at the funeral that he was glad the children would have "something special" from their mom when they got older.

Suggestions for Follow-Up

A key component of this assignment is for the family member who is the "holder" of the gifts to keep the items safely and to remember to give them to the children at the appropriate time. Families that are chaotic or do not keep track of items may have difficulty remembering or maintaining the items in a safe location. It is useful for the therapist to discuss this issue after the death of the patient. In some cases, several family members or friends need to be informed about the gifts so that this process can be completed with the children.

Contraindications for Use

Late into a terminal illness, patients are often unable to focus and function well. Medication for pain management can interfere significantly with this process. Patients need to be alert cognitively and emotionally clear to be able to use this exercise. Therefore, professionals have the difficult task of determining "when" to recognize the appropriate timing surrounding a terminal diagnosis to address a farewell directly. Clients who never reach this phase of accepting that they are dying (e.g., stay in the hopefulness of being cured) would not be suitable for this process. Family members who cannot write can also "dictate" the letter section of the exercise.

Readings and Resources for the Professional

Imber-Black, E., Roberts, J., and Whiting, R. (1988). *Rituals in families and family therapy.* New York: W.W. Norton.
Krieger, G. W. (1975).Terminal illness: Counseling with a family perspective. *Family Coordinator, 24*(3): 351-355.
Nadeau, J. W. (1998). *Families making sense of death.* Thousand Oaks, CA: Sage.
Robinson, W. D., Carroll, J. S., & Watson, W. L. (2005). Shared experience building around the family crucible of cancer. *Families, Systems, & Health, 23,* 131-147.
Saldinger, A., Cain, A., Kalter, N., & Lohnes, K. (1999). Anticipating parental death in families with young children. *American Journal of Orthopsychiatry, 69*(1), 39-48.
Seaburn, D. B., Lorenz, A., Campbell, T. L., & Winfield, M. A. (1996). A Mother's death: Family stories of illness, loss, and healing. *Families, Systems, & Health, 14*(2), 207-221.
Walsh, F. (1998). *Strengthening family resilience.* New York: Guilford Press.

Bibliotherapy Sources for the Client

Byock, I. (1998). *Dying well: Peace and possibilities at the end of life.* East Rutherford, NJ: Riverhead Books.
Carter, R. (2001). *Handbook for mortals: Guidance for people facing serious illness.* Oxford, England: Oxford University Press.
Kessler, D. (2000). *The needs of the dying: A guide for bringing hope, comfort, and love to life's final chapter.* New York: Harper Paperbacks.
Rando, T. A. (1988). *Grieving: How to go on living when someone you love dies.* Lexington, Massachusetts: Lexington Books.

Chapter 29

Aging Parents and End-of-Life Decisions: Helping Families Negotiate Difficult Conversations

Nathalie L. Kees
Jennifer T. Aberle
Christine A. Fruhauf

Type of Contribution: Handout

Objective

The goal of this chapter is to help adult family members make some of the difficult end-of-life decisions associated with having a terminally ill parent. A handout is provided to help adult family members discuss the issues related to transitioning from rehabilitative therapies to palliative care for an elderly parent who has suffered a massive stroke. The handout also functions as an aid for improving communication and collaboration between family members and health care teams.

Rationale for Use

As members of the "baby boom" generation (1946-1964) age, dealing with the difficult end-of-life decisions related to aging parents becomes a commonplace occurrence for many in this age group. Today, 13 percent of the United States population is over the age of sixty-five and by 2030 this will grow to approximately 20 percent (U.S. Census, 2000). The increase in our aging population not only has implications on medical and economic costs, but it will also have implications on the 50 million family members (National Family Caregivers Association, 2003) who are assuming caregiving roles and responsibilities for chronically ill, disabled, or aged family members or friends.

Communication among family members, as well as between family members and health care teams, is one of the primary challenges faced during these difficult times. The contextual frameworks and worldviews from which each member interprets and analyzes the situation greatly affect how they will articulate their hopes and desires for their loved one. In addition, health care teams may not always understand the unique wishes of the family based on these multiple viewpoints. Therefore, any attempt to intervene in order to avoid miscommunication is an important consideration. As counselors and therapists, one of our roles can be to provide creative and appropriate approaches for communicating during this time. In this way, understanding the diversity of lenses and multiple perspectives from which family members consider the situation is essential to good communication and helpful decision making for the well-being of the patient.

Mental health practitioners can help families develop and maintain open lines of communication during the most stressful transitions, aiding family members in becoming the best possible advocates within the health care and hospice systems for their ill and dying loved ones. It is important that therapists have the necessary tools to help family members gain information to understand their advocacy roles as well as cope with the complexities of these situations. When family members recognize the needs of their loved one and are aware of the ways in which these needs can be met, they are more likely to feel empowered toward making helpful and adequate decisions as well as promote collaboration with their loved one's health care team. Therapists can help aid this process by offering clients ways to gather this information, process it, and assemble a plan for carrying it out.

The handout provided was created to help one family negotiate the difficult decisions that needed to be made during the transition of a family member from rehabilitative care to hospice services. The handout provided clarity of purpose and focus for a conversation between family members and their mother's health care provider. These conversations can be both emotional and confusing for those involved. Having a clear focus to help direct questions and answers was very facilitative and allowed the best possible choices to be made for the family member.

This handout and its purpose of promoting open and specific information about the loved one's needs emerged from systemic and constructivist theoretical and contextual frameworks. Systems theory suggests that individuals and circumstances are influenced by multiple variables that simultaneously inform one another to produce certain outcomes and inputs for functioning, which in turn form a system. This intervention considers the relationships between multiple systems such as family, medical and health care, and social systems. The handout helps therapists offer clients ways to inform the systems (i.e., doctors, family members, clergy, social workers, etc.), as well as understand how systems are affecting them (i.e., medications, finances, support, etc.) in a manner that honors their unique situation and belief systems.

In addition, the intervention is founded on a constructivist conceptual framework which provides the foundation for building specific and individualized plans based on the dying person's needs, the families' views, beliefs, and values, and other factors influencing the families' decision-making processes. Accordingly, therapists can aid clients in understanding how they assemble and make meaning of information in order to bring forth strategies to help their loved one and themselves during this difficult time at the end of a family member's life.

Instructions

To help facilitate the discussion with the doctor, one of the family members (who also happened to be a licensed therapist) created the following handout of Helen's treatments so that the family could reach agreement with one another and with the doctor concerning Helen's transition from rehabilitative care to hospice services. The handout allowed each family member to have a written record of the decisions made during this meeting and it provided a focus for the types of questions that still existed in family members' minds.

A handout such as this could be developed, discussed, and revised with family members prior to meeting with health care professionals in order to insure agreement on the questions needing to be clarified and the decisions needing to be made. Therapists can help families decide who should be involved in the decision-making processes and how to involve family members who might be at a distance, perhaps using conference calls and faxing information beforehand.

Brief Vignette

Helen, the eighty-two-year-old matriarch of a large German-American, Midwestern family, suffered a massive and debilitating stroke. Up until the moment of the stroke, Helen and her eighty-four-year-old husband had been living independently in their home, actively engaged in life, community activities, and service work. The stroke left Helen paralyzed on her right side and unable to speak, write, or fully comprehend questions asked of her. Her adult children and their spouses rallied around Helen to provide care and support and to help their father as they worked together to make the difficult decisions that arose throughout the last months of Helen's life.

During the first week of Helen's hospitalization following the stroke, the family had to make a decision about the continued use of a feeding tube. Helen had a signed living will that stipulated that she did not want to be kept alive through artificial means. The family met alone and with hospital staff and doctors several times during the week to determine Helen's prognosis and whether or not the feeding tube should be discontinued. The decision was made to remove the feeding tube and Helen was moved to a nearby in-patient hospice facility the next day. After ten days in hospice, the hospice nurses suggested that Helen may not yet be ready for hospice and may benefit from attempting rehabilitative therapies. The family members, with the doctor's approval, decided to move Helen to the rehabilitative wing of the same health care facility. After two months of therapies, Helen's progress diminished and she became unwilling to participate in any additional therapy. The decision was made by the family to place Helen back under hospice care.

It was during this last transition from treatment to hospice services that the family began to struggle with the number of medications Helen was being given and which types of things Helen should continue to be treated for. The question of quality of life and comfort care measures verses interventions that may prolong Helen's life became a difficult one for the family members to agree upon. For example, while the family had agreed that Helen should not be treated for major infections that might hasten her natural process toward death, Helen had experienced several urinary tract infections during her time in the nursing facility. This is not uncommon, particularly during extended periods of catheter use. Family members disagreed on whether the continued treatment of a urinary tract infection would constitute a comfort care and quality of life measure or a treatment meant to extend Helen's life. The family arranged a meeting with Helen's doctor and used the following handout to help clarify this, and other questions, for all involved.

Instrument

Certainly, each family's situation will differ and each patient's treatments will be unique to the individual. However, the process this family was able to engage in concerning their mother's last days provides a helpful narrative for others facing these types of decisions, which, when in the midst of such painful circumstances, are never easy.

After two-and-half months of being confined to a hospital bed, recliner, and wheelchair, Helen was experiencing many of the common breakdowns of skin—itching, discomfort, and bedsores. Like many stroke victims, Helen was experiencing long bouts of crying, depression, and lack of appetite and was treated for these with an antidepressant containing an appetite stimulant. Helen was treated with antibiotics for the urinary tract infections that usually led to yeast infections from the antibiotic use. She was also treated for the yeast infections. Helen began experiencing severe anxiety and was given tranquilizers as needed. She had been on thyroid and blood pressure medications and eye drops for her glaucoma prior to the stroke and these protocols were continued during her time at the nursing facility. She had been receiving speech, physical, and occupational therapies while a resident at the facility.

Example Handout for Helen

Treatment for Comfort Care, Quality of Life, Prolonging Life

1. Steroid creams and antihistamines for bedsores and itching
2. Eye drops for glaucoma
3. Thyroid medication
4. Blood pressure medication
5. Diuretic for blood pressure
6. Antidepressant with appetite stimulant
7. Tranquilizers for anxiety
8. Tylenol and Tylenol 3 for pain
9. Antibiotics for urinary tract infections
10. Monistat for yeast infections
11. Therapies:
    Speech
    Physical
    Occupational

As a result of this meeting, the family and doctor decided that the blood pressure medication and diuretic would be stopped as soon as the speech, physical, and occupational therapists concluded their work with Helen, which occurred later that week. It was decided that any urinary tract infection would be treated for comfort care as needed without necessarily testing again. The same would be done for any yeast infections. The doctor was able to clarify for the family that treating urinary infections is a comfort measure and not a treatment to prolong life as it can take a good deal of time for a urinary infection to become life threatening. The eye drops and thyroid medications were continued as comfort and quality-of-life measures as untreated glaucoma and thyroid problems can cause pain and a good deal of discomfort. It was at this point that the family was also able to talk with the doctor about the types of pain medications hospice would be able to provide Helen so that she might rest comfortably during her last weeks. The family felt a great deal of relief at the end of this meeting and the doctor complimented the family on their ability to continue communicating and reaching agreement. She stated that this was not necessarily the norm in her many years of experience.

Suggestions for Follow-Up

As stated earlier, this handout can, and should, be modified to include different types of treatment for the diverse needs of older family members and their caregivers. To facilitate this, a general handout format is provided at the end of the chapter. A column has been added to this prototype to help family members determine who will be responsible for care and treatment for the debilitated individual as not all families will be able to access, or necessarily afford, round-the-clock nursing or hospice care.

All family members may want to be present during discussions with medical staff but one family member may elect to be the note keeper. This will allow all members present to ask questions, but may eliminate the need for all family members to feel pressured to take an active (i.e., record keeping) role in the caregiving process. This written record can then easily be shared with other family members living at a distance or those participating via conference call. Therapists must also be sensitive to cultural beliefs about end-of-life practices and will need to modify the handout accordingly.

Contraindications for Use

In order to ensure correct information and explanation of the type of medical care, it is recommended that this handout be used with the consultation of a physician and/or a care plan team (i.e., including nursing staff, social work, dietary, etc.). The handout may not be suitable for individuals who practice certain religions (e.g., Christian Science) as it may go against their belief systems. Further, this handout may be used with families who are providing care to terminally ill individuals regardless of age.

References

National Family Caregivers Association. (2003). Family caregiving statistics. Retrieved January 28, 2003, from http://www.nfcacares.org/.

United States Census Bureau. (2000). Population Finder Fact Sheet. Retrieved October 1, 2005, from http://www.census.gov/main/www/cen2000.html.

Readings and Resources for the Professional

Blank, R. H., & Merrick, J. C. (2005). *End of life decisions: A cross-national study.* Cambridge, MA: MIT Press.

Coppola. K. M., & Trotman, F. K. (2002). Dying and death: Decisions at the end of life (pp. 221-238). In F. K. Trotman & C. M. Brody (Eds.) *Psychotherapy and counseling with older women: Cross-cultural, family, and end of life issues.* New York: Springer.

Randall, F., & Downie, R. S. (1999). *Palliative care ethics: A companion for all specialties.* Oxford, UK: Oxford University Press.

Bibliotherapy Sources for the Client

Aging with Dignity. (2001). *Next steps: Discussing and coping with serious illness.* Tallahassee, FL: Author. www.agingwithdignity.org.

Buckman, R. (2005). *I don't know what to say: How to help and support someone who is dying.* Toronto, Ontario: Key Port Books.

Callanan, M., & Kelley, P. (1992). *Final gifts: Understanding the special awareness, needs, and communications of the dying.* New York: Bantam Books.

Concept Alliance, The. (1999). *These last words.* Fort Collins, CO: The Concept Alliance, LLP.

Funeral planning and grief support Web site: http://funeralplan.com/.

Haman, E. A. (2004). *How to write your own living will.* Naperville, IL: Sourcebooks.

Shenkman, M. M., & Klein, P. S. (2004). *Living wills and health care proxies: Assuring that your end-of-life decisions are respected.* Teaneck, NJ: Law Made Easy Press.

HANDOUT 29.1.
General Handout to Help Families Identify Needs, Discuss Issues, and Create Strategies for End-of-Life Decisions of Older Adults

Treatment for:	Comfort Care	Quality of Life	Prolonging Life	Who is Responsible
PAIN				
symptom/illness/treatments				
INFECTIONS				
symptom/illness/treatments				
BLOOD PRESSURE				
symptom/illness/treatments				
PRE-EXISTING CONDITIONS				
symptom/illness/treatments				
MOOD/MENTAL HEALTH				
symptom/illness/treatments				
THERAPIES				
symptom/illness/treatments				

Kees, N.L., Aberle, J.T., & Fruhauf, C.A. (2007). Aging parents and end-of-life decisions: Helping families negotiate difficult conversations. In D. Linville, K.M. Hertlein, and Associates, *The therapist's notebook for family health care: Homework, handouts, and activities for individuals, couples, and families coping with illness, loss, and disability* (pp. 211-216). Binghamton, NY: The Haworth Press.

BONUS SECTION: PROFESSIONAL DEVELOPMENT WITH ILLNESS AND LOSS

Chapter 30

Achoo!: Treating Clients When the Therapist Faces a Chronic Illness

Katherine M. Hertlein

Type of Intervention: Activity

Objective

When therapists face personal issues that may affect their therapy, they are often advised to seek support, increase their vigilance around their schedule, and establish and maintain appropriate boundaries. Therapists who face a chronic illness also have to adjust their schedules, boundaries, and seek support in much the same way. The objective of this activity is to provide couple and family therapists who are struggling with their own illness strategies for appropriately interacting with families.

Rationale of Use

The entirety of this book is devoted to families who are struggling with chronic illness, grief issues, and other health concerns that impact their family system and their interactions with one another. As practitioners, we have to be aware of the interplay of physical with mental health. Clients who seek our counsel are embedded within an environment where they struggle with identifying ways to maintain their emotional well-being, yet as educated clinicians, we are aware that the mind-body connection can be a very strong link in people and that their emotions may be regulated to some degree by their physical health, and vice versa.

Just as it is difficult for families to deal with these issues in the context of their relationships, couple and family therapists may also be struggling with diseases and illnesses of their own. Disease, chronic illness, and grief and loss are also issues that will affect the emotional well-being of the therapist. In situations where a therapist's well-being is compromised in some capacity, their clinical work may be compromised. In these cases, therapists have a responsibility to their clients to manage their illness so that it does not negatively influence their work with clients.

Biopsychosocial model. This chapter is primarily underscored by the biopsychosocial model. The biopsychosocial model emphasizes the interconnectedness among the physical, social, and psychological aspects of people. This same model underscores that of medical family therapy and recognizes the interplay of physical and emotional well-being contributing to a client's mental health (McDaniel, Hepworth, & Doherty, 1992). Specifically, medical family therapists look at how a patient's physical symptoms inform their issues in therapy.

In a departure from the medical family therapy lens, which primarily focuses on the patient, this chapter will explore the impact of a therapist's illness on the treatment he or she provides. Just as the medical family therapy field emphasizes the relationship between family systems and health on the part of the client, this chapter proposes that there also exists a significant relationship between family systems providers and their own personal health. Therapists with an illness, just like their clients, can be influenced in their clinical work by the existence of their illness. For example, one's therapy can be influenced by how tired they feel, the extent of their symptoms on a given day, etc.

Experiential family therapy. As a secondary framework, this intervention is influenced by Whitaker's experiential therapy. There are two other important experiential concepts included in this intervention: the battle for structure and the battle for initiative (Whitaker & Keith, 1981). In the battle for structure, the family and clients concede to accomplish the tasks in the way the therapist deems important. In this sense, the therapist sets the tone for treatment and the family/client follows what the therapist recommends in terms of prescriptions, interventions, etc. In what Whitaker describes as the battle for initiative, the therapist keeps the client or family on track with their already identified goals.

Whitaker believed that both a battle for structure and a battle for initiative were critical for a client's personal growth (Whitaker & Keith, 1981). Applied to this intervention, the therapist needs to provide this structure and initiative for himself or herself. The therapist has to be the one to decide how he or she will proceed with his or her daily life in light of the illness and is responsible for providing his or her own structure. Once this structure has been determined, the therapist can proceed with the initiative to meet his or her goals. This goal setting and establishment of a structure will promote safety and security. In this safe environment and the context of therapy, clients will better join with their therapist and be able to more effectively work within the safety and structure of the therapeutic relationship.

In this intervention, the therapist learns to manage the interplay of his or her own illness and his or her role as a therapist. The therapist considers himself or herself as part of the context of the environment. As such, therapists must consider the impact of their illness(es) on the systems of the families with whom they interact.

Self-of-the-therapist. One of the hardest things for therapists to do is to take care of themselves. Self-of-the-therapist is one of the critical concepts in one's development as a therapist. Therapists are encouraged to take the appropriate steps to do what they need to do in order to best care for themselves (Weiss, 2004). Some strategies that therapists use for caring for themselves include getting their own therapy, taking breaks from sessions and their work when they need to do so, and using of supervision.

Emotionally caring for oneself is part of the self-of-the-therapist; yet caring for oneself physically is also part of the task of the therapist in terms of watching their self-of-the-therapist. In terms of medical illness, when therapists get sick, they have to make themselves a priority. This may be difficult for some therapists to accomplish. For example, therapists might feel guilty for not "being there" for their clients. In other ways, it might be financially difficult for therapists to lose work or see clients. Therapists might be employed on either a full- or part-time basis. Those therapists who work part time might be paid hourly such that their salary depends on the number of clients they see. As such, it is not realistic for these therapists to simply stop seeing clients while they confront and manage their medical issue.

It is imperative that therapists put themselves in a position to learn how to manage their illness or issues of grief and loss and be able to provide effective service to their clients. This chapter outlines several strategies that therapists can use to manage their illness appropriately and to continue to provide the best care for their clients.

Instructions

Take care of yourself. Taking care of the self is critical for therapists in order to sustain their physical and emotional health. Just as we advise clients to care for themselves, there are several reasons that therapists should take their own advice when facing a chronic illness. First, taking care of oneself physically allows one to recover from illness. Therapists are not unlike workers in other professions and should model the behavior that they would like their clients to employ.

Second, therapists are of little value to clients if they are sick and not caring for themselves. When people experience illness, there may be fluctuations in their symptoms and periods of time where they are more tired than others; they may have difficulty concentrating; suffer from headaches; or other symptoms that can be debilitating during the course of a day. These symptoms can interfere with daily functioning and can influence the amount of resources and care that therapists are able to provide to co-workers and clients on any given day.

Taking care of oneself includes putting medical needs into an already existing schedule and routine, for example, by making time for appointments, making time in the day to take medications, etc. Depending on the situation, therapists experiencing illness might have some activities prescribed by their doctor to complete. These activities, whether they include exercise, taking medications, or going for treatments, may take a significant amount of time. Therapists should incorporate their doctor's recommendations into their daily routine.

Second, caring for oneself includes setting boundaries and limits regarding one's workload. Therapists, healthy or sick, may struggle with setting limits, yet this is important to maintain a healthy distance at work and provide the patient with some much-needed space to emotionally survive within a clinical environment. Weiss (2004) proposes several strategies for therapists to employ in setting boundaries and limits in their work. Some of these include learning to say no, screening clients more thoroughly, and actively delegating tasks. For therapists who work in an agency setting with multiple staff members, the therapist struggling with illness may consider asking an administrative assistant to assist with time-consuming tasks that interrupt the flexibility of one's schedule. For example, my former agency included an employee who offered to type intake reports for the therapists. Therapists feeling the crunch of duties and work may be best served by discussing with their supervisors and identifying "shortcuts" available during the duration of their treatment.

Other examples of limit setting might include not taking new cases and structuring the cases seen weekly to once every two weeks. Those therapists who work at an agency might consider limiting their involvement with other agency projects, such as committee work or presentations. These volunteering aspects of the job can wait until the sick therapist is in a better place, both emotionally *and* physically.

Make the covert overt. Because so much of their work addresses ambiguity and fears, therapists who become chronically ill might themselves experience feelings of fear or trepidation when considering who should know about the illness, how much it will affect their work, etc. Suffice it to say, the aspects of illness that the therapist thinks are invisible may not be. Therapists should consider being up-front with both clients and co-workers about the specifics of their condition.

Disclosure with co-workers. Co-workers, specifically those with whom the ill therapist is close, will likely be able to tell when the therapist is not "herself or himself" and not feeling well. Therapists who are up-front with their co-workers about their condition will have the benefit of co-workers understanding, support, and nurturing.

Disclosure with clients. Similar to co-workers, clients know when their therapists are not feeling well. Just as therapists are attune to their clients' moods, clients who know their therapist will recognize a difference in days when we are a bit "off" and not quite ourselves. It may be important for sick therapists to disclose some of their condition with their clients. One main reason for this is that clients may interpret the therapist's behavior as a result of the session rather than the illness. They may believe that this is an inappropriate interpretation, a belief which could impact the therapist-client relationship in a negative way. In some cases, it is important that the chronically ill therapist be completely open and up-front with clients regarding their illness.

Clients will worry. Part of a therapist's struggle may be because of the concern that the client will begin taking care of the therapist rather than the other way around. As mentioned, some clients may notice that something is different about their therapist. This difference can translate into a loss of safety and security within the therapeutic relationship. Therapists with this concern should find a way to disclose the information in a manner which conveys to the patient that the therapist's behavior is not a reflection of the session.

Gain support. Gaining support is critical to one's ability to manage an illness in addition to the day-to-day routines of life. Gaining support does not necessarily mean complaining about the illness or condition but rather letting others in the office know how they can provide support. Specifically, gaining support might include letting one's supervisor know about needs such as needing a more flexible schedule to incorporate a number of doctor appointments, treatments, etc. The staff at an agency can be very supportive and sincerely interested in therapists' emotional and physical well-being.

Maintain a flexible schedule. This is one of the critical parts of self-care. The therapist struggling with a chronic illness needs to have a schedule that is flexible and able to accommodate all of the appointments that he or she may need to make. There might be instances when, for example, a physician will request that laboratory tests be completed within a few days of an appointment. It is important that the therapist have the flexibility in his or her clinical schedule to attend these appointments.

Be proactive. A significant part of maintaining flexibility is being proactive. This means that the sick therapist maintains contact with his or her supervisors, colleagues, and clients in regard to scheduling. Co-workers and clients will look more favorably upon the therapist if appointments are scheduled at times when the therapist is certain to be available rather than having to cancel repeatedly for last-minute medical appointments. Scheduling clients every other week when it is certain the therapist can be present, rather than scheduling every week with the possibility of potentially canceling to accommodate the doctor schedule, may be the better and more professional option.

Be realistic. It is very important for the sick therapist to be realistic about the things to which he or she can and cannot commit. As much as we would like, there are times when we cannot do all of the things that we were able to do when we were well. It is important to learn to say "no" to projects that might get in the way of appointments and one's healing process.

Special concerns working with children. For those of us who have worked with children, we know that children are extremely perceptive, and can also pick up on small changes in a therapist's behavior or demeanor. Because of this, therapists who are ill are best advised to disclose their condition to young clients. This disclosure should be grounded in continuing to promote safety and security in the therapeutic relationship. If the therapist has determined that it is appropriate to disclose the condition to a child client, the discussion should be centered on the facts of the disease or illness, couched in the reassurances that the therapy will continue to the best of the therapist's ability and, if possible, continue as it has in the past. For children, the therapist should also provide a question/answer period as a way to continue to promote the safety and security already present in the therapeutic relationship.

Brief Vignette

Stacy was a thirty-six-year-old therapist who began to have difficulties breathing. She had been a therapist for ten years, and had no previous health problems. The onset of this illness was sudden. Her symptoms included daily low-grade fevers, nausea and instances of vomiting, chest pains, breathing problems, and dizziness. She also observed that she had an erratic heartbeat, constant migraines, chest pains, and periods of high blood pressure. As a result, Stacy sought answers from several physicians, and most were uncertain as to how her symptoms all fit together, and, more important, were unclear about treatment. They could treat the symptoms but not the larger problem.

These symptoms affected her work in the following manner. First, as a child therapist, due to her problems breathing, she was no longer able to run or engage in activities with her clients in the manner in which she was accustomed. Second, it was difficult for her to manage her schedule with her doctor appointments. As a result of the variety of symptoms, Stacy was at a doctor's office on a weekly basis and, in some cases, had to reschedule appointments because she had to be at the hospital for tests.

After the illness had continued for a period of three months, Stacy believed it was necessary for her to begin taking steps to treat this as a long-term illness. First, she spoke with her supervisor regarding her condition. She and her supervisor identified ways that she could avoid taking more cases onto her schedule. Stacy then informed the intake coordinator about her condition and asked to be released from getting intakes until the condition cleared. In addition, Stacy also met with one of her other supervisors at another site. Because of the nature of her job at that agency, she was required to be on-site on a regular basis. Due to the doctor's appointments, the therapist and her supervisor worked out another position for her within that agency.

Stacy then met with the agency director and told him about her condition. The agency director was able to offer his support and allow Stacy to revise her own schedule to accommodate her medical appointments. Her supervisor thanked her for being up-front about her condition and asked her to continue to keep him informed of any developments and changes in her health.

As her medical tests continued, her invisible symptoms became more visible. Her physicians, in attempting to uncover the cause of her symptoms, decided to place several monitors on her. These monitors were small but visible. It was at this point, realizing that her schedule would be altered and that she would have to explain the monitors, Stacy decided to reveal her condition to her clients.

The disclosures came at the beginning of the session. The clients noticed her monitors when they walked back with her to her office for the session. Stacy explained that she was having several symptoms, briefly described her symptoms, and explained the purpose of the monitors. For her child clients, Stacy told them that the monitors would be a part of session for several weeks, and therefore, they should have a name. Each family picked a name for the monitors. Stacy provided the children with an opportunity to ask questions and also gave them an open invitation to continue to ask questions in future sessions. Stacy reassured the children that she was continuing to seek medical care until she was well again. After making the covert overt and disclosing her condition, Stacy retuned to the business of therapy for the rest of the session.

Suggestions for Follow-Up

The suggestions for follow-up are based on each individual. The most important thing for therapists to remember in these cases is to make a continual assessment of their health situation. For example, if one's health situation becomes worse, the therapist may have to consider making more changes to their schedule. As the situation changes, the therapist is advised to keep his or her supervisor appraised of the health situation.

This intervention is not intended as a quick fix or one-time event. Instead, the instructions here are intended to be fluid, and used for making decisions as a therapist when facing chronic illness. Therapists experiencing chronic illness, much like therapists who are struggling with personal issues, may try to seek support as often as needed and continually throughout this process. Therapists struggling with illness are advised to make the covert overt as much as it will be appropriate in their cases and with co-workers. Finally, therapists should also continue to monitor how realistic their goals are as they consider accepting more workload responsibilities. If a sick therapist reduced his or her caseload and then discoverd that he or she can handle more, there is always the option to take on more cases. Conversely, if the decreased workload is still too difficult to manage, there is always the option to further reduce the caseload.

Contraindications for Use

This intervention is not to be used in cases where clinicians discover that they have a very serious illness. Under these circumstances, the therapist may want to think about focusing on her or his health long term, which can include taking a hiatus from clinical work altogether. As mentioned, there are special concerns related to disclosing to children. In some circumstances, the therapist can discuss her or his position with the parents and make a decision together about the appropriateness of informing the child of the condition. This intervention is particularly powerful when the therapist is working with a family where there is a member with a chronic illness.

References

McDaniel, S., Hepworth, J., & Doherty, W. J. (1992). *Medical family therapy: A biopsychosocial approach to families with health problems.* New York: Basic Books.

Weiss, L. (2004). *Therapist's guide to self-care.* New York: Brunner-Routledge.

Whitaker, C. A., & Keith, D. B. (1981). Symbolic-experiential family therapy. In A. Gurman & D. Kniskern (Eds.), *Handbook of family therapy* (pp. 187-225). New York: Brunner/Mazel.

Reading and Resource for the Professional

Weiss, L. (2004). *Therapist's guide to self-care.* New York: Brunner-Routledge.

Chapter 31

Building Your Home Project

Angela L. Lamson
Patrick L. Meadors

Type of Contribution: Homework task for the therapist

Many of the chapters in this book are directed at providing homework, handouts, activities, or interventions for individual, couple, or family clients. However, this chapter is dedicated to therapists who have experienced a medical trauma, severe illness, loss/death, or disability in their life and have an interest in providing clinical care in medical contexts or with families facing illness or loss. This task is intended for beginning therapists who recognize the importance of understanding and revisiting their self-of-the-therapist throughout their growth as a therapist.

Objective

Interacting with patients in medical environments can be difficult for some family therapists and overwhelming for others. Even therapists who feel comfortable providing care in medical environments will likely encounter a situation that sparks doubt on their personal or theoretical approach or regarding an intervention or assessment used in their provision of care. The objective of this homework assignment, called "Building Your Home Project" is intended to assist beginning medical family therapists in clarifying for themselves how their self-of-the-therapist links to their theoretical approach, interventions, or techniques used with patients, and how they evaluate or assess their level of effectiveness with patients.

Rationale for Use

Many beginning therapists learn about the critical components of therapy, such as how to assess for safety, complete a treatment plan, and gain an understanding of the policies and procedures required of them throughout their clinical experience. Unfortunately, a vital step that is often missing from the training for medical family therapy sites is clarifying how one's "self" interplays with theory, interventions, and evaluation of practice in a medical setting. This is best expressed by Harry Aponte (1994), who stated in his book *Bread and Spirit: Therapy with New Poor:*

> Therapy has long recognized the need for training of therapists to manage their personal issues in the context of therapy in ways that are not harmful to clients. Today's active thera-

pists involve themselves much more personally with clients than in previous generations. The extent to which therapists understand and have resolved their own stories will determine how sensitive they are to their clients' stories. If therapists are able to see and feel the pain of their own experiences and to accept the contradictions and inconsistencies of their attitudes and others, that will help them deal with similar feelings in their clients. (pp. 154-155)

How my {primary author} own foundation helped establish this homework assignment. As the daughter of a carpenter, I grew up observing my father add his unique touch to someone's future home or to a community hospital, bank, or nursing home. I remember learning at a very young age that no matter what his project, a solid foundation was the most essential element for all else to be successful. To outsiders, the foundation may not have been as noticeable as the beautiful home or building that stood upon it, but those who occupy the home or building understand the importance of that foundation. The occupiers understand that if the foundation were to deteriorate or become unstable, so would the structure that was built upon it.

It was through the indirect teachings from my father that I formulated my understanding to learn and teach about the "foundation" and "home" of family therapy. My belief is that our self-of-the-therapist is our "foundation" and this includes all that we are and all that we bring to our first steps as a family therapist. Our "house" is the theoretical orientation that we find our "foundation" sealing itself to. The "roof" of our house includes those techniques that best fit with our foundation and the "chimney" is the way in which we continue to evaluate our self-of-the-therapist as well as our progress with a patient and his or her family/larger system.

I have used this metaphor to teach graduate students about the importance of self and theory as they prepare for their future as therapists. In order for students to maximize their understanding of their "house" in the context of medical family therapy, I ask students to complete the assignment as detailed in the instructions section. Through this assignment we discuss their foundation by asking students to describe their definition of family, express values and beliefs, as well as explain their personal strengths and areas of growth. The students are asked to examine their foundation to further clarify and solidify who they will be when they enter the medical family therapy context.

Students are required to read and learn about family therapy theories and are asked to select or formulate a theory that best fits with their foundation. They are told that their foundation and house should feel like a seamless transition. The students are also informed that they may not be able to make a firm decision on a theory or "house" if their foundation feels unstable. For those who recognize instability in their foundation, many request to meet with a personal therapist or to meet with the clinical faculty to discuss their concerns. Although the challenge to find one's house can be very anxiety provoking for students, I request that they select one theory initially rather than selecting several to bounce back and forth between. I state that it is most common that people own one house not several and it may help them stay more focused on their foundation if they have just one house/theory to concentrate on.

Once the students have assessed their foundation and selected their house, they are then asked to put on the roof. The roof signifies the techniques that best fit their theory. Although many therapists or academics may disagree, my perspective is that techniques can be borrowed from many theories as long as the theoretical lens doesn't shift (e.g., a therapist that uses structural family therapy as his theoretical lens may include scaling questions in his approach but must understand the purpose of using that particular technique in therapy). The way that I teach about the roof is to say, *while people tend to have one house, they may find on a windy day that their neighbors' shingles have attached themselves to their house.* I challenge students to not simply select a technique, but to put it into a context of their "house" or theoretical framework. As most therapists know, not all techniques lend themselves to all theories.

Finally, I teach the students about the chimney. The chimney symbolizes the student's need to formally and informally evaluate their personal and clinical effectiveness. They are asked to describe how they will routinely evaluate their effectiveness with patients and how they will address any personal or professional struggles and strengths as they grow as a therapist.

The following section details how a student or clinician can complete the Building Your Home Project. It is important to note that the length of this assignment is not as relevant as the learning and knowing of one's self, theory, interventions, and evaluation of practice.

Instructions

This assignment is designed to facilitate a continuous process of integrating your personal beliefs, biases, strengths, and areas of growth with principles, strategies, and techniques into a congruent personal therapeutic style.

Think of the assignment like building a house: (1) You will start with your foundation (self-of-the-therapist), (2) assure that there is a transition or sealing point between your foundation and house (understanding why your theory matches your self-of-the-therapist), (3) build your house (theory), (4) a roof must then be added to complement the house (techniques), and finally (5) a chimney is created to support the ventilation of the house (effectiveness/flow of movement toward growth as a therapist).

1. The Foundation

Reflect on and document your self-of-the-therapist. This can include: how you define families, what brought you to medical family therapy, what strengths you bring to becoming a therapist, what areas of growth you bring to becoming a therapist, and what issues/situations may be a struggle or strength for you. Also note any personal or professional events or issues that have occurred in your life that may have a significant impact on your role as a therapist and how you have managed these experiences.

Among these events may be biological, psychological, social, or spiritual issues that have influenced your foundation. An example of a biological influence would be a disability, illness, or physical trauma that you may have experienced personally or via a family member/peer that has shaped your foundation. Psychological (e.g., personalities, coping strategies, or mental health), social (e.g., parental/familial relationships, peer relationships, communication patterns, etc.), and spiritual (e.g., value systems, beliefs, etc.) issues may also be delineated when forming your foundation.

2. The Transition from Foundation to House

Describe the major influences (i.e., life events, key figures or people, defining interactions or other important instances) that contributed to the development of your understanding and approach to family therapy. The components described in this section often provide the most insight into how you as a therapist understand and define family systems, the purpose of family therapy/medical family therapy, and health and illness issues.

Making a connection with your personal and professional values, beliefs, strengths, and challenges regarding medical treatment, collaborative versus directive care, and larger systems as it fits with your theoretical lens will be important to capture in this section. You should also explore the link between your (1) perspectives on health, (2) death, (3) medical diagnoses and treatment, (4) mental health diagnoses and treatment, (5) social factors, and (6) spirituality and your theory.

3. The House

Discuss the basic theoretical underpinnings of your approach including, (1) the nature of therapeutic assessment, (2) the process by which goals are established, (3) who determines the goals for treatment and how differences in goals are resolved, (4) what, if anything, would you share with your clients about your approach, and (5) what strengths and challenges you perceive you will encounter with your theoretical approach in a medical context i.e., what difficulties or strengths may arise when using your theory with particular populations (e.g., those who are just getting diagnosed versus those who are near death or patients who are children versus patients who are in later life) or how might patients or providers make sense of your theoretical approach.

4. The Roof

Describe the techniques that you frequently use in your approach to medical family therapy (e.g., externalization, miracle question, genograms, family sculpture, etc.) and their purpose. Consider techniques that would be used throughout the process of therapy and how they supplement your house and foundation. These techniques may differ based on the context (e.g., medical versus a non-medical environment, ability of the patient, level of collaboration with the patient's care team, and whether you are working with an individual, couple, or family).

5. The Chimney

Discuss how you plan to routinely assess your effectiveness as a therapist (in personal growth and patient/provider relationships) and what resources may assist you in assessing or analyzing your level of effectiveness. Describe how you will address strengths and challenges in your foundation, house, roof, and/or chimney, as well as areas of growth as a medical family therapist through collaborative relationships, knowledge in biopsychosocial care, and health care outcomes. This section should also include a personal and professional plan of care and plan for professional development (mini-time line).

[As you revisit the BYHP over time, note patterns of growth from your first draft to the latest version of your paper.]

Brief Vignette

It is essential that a therapist be confident in his or her foundation to ensure the stability of his or her clinical house. Now that the parameters of this activity have been delineated, it is important to demonstrate a practical example of the project. I (second author) will provide the foundation and background of my loss experience/self-of-the-therapist and then follow it up with the transition to my house, roof, and chimney to complete the construction of my theoretical home. (Note: Due to the length of the original document only segments of this project are detailed here.)

Foundation. In June of 1982, my father and mother were proud parents of two-year-old twin boys. My father decided to start cooking dinner on the grill. Little did I know, this decision would change our entire family's life path. Gas containers that were left in the garage spontaneously ignited trapping my brother and me in the flames. We were too young to understand what was happening, and the clothes we were wearing caught fire. My father remembers grabbing me and trying to take off my clothes to put out the fire and then he grabbed my brother. I was burned on 15 percent of my body and spent the next eight weeks in a burn unit and my brother was burned on 90 percent of his body and passed away three weeks into our treatment. This loss and the systemic changes that occurred as a result of this loss would have a lasting impact on my family and me.

At a familial level, the dynamics changed drastically at the time of the accident. Initially, I realized that I lost my twin and I constantly thought about how different things would be if my identical twin brother were still with me. My parents hadn't considered having more children after the death of my brother, but a year after the accident my parents were excited to bring home a beautiful baby boy and two years later, a beautiful baby girl. My parents exhibited unbelievable strength and resiliency in healing from the tragedy of losing a child and caring for an injured child.

Since my loss experience is ongoing, this traumatic experience will continuously shape the way that I view the impact of injury, illness, and loss on an individual and his or her family. This philosophy is inherent in the understanding of medical family therapy and the role of illness/injury within a family system. When I think about how an accident twenty-four years ago changed my life and my family's life completely, it provides me with a new perspective to view other people's illnesses and losses. It provides an appreciation of the role that every loss/illness experience will be unique to that person and his or her family as my family may have reacted differently to this loss than others who have experienced a similar tragedy. This understanding is crucial in the treatment of individuals and families as a medical family therapist.

Even though the components of a person's foundation can consist of a variety of materials, one of my materials is self-discovery. My self-discovery came during my second year of college as I regained authorship in my life. Up until that point, my father, an OB/GYN, had pushed me to attend medical school and I was doing poorly in all of my prerequisites required to apply. Since my loss experience, my entire life was built around not disappointing my father or seeing him hurt. It was at this point in college that I realized that I was not applying to medical school for myself, but rather to please my father. I knew my strengths in working with others and had strong motivation to help other people, but I began to gain ownership over my journey and my grades began to rise and my self-esteem subsequently rose. With a combination of regaining authorship in my life and the background within the medical field, I was naturally drawn to working as a medical family therapist. Clinically speaking, it became apparent following this realization that some of my future patients may have adopted narratives that they have not written and this can affect their functioning and leave them feeling helpless.

Transition from foundation to house. Since my loss experience is still present through visible scars, my interactions with others still shape my perceptions and path. For this assignment, it was important to venture to my past narrative and try to gain an understanding of when it was apparent that a person's narrative and interactions shape a person's perceptions. My first recollection of this component came in kindergarten, when my teacher asked me to leave the room while she proceeded to tell the class what had happened to me. When I returned to the room, every set of eyes was directed at me and the entire room was silent. At this point, I realized that I was different and remember wanting to be normal from that point on. This one interaction created an insecurity in myself that still affects my interpersonal relationships. Recognizing the impact of this experience on my own narrative will create an empathetic clinical ear for my patients who have negative interactions following a loss or illness. This exemplifies the sheer power that an unhealthy narrative can have on someone and how difficult it is to overcome such narratives. Ultimately, it contributed to my recognition of my theoretical home in narrative family therapy.

There are a variety of events that have facilitated change and discovery of the impact of these previously mentioned events has firmed the foundation of my house. I understand how my own life experiences (from losing my twin brother at the age of three, to how my parents decided to raise me, to my own personal relationships, to regaining authorship of my life) have allowed me to truly appreciate the narrative metaphor and the distinct power that a person's chosen path through life can have on his or her outlook and personal perception. Looking through my past, it is relatively simple for me to see how these events have affected my life course and shaped my interactions. My connection with these events serves as a springboard for working with my patients. Understanding how these events in my life facilitated change encourages me to work with clients who are in search of answers that that will in turn produce change.

While these events seem somewhat disconnected, it makes more sense to see them from the collaborative lens that is entrenched in the medical family therapy model. When examining my injury experience, there were multiple systems that needed to collaborate for the best treatment (school system, religious leaders, parental dyad, siblings, peers, medical personnel, and a medical family therapist). My understanding of how important each piece of this collaborative system was to my own care further motivates me to continually pursue collaborative care with and on behalf of patients.

House. Whenever you are looking for a house, it is common to explore all of your resources before you actually find a house that fits for you. Some people find a perfect house when they first start looking, but others look at all of the houses they can before making a decision that best fits them. There are times when it is necessary to make adjustments to your house but the structure usually stays the same. As previously mentioned, there were numerous factors that contributed to my understanding of families, and ultimately determining that narrative theory was the best fit for my clinical practice.

In regard to my "house," I will first describe my approach and some of the main principles of narrative family therapy and then discuss how this particular house is a perfect fit with my foundation. Narrative family therapy is an inherently strength-based approach that is built upon the principle that individuals adopt narratives about themselves that influence how they set priorities and find meaning in life. Concerns arise when oppressive stories dominate a person's life thereby engrossing them in a problem-saturated narrative that the individual finds difficult to escape. As a therapist, I can work with the client(s) as they deconstruct the problem-saturated stories and develop a healthy narrative to form a more strength-based story. The stories that we tell organize our experience and shape our behavior, thus the importance of deconstructing these unhealthy narratives and reconstructing healthy ones should not be ignored.

As a narrative therapist, the purpose behind my work is not to solve their problems, but rather to collaborate with my clients to change their lives through exploring and enriching their narratives. As a provider working from a narrative perspective, I would collaborate with the patient(s) in creating goals that are relevant to the individual or family's preferred path toward treatment. It is important as a narrative therapist to emphasize the notion of multiple realities and treat each individual as a human being, with a unique personal history, and help separate the individual from the dominant problem-saturated story he or she has internalized. This separation will leave room for alternative life stories and begin the process of building a healthy narrative.

I recognize that both strengths and challenges will be present when using narrative therapy in a medical context, especially as patients and I discuss the presence of their existing meaning making system. One of the challenges associated with my approach in the medical context is instilling hope that a preferred path is within their grasp despite the diagnosis of a debilitating illness. So many times individuals and families are consumed by an illness and the illness itself begins to preside as the dominant meaning for that family and its members, instead of fighting the illness together. One of the strengths of my approach will be the strength-based nature of narrative family therapy during a time when most of the patients may not be capable of seeing their life through that lens. Part of the therapeutic process would be to collaborate with the patient to allow him or her to see his or her life through the same strengths and ultimately gain control of the life that temporarily was consumed by the illness.

Once I found my theoretical house in narrative family therapy, it was important for me to assess how closely it fit with my foundation. If the wrong house is put on a foundation there are a variety of outcomes that can develop (i.e., the house could sink, fall apart, be unstable, etc.). You should never build a house without first examining the foundation and then finding the house plans that best fit.

When I learned about narrative family therapy, it became obvious what my approach was going to be. Narrative family therapy helped make perfect sense out of my own problem-saturated narrative surrounding my twin brother as well as the interactions between my father and me. Once I revisited my past experiences with my twin brother and discussed this traumatic event with my parents, I became knowledgeable about why certain insecurities still existed, why my parents tried so hard to shape me into what they wanted, and why my peer interactions in middle school were difficult. Coming to peace with my past narrative and externalizing that event gave room for me to start a new narrative. It also improved the relationship that I had with my parents as I began to understand their experience during that time. This became my "ah-ha" moment, as I knew that deconstructing my past narrative provided room for me to construct a new narrative. By understanding how my theoretical house was shaped by my foundation, it led to my understanding of families through a narrative lens. My house not only fit the foundation, but was molded by my past experiences and it truly led me to understand my own family as well as other families that I will see in my practice.

Roof. When it comes to the techniques that I will employ, there are so many different avenues that will fit with my approach. I will pull techniques from other theories and reframe them to serve a purpose in my house of narrative theory. One of the most influential and prevalent techniques in narrative therapy is asking questions that are designed to empower the client, help separate the client from the problem/illness, and create space for new narratives. The initial questions will focus on externalizing the problem/illness/injury from the individual or family. The next technique will focus on the deconstruction of the narrative, as it may be important to discuss societal factors that play a role in the client's narrative. For example, scaling questions from the solution-focused approach can often be used as one component of deconstructing the problem. Once you have united the family or individual against the problem, the reconstruction phase can begin. Numerous techniques can be employed from this point, from therapeutic letter writing, to use of certificates designed to empower the client, to asking questions pertaining to a unique outcome that the client has considered. All of the techniques surround the idea of creating and maintaining the new narrative with the clients, which is important for my patients who may be struggling to keep authorship of their life in the face of tragedy or illness. Once the client has designed and authored a new narrative it is typically important to involve family members or those close to the patient/client to ensure that the new narrative is maintained. My techniques will be centered around the main goals of therapy and based on the uniqueness of the client's narrative.

Chimney. One of the most important aspects of therapy is the debriefing process. I will be able to assess my effectiveness as a therapist through interactions with my colleagues, physicians, supervisors, and clients. It is acceptable within narrative family therapy to collaborate with the client and ask him or her what was helpful and what he or she thinks would have been more beneficial. This is one of the advantages of the collaborative stance of the therapist and client relationship in narrative therapy.

To take my assessment further, it may be important to ask specific questions of myself. To be effective as a narrative family therapist in a medical context, I believe it important that all of my questions to a client/patient serve a purpose relevant to the therapeutic path (knowledge pertinent to case/illness, deconstruction, or reconstruction). One method of evaluating my effectiveness is to retrace the session to ensure that I was focused throughout in obtaining the goals set for narrative therapists and stayed focused on the clients' needs. Overall, being in touch with the therapeutic process for each client will be essential to maintaining my clinical integrity.

There will be instances where I am stuck in therapy and collaboration with colleagues will serve as a vital piece of this assessment and evaluation process. When I am stuck, I plan on using other sources of information (i.e., journals, larger systems, etc.) and consult other clinicians about how to better reach my client. It is vital to me that I am providing the best care possible and I will never have too much pride to ask another therapist or medical provider for help. The best care of the patient is inherent in collaborative health care and continuous involvement of the interdisciplinary system of providers. This inclusion of mental health providers, physical health providers, and/or spiritual leaders as a part of the collaborative team will help me to extend a more comprehensive level of care.

Suggestions for Follow-Up

It will be important for therapists to review their Building Your Home Project after significant changes in their personal life, variation in theory, change in professional context, or after learning new clinical or evaluative approaches. Therapists may also find it helpful to review this assignment after a personal loss, illness, or disability in their home or with that of a patient. We recommend that beginning therapists review this assignment every three months and to update changes throughout the five sections as necessary. Many therapists have provided feedback on this assignment stating the significance of reviewing each section on an annual basis to maintain the integrity of their self and their practice with patients.

Contraindications for Use

The Building Your Home Project is not intended to be shared with patients but is a way to identify and build on one's personal and professional identity as a medical family therapist. This project is also not intended to be used by a supervisor to gain personal information from a therapist, but rather as a supervisory tool to address self-of-the-therapist, theoretical approach, interventions, or evaluation of personal/professional effectiveness. If personal conflict in the therapist's foundation cannot be rectified, he or she should seek mental or medical health treatment.

Readings and Resources for the Professional

Aponte, H. (1994). *Bread and spirit: Therapy with the new poor.* New York: W.W. Norton & Company.
Fontes, L., Piercy, F., Volker, T., & Sprenkle, D. (1998). Self issues for family therapy educators. *Journal of Marital and Family Therapy, 24*(3), 305-321.
McDaniel, S., Hepworth, J., & Doherty, W. (1997). *The shared experience of illness: Stories of patients, families and their therapists.* New York: Basic Books.
Torre, M. (2005). Self reflection: An important process for the therapist. *Perspectives in Psychiatric care, 41*(2), 85-88.
White, M. (1997). *Narratives of therapists' lives.* Adelaide: Dulwich Centre Publications.

Bibliotherapy Sources for the Client

www.FamilyTherapyResources.net
www.TherapistLocator.net

Index

Page numbers followed by the letter "f" indicate figures; those followed by "t" indicate tables.

Academic environment, influence of, 13, 169
Academic environment, persons with Asperger's Syndrome in, 107-109
Academic performance of bipolar disorder patients, 176, 178
Academic performance of diabetic patients, 92
Actions, barriers to, 54
Activities of daily living, 19, 20, 180. *See also* Day-to-day tasks
Acute care situations, 11
Adjustment
    to cancer, 167
    in diabetic adolescents, 92
    family cohesion impact on, 26
Adlerian psychology, 202
Adolescents
    Asperger's Syndrome in, 109
    bipolar disorder in, 175, 176
    diabetes in, 33-34, 43-45, 91-97
    families with, 38t
    grief and bereavement in, 208
    patient education for, 95
African-American culture, 60
African-American families, 62, 168
African-American students, 108-109
African American (term), 108, 109
African-American youth, diabetes in, 91
Afro-Caribbean culture, 60
Age, inquiring about, 6
Aggression in children, 81, 83, 176
Aging, physical changes associated with, 142
Aging parents, caring for, 115, 211-215, 216t
AIDS, 113, 114-115
AIDS Memorial Quilt, 119, 120, 121, 122, 123
AIDS patients
    case studies of, 34-36, 115, 121-122
    handouts for, 117-118
    quilting by, 120
Alcoholism and alcohol use, 21, 59, 176, 178
Alzheimer's Disease, 157-158
American culture, 167, 168

ANGELS (A Neighbor Giving Encouragement, Love, and Support), 92, 95-97
Anger
    in bipolar disorder-affected families, 176
    breathing, impact on, 71
    expressing, 57, 79, 80, 81
    illness as cause of, 41, 49
    managing, 28, 77, 78-80
    rating scale, 77, 78, 80, 81
    as stage of grief, 77, 201, 205
    suppressing, 54, 55
    at withdrawal of support, 56
Anger thermometer, 78, 80, 81
Angry feelings toolbox, 77, 78, 80
Animals, 169, 204
Anne (person with Asperger's Syndrome) (case study), 107-109
Anorexia, 141, 144
Anticipatory grief, 119, 121
Antidepressants, 144
Antiretroviral treatments, 113
Anxiety
    in AIDS patients, 122
    breathing, impact on, 71
    over chronic illness or disability, 41, 69
    cycle, breaking, 149
    in eating disorder patients, 143, 144
    managing, 75, 81
    normalization of, 75
    in persons with Asperger's Syndrome, 104, 108, 109
    reducing, 73, 75
    in stroke patients, 213
    symptoms exacerbated by, 70
Aponte, Harry, 225-226
Arguments, 15, 16
Art, collaborative, 119, 120, 121
Art play therapy, 74
Art in therapy, 54, 78, 119, 120-121, 188-189, 195-196, 198. *See also* Collages and collage-making; Drawing; Painting; Quilting
AS meltdown incident, processing, 107, 109
Asperger's Syndrome, 103-109, 105f

The Therapist's Notebook for Family Health Care
© 2007 by The Haworth Press, Inc. All rights reserved.
doi:10.1300/5420_32

Assertiveness, 152
Assessment instruments and tools, 31, 168, 169, 170, 171, 172
Assessment models, 158-162
Assistance, allowing, 20
Assisted living environments, interviews conducted in, 5
Asthma patients
    African American, 62
    family relationships of, 51-52
Attachment disorder, 81
Attention deficit disorder, 21
Attention deficit hyperactivity disorder (ADHD), 104
Auditory information processing, difficulty with, 106
Authorship of own life, regaining, 229
Autism, 83, 85-86, 104, 105

Backup arrangements for breakdown, 179, 182f
"Basic Ecological Concepts" (handout), 132, 136
Beauty, standards of, 143
Behavior
    modifying, 77, 84-86, 89f
    problems, 83, 84-86, 89f
    symptoms, physical, impact on, 7
    target, 131
    understanding, limited of others', 106
Behavioral diagnostics interview, 85
Belief system
    about medical care, 215
    of caregiver, 160
    impact of, 212
    inquiring about, 3
    resiliency, role in, 168
Beliefs
    about diet and exercise, 133t
    about illness, 4-5, 61
    about medical care, 227
    cultural, 132
    sources of, 134, 136, 138t
    of therapists, 226, 227
Bereavement. See Grieving process
Bereavement overload, 119
Betrayal, 114, 117
Beverages, portion sizes of, 126, 127-128, 130
Beverly G. (case study), 204
Bicycle (metaphor), 179, 182f
Big, Hairy, Audacious Goal (BHAG), 94, 101
Binge drinking, 178
Binging, 150-151, 154f
Biological influence, 227
Biological problems, psychosocial implications of, 3
Biomedical information, 6-7
Biomedical well-being, theories on, 6
Biopsychosocial (BPS) model, 31, 53, 74, 219-220
Biopsychosocial-Spiritual (BPSS) Interview method, 3-11
Biopsychosocial-spiritual lens, 195, 196
Bipolar disorder, 104, 175-180

Birth place, 6
Bishop (sister of asthma patient) (case study), 51-52
Blankets, 202, 203-204
Bleeding, heavy, 69
Body image
    case studies, 144
    concerns, assessing, 147
    conflict over, 141
    cultural influences on, 142, 150, 151
    eating, link to, 143
    professional help for problems of, 145
    purging, link to, 154f
    of women, 149
Body response to illness/injury, 7
Bowel movements, 86, 89f
Brack and Bev G. (case study), 197-198
Bread and Spirit: Therapy with New Poor (Aponte), 225-226
Breakdown, backup arrangements for, 179, 182f
Breast cancer patients, families of, 42, 167, 168, 169-171
Breath, holding, 69
Breathing, 69, 70, 71
Breathing techniques, 28, 67
Brief therapy, 159
Bronfenbrenner's ecological model, 14, 131, 132
Bruising, 69, 70
Bubble intervention, 67, 68, 69, 70, 71
Bubble wrap exercise, 79, 80
Bulimia, 141, 144, 149, 150, 151, 152
Bumper sticker (concept), 59, 60
Burden, perception of being, 45
Burn out, 49

Cancer
    discussion groups addressing, 59
    fear of, 70
    journey with, 167-168, 169-172
    terminal, 190, 208-209
Cardiac arrhythmia, 144
Caregiver as herself, 159, 160, 165f
Caregivers
    of aging parents, 211, 213, 215
    of AIDS patients, 114, 115, 117-118
    burnout of, 49, 118
    of dementia patients, 157-158, 159, 160-163
    guilt of, 49
    isolation, feelings of, 41
    mental health of, 158, 159
    perspective of, 61
    physical health of, 25
    role of, 54, 60
    stress in, 157-158
Caretaker, child as, 187-188, 189
Cars as metaphor, 177-178, 179-180, 182f, 183
CBPR (community-based participatory research), 91, 92, 95, 96, 97

Cerebral palsy, 84
Cerebral palsy patients, sibling relationships of, 28
Challenges, dealing with, 169, 171
Change
    adapting to, 168
    as constant, 78
    energy for, 158
    experience with, 170
    investment in, 92
    resistance to, 106
"Check up" (on coping skills), 29
Chelation therapy, 83
Childless couples
    life cycle variations of, 36
Children
    aggression in, 81, 83, 176
    anger management in, 77-81
    Asperger's Syndrome in, 103, 107
    bipolar disorder in, 175, 176
    of cancer patients, 74-75, 171-172
    as caretakers, 189
    couples with, 35, 36, 38t
    developmental disabilities in, 83-87
    diabetes in, 80-81, 91, 92
    with disabilities, 49, 192
    inquiring about, 6
    loss, experience of, 187-192, 228-229, 231
    with terminally ill parents, 207-209
    working with, 222, 223, 224
Children of divorce, diabetic, 33-34, 43-45
Chimney (metaphor), 226, 227, 228, 231-232
Chronic illness. *See also specific illness, e.g.:* AIDS
    family challenges of, 41
    social support in managing, 19-22
    therapist experience of, 219-224
Chronosystem, 136, 138t
Church, visualizing, 198
Church friends, 21
Cirrhosis (liver disease), 9
Citizen Health-Care Model, 93, 94, 95, 96-97, 101
Clark, Jessica (diabetic) (case study), 80-81
Clients, disclosure with, 221-222, 223
Closeness, family, demonstration/depiction of, 14-15, 16
Closeness, family, perspectives on, 168
Closing interview, 8-9
CMWC (Contextual Model of Women Caregivers), 159-162, 165f
Co-workers, disclosure with, 221, 224
Cognitive-behavioral therapy, 77, 159
Cognitive limitations, 42
Cohesion of family, 13-14, 26
Collaborative health care, 232
Collages and collage-making, 61-62, 120, 122
Colleen (Non-Hodgkin's Lymphoma patient) (case study), 55-57
Comfort foods, 127
Common Threads (film), 121
Communication
    among aging parents' family members, 211-212, 214
    in AIDS patients and support networks, 119
    barriers to, 54
    in bipolar disorder-affected families, 175-176, 177
    in children, 74, 77, 79, 81, 171-172, 188, 189, 190-191
    about diet, 126
    marital, 36
    patterns of, 227
    in persons with Asperger's Syndrome, 106, 107
    skills, interpersonal, impaired, 106
Community-based participatory research (CBPR), 91, 92, 95, 96, 97
Community homes, interviews conducted at, 5
Community leaders, 93-94
Comorbid conditions of AIDS patients, 115
Conduct disorder, 81
Confidentiality, maintaining, 8, 11
Confidentiality of AIDS patients and families, 121, 123
Confusion, 108, 175
Connectedness, 67, 68
Consciousness, loss of, 144
Constipation, treatment for, 86, 89f
Constructivist conceptual framework, 212
Consumer culture, 142
Contextual Model of Women Caregivers (CMWC), 159-162, 165f
Control
    for eating disorder patients, 150
    as family interaction dimension, 68
    lack of, feeling, 154f
    loss of, 56
    sense of, 67, 70
Coping skills
    for bipolar disorder-affected families, 175, 176
    developing, 25, 26-29, 43, 77
    maladaptive, 27, 29, 205
    and strategies, 160, 163, 165f, 227
Corey (diabetic) (case study), 43-45
Cosmetic plastic surgery, 142
Couple relationship, loss or diagnosis impact on, 195, 196-198
Couple relationship, maintaining, 57
Couples therapy, 55, 57
Course of disease, 31, 114
Criminal arrest, 109
Crisis intervention, 35
Crisis management mode, 7
Crisis plans for bipolar disorder-affected families, 176, 179
Crisis stage of illness, 114, 117, 167, 168, 169
Criticism of ill family members, 176, 177, 178, 180
Cross-generational coalitions, 14
Cultural beliefs about end-of-life practices, 214
Cultural meanings on food and eating, 132
Cultural sensitivity, 60, 62

Cultural values, 136, 138t
Culture
    as constant, 60
    identifying, 160
    perceptions of, 162
Cure, race for, 4

Daily activities, 19, 20, 180
Dark, fear of, 74-75
Day-to-day tasks, 59, 114, 115
Deaf persons, 9
"Death denial" culture, 187
Death and dying
    activities related to, 122
    of AIDS patients, 114, 115, 118, 120, 121, 122
    apprehension in, 114
    of child, 196, 197-198
    children's perception of, 188, 191
    expected *versus* unexpected, 201
    feelings and emotions regarding, 191
    meaning ascribed to, 4-5, 118, 132
    of parent, 169-170, 171, 207-209
    of pets, 204
    preparation for, 171, 207-209, 214
    relationships enduring beyond, 121
    resiliency following, 171
    responses, personal to, 123
    therapist encounter with, 225
    thoughts of, 176
Decision making
    democratic, 94, 97
    dietary, 125, 126
    end-of-life, 211, 212, 213, 214, 216t
    self-directed, 53, 57
Deep breathing, 70, 71
Deficits, focusing on, 106-107
Delegating tasks, 221
Dementia patients, 157-158, 159, 160-161, 162-163, 165f
Democratic partnership, 92, 97
Democratic planning, 94
Demographic information, obtaining, 6
Denial
    resiliency, role in, 168
    as stage of grief, 201
    in terminally ill, 209
Depression
    in AIDS patients, 122
    in bipolar disorder patients, 175
    breathing, impact on, 71
    in caregivers, 158, 159
    cycle, breaking, 149, 152
    in diabetic patients, 92, 132
    in eating disorder patients, 143, 144
    feelings of, 41
    in persons with Asperger's Syndrome, 104, 108, 109
    as secondary illness, 19, 21, 69, 70, 213

Developmental Changes, Challenges, and Opportunities: A Tool for Family Education, Coping, and Adaptation, 31, 32-33, 34, 35, 36, 38t-39t
Developmental disabilities, 9, 83-87, 103, 106, 109. *See also* Asperger's Syndrome; Autism
Developmental family psychology, 14
Developmental stage, illness impact affected by, 32, 35
Developmental stage of caregivers, 160
Developmental tasks, 32
Diabetes
    in adolescents, 91-97
    in children, 91, 92
    dietary aspects of, 125-128, 131, 132, 133
    management of, 131-134, 152 (*see also* Self-care of diabetics)
    overview of, 91, 131
Diabetic patients, case studies of
    adolescents, 33-34, 43-45
    adults, 21-22, 62, 127-128, 132-134
    children, 80-81
Diagnosis of illness
    AIDS, 114, 117
    cancer, 167, 169
    couple relationship, impact on, 195, 196
    history, 6
Dialysis, 70
Diaphoresis, 67
Diaphragmatic breathing, 68, 70, 71
Dietary education, 126, 127-128, 130
Dieting, levels of, 142, 143, 147
Disability
    characteristics of, 31
    in children, 49, 192
    emotions regarding, 26
    externalization of, 50
    family challenges of, 41
    influence of, 227
    life cycle impact on, 32
    managing, 54
    meaning ascribed to, 4-5
    reciprocal impact of, 31
    therapist experience of, 225
Disappointment, 49, 57
Discovery, 159
Discrimination, anti-gay, 113
Disease, characteristics of, 31
Disease management in adolescents, 92, 95
Disenfranchised populations, HIV/AIDS patients in, 119
Distrust in HIV/AIDS-affected couples, 113
Divorce as life cycle variation, 36
Divorced parents, 21-22
"Doctor's Bag" (concept), 26, 27-29
Door, closing (metaphor), 195, 196
Down syndrome, 9

Drawing
    as anger release, 79, 80
    stress relief, role in, 26, 28
    of symptoms, 68-69
    in therapy, 120, 188, 189, 190-191, 195, 196
Drug use, 176
Dyspnea, 67

Eating disorder patients, case studies of, 143-144, 150-151
Eating disorders, 92, 141-145, 147, 149, 150
Ecograms, 169, 170, 171, 172
Ecological concepts, 136-139
Ecological model, 14, 131, 132, 134
"Ecological Risk and Resilience" (handout), 132, 137, 138t
Ecomap, 169
Ecosystems, 14
Effectiveness, evaluating, 225, 226, 227, 231-232
Embarassment, 109
Emotional capacity, illness impact affected by, 32
Emotional closeness, establishing, 45
Emotional comfort, 202
Emotional impact of illness or loss, 197
Emotional limitations, 42
Emotional overload, assessing for, 45
Emotional resources, 19, 20
Emotional scarring, 107
Emotional support
    for bipolar disorder patients, 179
    feeling, 21
    for gay couples, 114, 118
    through support groups, 26
Emotional well-being impact on mental health, 53
Emotional work, 168
Emotional Work Scale, 168, 170
Emotions and feelings
    AIDS-associated, 123
    controlling, 53, 54
    about death, 191
    about eating and body image, 143
    expressing, 42, 50, 51-52, 77, 81, 120, 126, 188, 202
    about illness, loss, or disability, 26, 27
    managing, 28, 29, 42, 50, 120
    negative, 49, 50, 51-52
    openness regarding, 4
    pictures of, 51
    polarizing, identifying, 55-56
    positive, 49, 50, 177
    symptoms, physical, impact on, 7
    understanding, limited of others', 106
Empathy, 3, 42-43, 104
Employment
    of persons with Asperger's Syndrome, 107
    status, 6
    of women, 149, 150, 151-152
Encopresis, 83
End-of-life stage, 39t, 211-215, 216t

Enuresis, 83
Estate planning, 118
Ethnic minorities, diabetes in, 91, 132
Ethnicity, 60
Executive function challenges, 105, 106, 109
Exercise
    beliefs about, 133t
    for bipolar disorder patients, 179
    for chronically ill, 21, 221
    in diabetes management, 22, 131, 132, 133
    excessive, 143, 144, 147, 149
    walk, taking, 26, 27, 28
Exiles (internal system parts), 53, 54, 55, 56
Exosystem, 14, 131, 136, 138t
Expectations, rigid, 106
Experiences, understanding one another's, 42
Experiential family therapy, 26, 220
Experiential family therapy model, 202
Extended (nonhousehold) families of color, 60
Extended (nonhousehold) families of gay persons, 114, 115
Externalization, use of, 73-74, 75
Externalization of illness or disability, 50, 231
Extramarital affairs, 35

FACES-III, 168, 170
Facilitated Mirroring, 104, 105-107, 105f, 109
Faith role in illness management, 9
Families, psychosocial functioning of, 59
Families of color, 59, 60, 62
Families and Democracy Project, 93
Family
    adjustment and adaptation response model, 68
    bumper sticker (concept), 59, 60
    communication, encouraging, 50
    definition of, 60, 169, 226, 227
    development, 31, 61
    dynamics, illness-related, 55
    figures, symbolic representation of, 15, 16
    fleet (metaphor), 180, 183
    functioning, 125, 196
    genograms, 41, 42, 44-45, 169
    identity, 59, 60
    interactions, dimensions of, 68
    legacies, stressful event, dealing with, influence on, 42
    needs, vehicles meeting, 183
    organization, pre- and post-illness, 42
    of origin *versus* family of choice, 119
    paradigm, 168
    as patient, 62-63
    play, 67, 69
    reorganization, facilitating, 41
    room representing, 196
    song title (concept), 60, 61
    structure change, measuring, 13
    views of, assessing, 13-14

Family Crisis-Oriented Personal Evaluation Scale
    (F-COPES), 168, 170
Family FIRO Model, 68
Family focused treatment (FFT), 176-177
Family life, illness impact on, 61-62
Family life, impact on diabetic patients, 125
Family life cycle, illness impact on, 32, 36, 113-114
Family life cycle, stages of, 38t-89t
Family members, connection between, 26
Family members, illness history of, 7
Family-oriented diabetes management, 125-128
Family relationships
    and bipolar disorder, 175-176, 177
    illness impact on, 59, 61, 62, 63, 169
    parental relationships, 227
    transition impact on, 14
Family stress theory, 19, 68
Family system
    assessment of, 13-17
    of caregivers, 161, 165f
    disengagement of, 41
    and health, 220
    issues, addressing, 7
Family Systems-Illness Model, 113-114, 117-118
Family systems theory, 68
FAST (Family System Test), 13-17, 14f
Fast-paced life, 143
Fear
    in children, 67, 68, 69, 70, 73, 74-75
    desire to control, 54
    diabetes-related, 132-133
    HIV/AIDS-related, 113, 117
Feedback for eating disorder patients, 151
Feeding problems, 83
Female caregivers, 157-163
Feminist perspective, 149-150, 167
Firefighters (internal system parts), 53, 54, 55, 56
Fishbowl technique, 61
Focus, shifting, difficulties in, 106
Focused noticing, 169
Food
    and eating, cultural meanings regarding, 132,
        133-134, 133t
    intake, restricting, 150
    refusal, 85, 86, 89f
    relationship to, 143, 144, 147
    rituals, 143
Foundation (metaphor), 226, 227, 230-231
Friends, room representing, 196
Frustration, 41, 49, 175, 176, 178, 179
Future plans, illness impact on, 161, 165f

Gay couples, 113-115, 115, 117, 118
Gay persons, case studies of, 115, 121-122, 132-134
Gender roles, 136, 142-143, 149-150, 159, 165f
Generational roles, shifting, 39t

Genograms, 134, 169, 170, 171, 172. *See also* Family:
    genograms
Gifts from terminally ill, 207-209
Gina (diabetic) (case study), 21-22
Globalization, 141, 142
Goal-directed activities, 176
Goals, developing, 134, 220, 228
Goals, monitoring, 224
Gonzales family (case study), 34-36
Grieving process
    in adolescents, 208
    AIDS-associated, 113, 114, 117, 118, 119, 121, 123
    in children, 187-192
    at end of life, 39t, 207
    family experiences, sharing, 189, 191
    managing, 220
    meaning-making activities in, 119
    mementos as aid in, 201-205
    for parental death, 169-170
    stages of, 77, 201, 203, 204, 205
    therapist, impact on, 123
Group selection process, unstructured, 108, 109
Group sharing, 107
Group within a group model, 61
Guillain-Barré syndrome patient (case study), 9-10
Guilt, feelings of, 45, 49, 115
Gustatory hyper- or hyposensitivity, 106
Gym membership, 133

Hallucinations, 176
Hargrave, Terry, 201
Hargrave's factors of grief, 203
Harlem community, 59, 60
Harm to others, risk of, 7
Headaches, 69
Healing, shared experience of, 43
Health, room representing, 196
Health behaviors, changing, 133
Health care, improving, resource for, 101
Health care, lack of, 60
Health and healing, traditions of, 101
Health issues, expertise with, 94
Health issues, identifying, 93
Health outcomes, family functioning impact on, 125
Health outcomes, social support impact on, 19
Health problems, assessing and remedying, 84,
    86-87, 89f
Health problems, factors contributing to, 83
Health status
    information on, 6
    loss impact on, 197
    meaning ascribed to, 5
Healthy Families Project, 60, 62
Healthy relationships, ability to choose, 22
Heart palpitations, 67
Helen (stroke patient) (case study), 212-214
Help, seeking, 162, 163, 165f

Helplessness, 41, 49, 118, 154f, 175
Hemophilia, 69-70
Hierarchy of family, assessing, 13-14
Hispanic youth, diabetes in, 91
Historical and societal influences, 161-162, 165f
HIV, 4, 113, 114-115
HIV-positive gay men, 120
Holiday rituals, 170
Home project, building (metaphor), 226, 227-232
Hopelessness, 41
Horace (gay man) (case study), 121-122
Hospice, interviews conducted at, 5
Hospice care, 118, 208, 209, 212, 213
House (metaphor), 226, 227-228, 229-231, 230
Household, composition of, 6
Household management, discussions about, 15, 16
Hurt, desire to control, 54
Hyperactivity, 176
Hyperventilation, 69

IFS (internal family systems theory), 53, 54-55
Illness
    emotions regarding, 26, 41-42, 55, 56
    externalization of, 50, 231
    family beliefs about, 61
    family life, impact on, 61-62
    family relationship impact on, 59, 62, 63
    history of, 7, 42
    life cycle impact on, 32
    life cycle of, 32, 36, 61, 113, 114
    managing, 54, 61, 220, 221
    meaning ascribed to, 4, 8, 119, 168
    in more than one family member, 60
    partner's, response to, 160
    putting in place, 42, 43, 45, 47f, 62
    reciprocal impact of, 31
    reminder, 62
    symbols of, 55
    therapist experience of, 225
    trajectory of, 160, 165f
Illness experience
    differing of family members, 41-42
    factors affecting, 31
    interviewing about, 6
    and life cycle, 32
Illness story, personal, sharing, 41, 42-43, 44-45
Imagery, utilizing, 54
Immigrants, case studies of, 34-36, 69-71
Inadequacy, sense of, 56
Inattentiveness, 84
Incapacitation, level of, 31-32, 41, 114
Inclusion (family interaction dimension), 68
Individual, characteristics of, 136, 138t
Individual, control of, 53
Infidelity, 35, 114, 117
Information, generalizing, difficulty in, 106
Initiative, battle for, 220

Injury, experience of, 6
Inpatient rehabilitation units, interviews conducted at, 5
Instructions, difficulty following, 106
Insurance information, 6
Integration of crisis, 168
Intellectual capacity, illness impact affected by, 32
Intentions, limited understanding of others', 106
Interdependence, 168
Intergenerational family genograms, 169
Intergenerational impact of illness, 32
Intergenerational policy, 162, 165f
Internal family systems theory (IFS), 53, 54-55
Internal system, 53
International resources, 136
Interpersonal boundaries, shifting, 168
Interpersonal interactions, skills for, 77
Interpersonal relationships, injury impact on, 229
Interpersonal relationships of persons with Asperger's Syndrome, 107
Interventions
    identifying important, 10
    implementing, 92
    tools, 31
Interviews, initial, 3, 5-11
Interviews, third parties present during, 7, 8, 11
Intimacy (family interaction dimension), 68
Irritability, 84-85, 175, 176
Isolation, 41, 113, 118, 120, 121, 125

Jane (bulimia patient) (case study), 150-151
Janna (bipolar disorder patient) (case study), 178-179
Jennifer (bereaved granddaughter) (case study), 190-191
Jessica (diabetic) (case study), 80-81
Jobs, changing, 170
Joe and Dave (gay couple) (case study), 115
Journal, writing in, 16, 27, 28
Juice, portion sizes of, 126, 127-128, 130
Julio (von Willebrand's patient) (case study), 69-71

K-car (metaphor), 178, 179, 182f
Kidney function, losing, 70
Kinship networks, 169
Kubler-Ross, Elizabeth, 201
Kubler-Ross stages of grief, 203, 204, 205
Kvebaek Family Sculpture Technique, 14-15

Latino culture, 60
Laurel (sibling of cerebral palsy patient) (case study), 28
Laxatives, use of, 149
Leaders, community, 93-94
Learning communities, 94
Learnings as community property, 94

Legal issues affecting gay couples, 113, 114, 115, 117, 118
Lesbians, case studies of, 132-134
Lethargy, 84-85
Life cycle, death timeliness in, 201
Life cycle, illness and disability impact on, 31, 32, 113-114
Life events, 161, 165f, 227
Life experiences, breakdown of, 104
Life experiences of women, 158
Lifestyle
   altering, 41
   choices, revealing, 114, 117
   diabetes impact on, 127
   healthy, motivation to adopt, 96
   modern, 143
   requirements of chronic illness management, 19
Light sensitivity, 106
Listening, active, 177
Literal meanings, adherence to, 106, 109
Liver cancer patient (case study), 208-209
Living wills, 213
Loss
   children's experience of, 187-192, 228-229, 231
   couple relationship, impact on, 195, 196-198
   dementia patients' experience of, 161, 165f
   diabetes-related fear of, 128
   emotions regarding, 26
   at end-of-life stage, 39t
   feelings of, controlling, 54
   HIV/AIDS-related, 113, 118, 123
   impact, factors affecting, 201-202
   managing, 220
   potential of family member, 4
   preparation for, 47f
   spousal illness as cause of, 157, 158, 160, 165f
   sudden *versus* gradual, 201
   of support system, 55
   therapist experience of, 225
Love, vehicles meeting need for, 183
Low-income families of color, 59, 60, 62

Macrosystem, 14, 136, 138t
Managers (internal system parts), 53, 54, 55, 56
Mania in bipolar disorder patients, 175, 176
Manic-depressive illness (bipolar disorder). *See* Bipolar disorder
Mapping of past challenges, 169
Mark (son of cancer patient) (case study), 74-75
Marriage
   communication in, 36
   discord, premorbid, 45
   life cycle stage of, 38t
   problems in, 55-56
   room representing, 196
   status, inquiring about, 6

Martin (developmentally disabled boy) (case study), 85-86
Meadors, Patrick L. (therapist) (case study), 227-232
Meal planning, 126, 127, 128
Mealtimes, 125, 127
Meaning-making activities, 119, 122, 123, 157
Meaning-making strategies, 158, 159, 163
Media, influence of
   as exosystem element, 136, 138t
   exploring, 132, 133, 139f, 162
   female sexuality standard, 142
Medical family therapy
   approach to, 228, 229, 230
   entering into, motivation for, 227
   goals of, 68
   house metaphor in, 226
   physical and emotional connectedness in, 219-220
   professional identity in, 232
Medical providers
   familiarity with, 26
   relationship with, 6, 9
   symbolic representation of, 15
Medical support, 162, 165f
Medical system, influence of, 169
Medical system, mistrust of, 59
Medications
   adherence to, 152
   for aging patients, 213-214
   changing, 87
   current, 6
   managing, 179, 221
   psychotropic, 176
   side effects of, 42
Mementos, creating, 202-205, 207-209
Memorial quilts, 119, 120
Memories, personal, sharing, 202
Menopause, 142
Mental health
   loss impact on, 197
   physical and emotional well-being interplay on, 53
   social interest as cornerstone in, 202
   therapist's issues of, 227
Mental illness and chronic illness, 63
Mental retardation, 83, 85-86
Mentorship, 97
Mesosystem, 136, 138t
Metacommunication, skills at, 169
Michael (diabetic) (case study), 33-34
Microsystem, 14, 136, 138t
Mind-body connection, 219
Mind-body medicine, 71
Mistakes, fear of, 107
"Model letter," 20
Mood instability, 175, 176
Mother-daughter relationships, illness impact on, 62, 178-179
Motivational strategies in self-care, 131
Motivations, limited understanding of others', 106

Moving, 170
Multiple Family Discussion Group (MFDG), 59, 63
Multiple sclerosis, 196
Multiple sclerosis patients, family relationships of, 15-16
Multitasking, difficulties in, 106
Muscle tightness, 69
Music, cultural heritage of, 60
Music, listening to, 27
Mutual Storytelling Technique (MSTT), 188

NAMES Project, 120, 121, 122, 123
Narrative family therapy, 49-50, 73-74, 134, 229, 230, 231
Narrative therapy, 159, 169, 188, 195
National Eating Disorders Association, 144-145
National resources, 136
Native American youth, diabetes in, 91
Nausea, 67, 70
Negative emotions, 49, 50, 51-52
Negative Feelings Box, 50, 51, 52
A Neighbor Giving Encouragement, Love and Support (ANGELS), 92, 95-97
Neuromuscular disease, 32
Neurotypical translator (therapist), 104, 105, 105f, 107
New England family (case study), 167, 169-171
Nicole and Jordan (case study), 15-16
Nightmares, 176
Non-English speakers, patient education of, 36
Non-Hodgkin's Lymphoma patient (case study), 55-57
Nonverbal communication, impaired ability to provide, 106
Nosebleeds, 69, 70
Numbness, 67
Nursing homes, interviews conducted at, 5

Obesity, 142
Occupation, inquiring about, 6
Olfactory hyper- or hyposensitivity, 106
'One illness per family' model, 60
Onset of disease, 31, 114
Osteoporosis, 144
Outcomes
    of diseases, 32, 114
    of interventions, 92
    justifying, 93

Pain
    breathing, impact on, 71
    in children, 67, 68, 69, 70
    meaning ascribed to, 4
Pain-fear-hyperventilation cycle, 68
Painting, 195, 197
Palliative care, 118
Palpitations, 69

Paper ripping, 79, 80
Parent-child relationships, 231
Parental/familial relationships, 227
Parenting
    difficulties, 45
    illness impact on, 35, 36
    role, 55
Parents
    of disabled children, 49
    family member illness impact on, 25
    terminally ill, 207-209
"Partners in Diabetes" (initiative), 95
Passive-aggressive behavior, 56, 57
Patient
    education, 36, 95 (see also Psychoeducation)
    information concerning, 8-9, 10
    perspective of, 61
    role of, 54, 60
Patient-doctor communication, 152
Patriarchal society, 149-150, 151
Peer interactions, 231
Peer relationships, 227
"Personal Ecology Worksheet" (handout), 132, 139f
Perspective, lack of, 104, 106
Perspective-building, 106, 107, 109
Pervasive developmental disabilities not otherwise specified (PDD-NOS), 109
Pets, 169, 204
Physical changes following loss, 196
Physical exertion as anger release, 78-79, 80-81
Physical health. See Health
Physical limitations, 42
Physical well-being impact on mental health, 53
Pickup truck (metaphor), 179
Pillow, shouting into, 79, 80
Pillows, 202, 203, 204
Plastic surgery, 142
Play dough, 28, 126, 127
Play therapy, 74, 77, 79, 80, 171-172, 188
Polarizations, identifying, 54
Political correctness, 108, 109
Portion sizes, 125, 126, 127, 128, 130
Positive emotions, 49, 50, 177
Positive Feelings Box, 50, 51, 52
Poverty, 114
Practical resources, 19, 20
Prayer concern lists, 21
Presenting problem, cyclical nature of, 149, 150-151
Prioritizing, difficulties in, 106
Privacy, 8, 121
Problem solving
    abilities, 168
    in art therapy, 203
    community-based, 92, 96
    in family-focused treatment, 177
    Healthy Families Project techniques, 62
    self-reliance in, 78
    vehicles meeting need for, 183

Problems, documenting, 84
Professional expertise, using, 94
Progression of disease, 160, 165f
Property destruction, 83
Provider/consumer model, traditional, 95, 97
Psychiatric disorders, comorbid in persons with
    Asperger's Syndrome, 104-105, 109
Psychiatric disorders, premorbid, 45
Psychiatric problems in diabetic adolescents, 92
Psychoeducation
    in discussion groups, 63
    family reorganization, facilitating through, 41
    identifying important, 10
    and illness experience sharing, 42, 43
    source materials, 36
    tools, 32-33
Psychological aspects of diagnosis or loss, 196-197
Psychological aspects of illness, 3, 7, 9
Psychological influence, 227
Psychological well-being, theories on, 6
Psychosocial problems, 3, 113
Psychotropic medication, 176
Public policy, 136, 138t, 162
Purging, 149, 150, 154f, 155f

Questioning skills, developing, 5, 10
Quilting, 119, 120-121, 122-123
Quilts, premade, 204, 205

Race relations, 136
Racial minorities, diabetes in, 91
Rages, 176
Rapport, building, 5-6, 10
Reactions, limited understanding of others', 106
Reading ability, impaired, 106
Realistic options, investigating, 177
Reality, perceptions of, distorted, 176
Reality construction, 172
Recreational activities, 6, 170
Reflection, post-interview, 10
Reframing, 195
Rehabilitation units, interviews conducted at, 5
Rehabilitative care, 212, 213
Rejection, feelings of, 56
Relational changes, 151-152
Relational distress, breaking cycle of, 149
Relational hardiness, 168
Relationships
    balanced/fulfilled *versus* unbalanced/unfulfilled,
        201
    body image impact on, 143
    dementia patient-caregiver, 159, 161, 162, 163, 165f
    influences of, 133-134, 133t, 139f
    positive, building, 104
    types, impact on loss experience, 201

Relaxation techniques, 28, 67, 151
Remarriage as life cycle variation, 36
Resilience (strength) factors, identifying, 132, 133t,
    134, 137, 138t
Resiliency
    construct of, 167, 168, 169, 171
    legacy of, 169
    loss, dealing with, 207, 229
    theory, 19
Resources
    assessing, 159, 160, 162, 165f, 171
    internal, 160, 165f
    as legacy, 170
    recognizing and augmenting, 158
Respectful behavior in family, 16-17
Responsibilities, shifting, 114, 168, 171
Restaurants, 127, 128
Reverse hierarchies, 14
Rick and Lori (case study), 127-128
Risk (vulnerability) factors, identifying, 132, 133t, 134,
    137, 138t
Roles
    assessing, 160
    conflict of, 55, 158, 159
    gender, 136, 142-143, 149-150, 159, 165f
    generational, 39t, 62
    HIV/AIDS impact on, 113, 117
    multiple, 54, 60, 157, 158
    perceptions of, 162
    shift in, 39t, 62, 151-152
Rolland's Family Systems-Illness Model, 113-114,
    117-118
Rolland's typology of illness, 43
Roof (metaphor), 226, 227, 228, 231
Rooms as metaphor, 196, 197-198
Rugged individualism, 168
Rumination, 83

Sadness
    image of, 56
    managing, 81
    quilt representing, 121
Safety, assessing for, 225
Scatterplots, 83, 84-87, 89f
Schedule, flexible, maintaining, 222, 223
Schizophrenia, 59, 104
School absences in diabetic patients, 92
Schools, changing, 170
Scribbling, 79, 80
Sculpting, 169, 195, 196
Sealing point, 227
Second order systemic change, 151-152
Secondary illness, chronic illness accompanied
    by, 19
Seizure disorder, 84, 85-86
Seizures, 86, 89f
Selene (diabetic) (case study), 132-134

Self
    development of, 53
    image of, 54
    integration of, 54, 55, 56-57
    internal system part, 53
    leading of, 56, 57
"Self-Assessment for Eating and Body Image Concerns Handout," 143, 147
Self-assessment tools, 142, 143, 144, 147
Self-awareness, building, 104, 105, 143
Self-care
    of caregivers, 160, 162
    of chronically ill, 21, 22
    of therapists, 220-221, 222
Self-care of diabetics
    adolescents, 33, 34, 44, 45, 92, 95
    family support role in, 126, 127, 128
    systemic aspects of, 131, 132
Self-censorship, 55
Self-deprecation, 150-151
Self-disclosure of therapists, 189, 190-191, 221-222, 223
Self-discovery, 229
Self-empowerment, 73, 75
Self-esteem, 92, 151-152
Self-exploration, 159
Self-expression, 188
Self-harm, 7, 83, 85, 86, 89f
Self-help, 78, 131, 145
Self-help literature, 134, 144, 145
Self-leading, 55
Self-of-the-therapist, 220, 225, 226, 227, 228, 232
Self-reflection, 158, 159
Self-regulation, 104, 107, 109
Self-respect, 57
Self-stimulation, 83
Self-sufficient recovering person *versus* dependent person, 54
Self-talk, positive, 151
Self-understanding, 54
Self-worth, 151
Semi-private rooms, 11
Sensory integration dysfunction (SID), 105, 106, 109
Shared experience building, 41, 42, 43, 45
Shock, AIDS diagnosis-related, 114, 117
Short stories, writing, 56
Shortness of breath, 69
Siblings
    bubble intervention, cueing, 68, 70
    family member disability impact on, 28
    family member illness impact on, 25, 51-52
    loss of, 228-229, 231
Single-parent families, case studies of, 167, 169-171
Single-parent families, life cycle of, 36
Sleep disorders, 83
Sleep patterns, fluctuation in, 176
Smith, Mark (son of cancer patient) (case study), 74-75

Social behavior, difficulty understanding and modeling, 106
Social change, 94
Social-class marginalization, 60
Social-cognitive deficits, 105, 106, 109
Social confusion, 108
Social conscience quilts, 120
Social construction, 161-162
Social contacts, helping persons with limited, 22
Social/environmental aspects of illness, 3, 7-8
Social exclusion, 109
Social influences, 159, 161-162, 165f, 227
Social interactions, body image impact on, 147
Social interactions of bipolar disorder patients, 176
Social relationships, loss impact on, 197-198
Social resources, increasing, 21-22
Social support network
    actions within, 54
    illness impact on, 7
    sense of, establishing, 5
Social support system
    assessing (support persons), 20, 21-22, 162, 170
    of caregivers, 158, 165f
    in chronic illness management, 19-22
    diagram of, 170
    for eating disorder patients, 151
    for gay couples, 114, 117
    grief, dealing with, 202
    loss of, 55
    stressful life events, adapting to, role in, 19
    system, questioning about, 8, 9
    at workplace, 222, 223-224
Social unconscious, 138t
Socializing, vehicles meeting need for, 183
Societal and historical influences, 161-162, 165f
Societal structure, 136
Sociograms, 134
Solution-focused family therapy, 78, 134, 231
Spiritual aspects of illness, 3, 4-5, 8, 9
Spiritual resources, 162, 165f, 170
Spirituality
    attentiveness to, 3
    diagnosis or loss impact on, 197, 198
    influence of, 227
    thoughts on, health experience impact on, 8
Sports car (metaphor), 177-178, 179, 182f
Spreading the affliction intervention, 177
Stability, vehicles meeting need for, 183
Stacy (therapist) (case study), 222-223
Starvation, impact of, 144
Steinglass model, 59, 60
Stepfamilies, chronic illness in, 33-34, 43-45
Stepparent-stepchild relationships, 33-34
Stereotypes, 161, 162, 165f
Sticky balls, 79, 80
Stigma, anti-gay, 113, 114, 117, 119
Stigmatization of bipolar disorder patients, 176, 177
Stomachaches, 69

Stories, changing, 195, 230, 231
Story squares activity, 188-189, 190-192, 194f
Strategic orientation, 159
Strength-based psycho-therapeutic modalities, 106-107, 230
Strengths
   building, 179, 182f
   externalizing, 73, 74, 75
   inherent, 78
   personal, 226
   resilience factors, identifying, 132, 133t, 134, 137, 138t
   spiritual sources of, 162
Stress
   of caregivers, 157-158
   coping with, 168, 176
   family-related, 125
   feelings of, 49
   managing, 25, 26
   reducing, 20, 21, 25-26
   relieving, 79
   unconscious coping mechanisms, 143
Stress ball, 27, 28
Stressful life events, 19, 42
Stressors, 8
Stroke, 211, 212-214
Structural family therapy, 14, 226
Structure, battle for, 220
Struggling well (concept), 168, 171
Substance use and abuse, 114, 117, 176. *See also* Alcoholism and alcohol use
Suicide
   acts of, 176
   ideation of, 29, 205
   thoughts of, 108, 109, 176, 178
Superhero activity, 73, 74, 75
Support, benefits of, 56
Support, withdrawal of, 56
Support groups
   for adolescents with diabetes, 92, 95-97
   for AIDS patients, 118
   stress management, role in, 26
Survivor guilt, 115
Susan (eating disorder patient) (case study), 143-144
Symbolic-experiential therapy, 14-15
Symbolism, 54-55
Symptoms
   anxiety exacerbating, 70
   of dementia patients, 161, 165f
   depicting, 68-69
   fear exacerbating, 67, 69
   functioning, daily, impact on, 221
   managing, 67, 68, 69
   psychosocial components of, 70
   questioning about, 6, 7
   stress impact on, 25-26
   symbolic representation of, 15-16
   terminal-stage, 114, 118
   therapy issues, connection with, 53

Systemic orientation, 159
Systems, multiple, 13, 169

Tactile stimuli, over- or under-reaction to, 106
Talk, social support through, 20
Tank (metaphor), 179
Tantrums, 85, 86, 89f
Techniques in therapy, 226, 227, 231
Temperature changes, 67
Terminal stage of illness, 114, 118, 119, 121-122, 207-209
Terminally ill, case studies of, 208-209
Theory, building, 226, 227, 228
Theory of mind (ToM), 104, 106
Therapies, effectiveness, assessing, 83-84
Therapies, traditional, limitations of, 104
Therapist-client relationship, 221-222
Therapists
   illness of, 219-224, 225
   injury or loss of, 225
   self-disclosure of, 189, 190-191
The Therapist's Notebook for Lesbian, Gay, and Bisexual Clients (Whitman and Boyd), 123
Therapy skills, identifying important, 10
Thinking, symptoms, physical, impact on, 7
Thoughts
   illness or loss impact on processes, 197
   modifying, 77
   negative, 69, 150-151, 154f
   polarizing, identifying, 55-56
Three-generation African American family (case study), 62
Throwing, safe, 79, 80
Time commitment, 59
Tingling, 67
Touched with Fire (Jamison), 179
Transitions, difficulty coping with, 106
Transitions, experience with, 170
Trauma, internal system parts that have experienced, 53
Trauma, therapist experience of, 225
Treatment compliance, 152
Treatment plan
   for AIDS patients, 114, 118
   completing, 225
   developing, 10
   tools, 31, 33
Truck (metaphor), 179, 182f
Trust, establishing, 4, 5
Tuskegee Syphilis Study, 59
Type 1 diabetes, 91
Type 2 diabetes, 91, 131, 132

Underserved populations, HIV/AIDS patients in, 119
Unwanted house guest, illness as, 59

Validation, 62
Value systems, 227
Values, expressing, 226
Verbal communication, alternatives to, 29
Violence, 176
Vision disability, 192
Vitamins, 83
Vomiting, 83, 150, 155f
Von Willebrand's disease patient (case study), 69-71

Walk, taking, 26, 27, 28
Weaknesses
    focus on, 106-107
    identifying, 132, 133t, 134, 137, 138t, 182
Weight concerns, 149
Weight-control practices, dangerous, 141
Weight gain, 141
Weight loss, 145
Weight management, 127, 128, 143
Wellness, symbols of, 55
Wellness, willingness to make changes toward, 4-5
Wheelchairs, 29

White middle-class families, 59, 62
Window (metaphor), 195-196, 197, 198
Women's health, 141-145, 149-152
Women's worldview, 158
Work, illness impact on, 219, 220
Work environment, influence of, 13, 169
Workload, boundaries and limits on, setting, 221, 224
Workload, sharing, 171
World view
    adopting new, 32, 43, 47f
    altering, 41
    of family, 168
Wrench (concept), 150, 151, 152, 155f
Writing in therapy, 16, 28, 56, 188
Writing role in coping, 27
Written coping skills, 28
Written messages for children, 208

Young adults, life cycle stage of, 38t
Youth, eating disorders in, 141
Youth, idealized image of, 142